T0094212

ETHICALLY CHALLENGED

Ethically Challenged

+ + +

PRIVATE EQUITY
STORMS US HEALTH CARE

LAURA KATZ OLSON

JOHNS HOPKINS UNIVERSITY PRESS | *Baltimore*

© 2022 Johns Hopkins University Press
All rights reserved. Published 2022
Printed in the United States of America on acid-free paper
9 8 7 6 5 4 3 2 1

Johns Hopkins University Press
2715 North Charles Street
Baltimore, Maryland 21218-4363
www.press.jhu.edu

Library of Congress Cataloging-in-Publication Data

Names: Olson, Laura Katz, 1945– author.
Title: Ethically challenged : private equity storms US health care / Laura Katz Olson.
Description: Baltimore : Johns Hopkins University Press, 2022. |
    Includes bibliographical references and index.
Identifiers: LCCN 2021011728 | ISBN 9781421442853 (hardcover ; alk. paper) |
    ISBN 9781421442860 (ebook)
Subjects: MESH: Delivery of Health Care—ethics | Health Care Sector—ethics |
    Investments—ethics | Private Sector—ethics | United States
Classification: LCC R724 | NLM W 84 AA1 | DDC 174.2—dc23
LC record available at https://lccn.loc.gov/2021011728

A catalog record for this book is available from the British Library.

*Special discounts are available for bulk purchases of this book. For more information,
please contact Special Sales at specialsales@jh.edu.*

For my daughter, Alix, and grandchildren, Zinn and Gray

I owe a great professional and intellectual debt to Eileen Appelbaum, the coauthor of *Private Equity at Work*, who inspired me to take on the task of writing this book. Eileen has been most generous with her time and insights. She not only read the text but introduced me to a world of dedicated investigators and activists who look at private equity investments with a critical eye.

Many people shared their opinions and knowledge as I wrote, and they helped make this book a reality. I am particularly grateful to friends and colleagues who commented on various portions of the work, especially Gayle Binion, Stephen Bronner, Brian Fife, Holona Ochs, and Karen Pooley, as well as Josh Kosman, author of *The Buyout of America*. I owe special thanks to Deborah Stone: she painstakingly evaluated the manuscript and gave detailed comments and suggestions that contributed materially to the final product. She has been a great friend and mentor over the years.

I am indebted to the several founder-owners willing to share their post–private equity buyout experiences with me, which added lived perceptions to my story. Experts in the various health sectors, too, imparted valuable specialized information and technical know-how. These individuals gave freely of their time.

I want to thank Lehigh University for subsidizing the private databases that rendered this research possible, two awards from the university's faculty research grant program, another from the Department of Political Science's Neidell Faculty Development Fund, and my distinguished professorship endowment. My heartfelt thanks to Lehigh's Library and Technical Services team for instant interventions in resolving computer glitches, even those of my own making.

Others have contributed, if indirectly, to this volume. My forever friends and confidants—Anna, Betty, Bobby, Bruce, Janice, Marilyn, Phyllis, Sandy, and ViviAnn—bring joy to my life and a caring space apart from work. Special cousins Carol and Sharon have offered me emotional sustenance and sisterly love. My long walks with Judy Lasker over the years have provided both camaraderie and advice of all sorts. My political science comrade John Ehrenberg has nourished me professionally and personally.

I appreciate the efforts of Johns Hopkins University Press editor Robin W. Coleman, who shepherded the book so supportively and effectively. I couldn't have written this book without the ongoing encouragement and unstinting backing of my husband, George, who read several drafts of the manuscript and endured my obsessive chatter about the private equity industry. I appreciate the ongoing moral support, sense of humor, and always perceptive ideas and observations of my daughter, Alix, an assistant professor at Emory University's Oxford College. It is to her and my grandchildren, Zinn and Gray, that I dedicate this book.

Of course, the opinions, conclusions, and errors are mine alone.

ETHICALLY CHALLENGED

Hiding in Plain Sight

PRIVATE EQUITY (PE) firms have put their claws into all aspects of our lives, including what we drink (Dr Pepper), where we sleep (Motel 6), how we communicate online (Skype), where we obtain office supplies (Staples), and the way we power our electronic gadgets (Duracell batteries).[1] Now, with its voracious appetite, PE is encroaching on our health, well-being, and even our dying. If you are addicted to opioids, do not be surprised if PE owns your treatment center; if you are injured, PE's helicopter is likely swooping you up at a crash site. It can own your dermatologist, dentist, ophthalmologist, or gastroenterologist. You may be at its mercy in the hospital emergency room or at the dialysis center because your kidney has failed.

As Nicole Aschoff suggests, the PE "business model is simple and brutal."[2] Its toolkit relies on piling up massive debt on investment targets and requiring them to pay it off. The financial buyers seek well-functioning enterprises with a steady stream of cash and squeeze their portfolio companies to optimize the flow. Giant amounts of debt, the foundation of PE's pecuniary advantage, has been the downfall of many favored businesses in recent years, most notably Toys "R" Us, Gymboree, Necco (maker of Sweethearts and Necco wafers), Payless ShoeSource, Bumble Bee tuna, J. Crew, and Neiman Marcus.[3] General partners (GPs) conveniently insist that they rejuvenate distressed companies when the reality is that they are mainly interested in robust enterprises. If they do purchase troubled places—which another shop may have milked[4]—it is at fire sale prices, and they exploit the enterprise again. PE's primary function is to generate value for itself by buying and selling businesses.

The Neoliberal Turn

Since the mid-1970s, the United States (like much of the industrialized world) has experienced the rise of neoliberalism, whose logic centers on privatization, deregulation, and competition intertwined in an inextricable web of perpetual capital accumulation. Neoliberals seek to hand over formerly state-run services to private players, with few restrictions. In their view, entire industries, from the production of coal to investment banking to human services, must be free from government interference. According to neoliberal reasoning, the rivalry among companies for profit will achieve greater efficiency, reduced costs, and improved quality of products or services, all without burdensome bureaucratic roadblocks. The market and its values take precedence over individual health and well-being, the environment, and glaring disparities of income. Even more, neoliberalism assumes that social well-being will improve commensurately with greater penetration of the market into the public realm.[5]

Neoliberal views have percolated throughout every aspect of the US economy, polity, society, and culture. As David Harvey puts it, neoliberalism "has become incorporated into the common-sense way many of us interpret, live in, and understand the world."[6] Its rationales have seeped into our vocabulary.[7] For example, frail elders and prisoners have become "market commodities," morality is conflated with commercial accomplishments, streamlining a business is tantamount to undercutting the workforce, and sponsorship is synonymous with ownership.

The economization of US society led to the financialization of everything, especially when "capital accumulation was released from regulatory and redistributive restraints."[8] The amassing of assets has turned into both a means for investment and a goal unto itself. Product, in other words, is secondary to money. Political institutions have become subservient to finance as well. According to these logics, the role of the state is to create underlying social and economic conditions that enable and promote investment, capital accumulation, growth, and profit making. Tax policy is used to advance the interests of entrepreneurs rather than the population at large.

The Rise of Private Equity Firms

The advent of the neoliberal order and its restructuring of the US political economy coincided with the emergence of private equity in its shadow. Financialization took root and surged during the 1980s, and PE has been riding on that wave ever since. Buttressed through eased regulations and preferential tax treatment, the financiers have steadily advanced their tentacles into ever more market sectors, from manufacturing and retail to business and monetary products, energy, and information technology. Eventually, they gravitated toward human services, such as health care, where in some cases they created markets that had not previously existed.

Private equity's business model can be characterized as a later stage of neoliberalism, one that takes its rationale to greater extremes; it is neoliberalism on steroids. Supersized earnings for PE and its shareholders are front and center, with no pretense otherwise. Nothing else matters. The profit motive guides everything in both word and deed. At a PE conference I attended in 2019 hosted by the Wharton School, the entrepreneurs discussed their buyout priorities, value-enhancing strategies, return on investment, and other metrics; not once did anyone mention the impact of their playbook on individuals or society, at least not at the sessions I joined.[9]

Many modern corporations, on the other hand, are sensitive to possible reputational damage, and they may consider (or at least pay lip service to) additional concerns, such as good will, the image of their product(s), the long-term sustainability of the business, their employees, and the well-being of the communities in which they reside. Media-savvy executives may strive to protect their corporate image by engaging in public relations campaigns that attempt to appease socially conscious consumers who are concerned with the environment, global warming, animal testing, and the like. A few engage in charity work or serve a limited number of low-income clients, sometimes at a loss. In 2019, the Business Roundtable went so far as to revise its "purpose of a corporation" statement: instead of advancing only the interests of stockholders, the high-level executives agreed that they should consider the needs of labor and suppliers, protect the environment, and "foster diversity and inclusion, dignity and respect."[10] Obviously, these are hollow words without concrete proposals on how they intend to achieve such exalted principles and translate them into action. But the PE industry does not even pretend to take these matters into account. This is not to say that big business has been the paragon of virtue, nor that other goals are allowed to overshadow the bottom line. However, non-PE companies have long-term interests that PE does not.

While corporate America is concerned with building its assets for shareholders, private equity is more about extracting money from the businesses it owns. Public corporations have declining government regulations, private equity firms none. Unlike publicly traded companies, PE has no accountability to anyone other than its investors, and most aspects of its financial operations are shielded from view. Private equity lives in a darkly curtained world, protected from external scrutiny.

Neoliberals favor short-term market contracts over long-term agreements mainly because of their greater tractability, especially regarding labor. PE-land is neoliberalism in overdrive and is exemplified by transient affiliations with portfolio companies, allowing GPs to manipulate their workforce at will. Furthermore, Harvey notes, "The preference for short-term contractual relations puts pressure on all producers to extract everything they can while the contract lasts."[11] The PE model is built on acquiring businesses, squeezing out the most money in the briefest time frame possible, and then putting the assets up for sale again. Actual allegiance to a particular company would be considered quaint.

Operational standardization is another component of neoliberalism that private equity firms take to extremes. Neoliberals argue that there are best business practices that should be adhered to, regardless of industry. Such separation of product from procedure is only possible because they accept the premise that all enterprises should seek competitive advantage in the marketplace and keep to the same metrics (i.e., profit margins, internal rates of return, and work flow), overshadowing everything else.[12] PE-owned companies commonly have CEOs and boards of directors populated by officials who are experts in management and its techniques but who have little knowledge about or interest in the specific goods or services they are overseeing. Thus, a finely honed technique for manufacturing packaged foods may be applied to serving human needs, such as health care. Integral to their modus operandi, the buyout shops are seeking not just respectable returns on their investments but rather outsized earnings. They do not even produce anything; they are the embodiment of financialization at its worst or, as Brown puts it, neoliberalism's growing replacement of productivity with financial activity.[13]

Untrammeled competition, another catchphrase of neoliberal reasoning, regularly culminates in monopolies and their local, regional, national, and on occasion international control over specific goods and services. Through its "roll-up" acquisition strategy in the fragmented health care sector, PE has been a leading force in intensifying consolidation. GPs, who strive for domination in a particular niche, claim that they are maximizing efficiency and controlling costs; in reality, by cornering a market, their portfolio companies can, by design, offer inferior products at arbitrarily inflated prices. The already bloated cost of medical services in the United States has been magnified by PE's intemperate pursuit of the neoliberal agenda.

Neoliberal rationalization has elevated efficiency to a high-ranking status in the US hierarchy of values, surmounting human needs and moral codes of behavior. However, a market could—and should—be viewed as malfunctioning if it runs cost-effectively but promotes inequality of income and wealth, deprives segments of the population of basic needs such as health care, and tramples on the well-being of sick, disabled, elderly, and other vulnerable people. In this book I show that private equity's unbridled invasion into health care services has contributed considerably to these deleterious effects. It has been a formidable force in the prodigious and rising concentration of wealth in the upper echelons of society as well. As Jason Kelly makes clear, "Even among Wall Street companies, PE stands out as a symbol of inequality in the U.S."[14] Business professors Steven Kaplan and Joshua Rauh have found that the foremost GP barons are a mounting share of the richest 400 individuals in the country. Their research shows that "there are more private equity managers who make at least $100 million annually than investment bankers, top financial executives, and professional athletes combined."[15]

Neoliberals tout choice as one of the key elements of societal well-being offered by market competition. In health care today there has been a shift toward patients as consumers, shoring up that notion. For PE, which is primarily concerned with maximizing patient volume, this has meant catering to mindless consumerism. PE-owned health care companies often appeal to customer preferences for the trappings of medicine (convenience, telemedicine, remote patient monitoring, online appointments), modern facilities (impressive buildings, shiny offices), or beautiful outdoor surroundings in such sectors as alcohol and drug rehabilitation. On the other hand, the PE firms neglect less visible but more important aspects of medical care, for instance first-rate training of personnel and up-to-date equipment. Clients may "prefer" certain conveniences, a shopping mall–type of experience, expeditious services, or unlimited food choices during a hospital stay, but their proclivities may not always reflect the ingredients of high-quality care. Besides, choice is a misnomer in much of the medical world. Vulnerable patients generally have little information about fees and are not in a condition to shop around in any case.

The new economic order has had destructive repercussions for the population as public programs have been scaled back. The unraveling of the welfare state and its protections has furthered the aims of neo-liberalism by opening markets in new sectors, especially those that traditionally have been publicly provided or were primarily in the domain of nonprofit agencies. PE has increasingly taken advantage of vast gaps in caring services by expanding for-profit offerings. However, GPs do not expend their own capital in lieu of government funding. To the contrary, they enrich themselves while gorging at the public trough of Medicare, Medicaid, veterans' assistance, and other state resources. Of course, PE takes full advantage of commercial payers whenever it can. The entrepreneurs are only stingy with their own money, relying on limited partners to provide the bulk of the capital for their acquisitions.

Who are these investors? A significant portion of the capital for PE investments derives from state and local pension funds.[16] PE firms have drawn together an iron triangle of stakeholders that is full of ironies and contradictions as it entangles workers' assets and small business owners in its moneymaking web of activities. The adage "What is good for the country is good for General Motors—and vice versa" has, for them, metamorphosed into "What is good for private equity is good for retired and soon-to-be-retired employees." Unfortunately, when a company collapses under PE ownership, the labor force usually gets short shrift, losing jobs as well as retirement income and health insurance; pension funds are complicit in provoking the insolvency. For ongoing enterprises, their capital abets staff reductions, the confiscation of benefits, and the reduction of other safeguards for the residual personnel. As PE streamlines its newly acquired firms, wage earners are viewed as disposable commodities. Public pension fund administrators mainly turn a blind eye to these inconvenient downsides as they harvest what they view as hefty earnings.[17]

The third piece of this iron triangle of PE firms and workers' retirement money takes its cue from neoliberalism's "new managerialism," which fuses ownership and management by paying top corporate executives in stock options: "Stock values rather than production then become the guiding light of economic activity."[18] For PE, this takes the form of offering the founders of small and middle-size establishments not only high market valuations worth a million dollars or more but a relatively modest equity stake in future gains. These owners can get swept away with euphoria by the potential riches from the sale of their business and other lucrative enticements, such as bonuses. Some of them part with businesses that they have built up for years with a labor of love and out of authentic concern for the population they serve. In some cases, the pressures of the neoliberal economy—such as overwhelming bureaucratic obstacles or insurance company intransigence over reimbursements—force them to give up their firms. In any event, GPs can be like snake oil salesmen, promising more than they intend to deliver. In turn, founders become aligned with the values, practices, and metrics of their new PE owners; every move is weighed against return on investment. Those who cannot hack it are thrown aside—or leave of their own accord.

The Iron Curtain

My friends and relatives inevitably ask "what is private equity?" when I tell them about my research. Or they just stare at me uncomprehendingly, with furrowed brows. It is an uncanny ability of the PE industry to infiltrate every aspect of our daily lives while simultaneously remaining unknown. Secrecy is a hallmark of the private equity industry, and it rigidly sticks to its code of silence with pride. One observer asserts that GPs "are modern day Wizards of Oz—the men behind the private-equity curtain."[19] At the 2019 Wharton Twenty-Fifth Private Equity and Venture Capital Conference in New York City, attendees, including myself, were advised at every session—sometimes twice—that all discussions were "off the record."[20]

Such confidentiality, along with lax regulatory control, translates into a lack of accountability, scrutiny, and transparency; PE-owned firms are far less transparent than publicly traded businesses. And it is considerably more challenging to monitor PE-owned companies, even when the various enterprises acquire a significant percentage of their revenue from government sources. This is especially the case with health care, where Medicaid and Medicare pick up much of the tab for services ranging from at-home assistance and physician appointments to nursing homes and hospitals.

At least, publicly traded entities must file with the Securities and Exchange Commission (SEC) and disclose the information they provide, which is available for anyone to inspect. Since the enactment of the Dodd-Frank Act in 2010, GPs must register their shops with the SEC and report certain limited information about their funds, mostly related to debt. But unlike public companies, the SEC allows that material to remain confidential. And they do not have to disclose any data pertaining to the income of their senior leaders, which companies they hold in their portfolios, or financial details about them. Worse still, PE managers do not have to notify the employees, vendors, or other affected parties that a private equity firm has taken over.[21]

Despite this, the alternative investment market seemingly is emerging from the shadows as PE has finally caught the attention of policymakers, mainly a few Democrats in Congress. Hearings have been held and legislation proposed, although it is highly unlikely that any restrictive laws will be enacted soon. Since PE is still shrouded in utmost secrecy, the full exposure of its financial maneuvers and the considerable damaging externalities they generate has a long way to go.

Looting Health Dollars

When asked why he robbed banks, Willie Sutton famously said, "Because that's where the money is." The looting of health markets by PE has a similar ring. In 2020, the US health care sector reached 18 percent of gross domestic product (GDP), or $4 trillion. Unquestionably, that is where the money is. The primary driving force of mounting costs, even beyond the consumer price index, has been rising prices and not just demand.

The nation's limited attempts to control exorbitant health expenditures have been like putting a hand into a political hornet's nest of special interests. Strategies such as managed care and health savings accounts have fallen far short as well: prices continue to soar, rendering essential services increasingly unaffordable for the uninsured. Public program outlays have swelled as have commercial plan premiums. Overall, the United States suffers from a malfunctioning health system that fails to offer all Americans access to timely, good-quality, and affordable care; it rations services based on ability to pay, rather than need.

Even people with health care coverage may experience underinsurance and burdensome medical bills. Rising deductibles and coinsurance have enlarged patient shares of expenses, exacerbating the situation measurably. The former CEO of GoFundMe, Rob Solomon, points out that fully one-third of the billions raised on his site is for essential medical needs.[22]

Beginning in the 1980s, deregulation and the concomitant shift from nonprofit to commercial ownership in many health areas played a sizable role in augmenting prices. These profit-driven companies emphasized revenue maximization, not cost controls.[23] Today the situation has worsened: the PE industry—capitalism in overdrive—weighs down its health companies with enormous debt while pushing for extra-large earnings. Faceless PE shops take an oversized bite into US health dollars, transferring substantial public and private money for medical needs into the pockets of financiers who do not provide any health services per se.

Whatever PE shops take over is reconfigured in their own image, engendering new language, knowledge, form, and content. This book documents, for example, that they may add more treatment centers across the nation, but the therapies tend to be based on private equity's financial needs and imperatives. PE is undermining the rights of vulnerable people to receive the best possible care: children on the autism spectrum; teenagers with eating disorders; people addicted to alcohol and drugs; kids needing dental work; and the elderly seeking to die in peace, to name a few examples. The doctor-patient relationship, which has long been adapted to neoliberal logic, is increasingly sculpted to PE's extreme economic orthodoxy.

In this book I delve deeply into the industry's involvement in the health care sector and its impact on individuals and society. PE expert

Ludovic Phalippou, author of the textbook *Private Equity Laid Bare*, writes that private equity methods may not be appropriate in all industries. Undoubtedly, health care is one of the more unsuitable market sectors because it affects essential human services. Accordingly, the caring and health domains raise issues pertinent to private equity strategies that the financialization of the toy and candy industries does not. Can we really afford, as a nation, to have dental and physician practices, homecare agencies, or autism treatment centers collapse like Toys "R" Us?

There are several caveats to my story. First, this book encapsulates the period from the 1980s to the end of 2020. By the time it is published, many if not most of the buyout shops will have cast off assets, moving on to their next conquests. They are like chameleons, fully capable of adapting to changing economic and social conditions, including the financial consequences of the COVID-19 pandemic. These pages capture the past and recent iterations of the PE structure, strategies, and procedures. Bryan Burrough and John Helyar warn at the end of their celebrated book, *Barbarians at the Gate*: "Be assured . . . that the Barbarians are out there just beyond the gates, licking their wounds, biding their time, waiting for the next chance to storm the gates."[24] Nowadays, that next chance may well be a newfangled version of themselves.

Second, given the degree of confidentiality surrounding the PE world, it was challenging for me to acquire complete, accurate specifics, and often I could not obtain any documentation whatsoever. As one expert on the industry puts it, "Because of its pathologically compulsive quest for secrecy and the diverse and complex features of its deal making, private equity cannot be conceived in its entirety."[25] Transaction details, returns on earnings, and other financial data are strictly confidential. It is particularly difficult to uncover dividend recaps, a major means for PE to feather its nest at the expense of portfolio companies. Thanks to extensive funding by my university, I had access to a comprehensive database (*PitchBook Data, Inc.*) that provides unique and indepth information on individual corporations, their ownership history, and a wide range of PE deals and acquisitions, including health services. Unless otherwise cited, the particulars herein derive from this source.

I interviewed scores of founder-owners whose agencies or professional practices had been sold to private equity shops. Nonetheless, full information about their views, experiences, and the effects on prior businesses were considerably hampered by the nondisclosure agreements nearly all of them had to sign. Several former proprietors spoke to me in guarded language, others anonymously, and many not at all. Furthermore, a preponderance of previous owners could not be located—apparently, they either left no forwarding address or the PE-owned company withheld contact information from me. I did what I could to penetrate the inner workings of the private equity industry and, as Carl Bernstein has advised, attempted to unearth "the best obtainable version of the truth."[26]

Third, health services encompass diverse domains ranging from information technology to pet care. I have selected for analysis only a few of these subfields. Although I endeavored to separate these services into individual chapters, PE portfolio companies frequently traverse several areas. For instance, homecare operators can also run hospices, nursing homes, and other elder care enterprises. Ground ambulances have been amalgamated with emergency medical helicopter services. There are no sharp lines that can be drawn in most cases.

Fourth, the geographic reach of a PE firm can be long, stretching across every continent. I have confined my narrative to the United States.

Overview and Organization of the Book

In chapter 1, I describe the essential elements of the private equity toolkit, including its use of debt to siphon outsized profits. I argue that the industry has been carefully crafted to meet its own pecuniary needs, without regard to its portfolio companies, labor, the community, or anything else that stands in its way. The goal is to squeeze as much money as possible out of its purchases and enhance their value for resale. Through financial wizardry, along with assorted fees and dividends charged to the portfolio companies, PE has generated the most lucrative Wall Street enterprise in the world, which is propped up mostly by public pension assets.

I detail alternative tactics used by the PE industry for its rapacious value-building objectives, such as leveraged buyouts, growth equity investing, acquisition and consolidation, and secondary buyouts, where enterprises are tossed back and forth like volleyballs. I show how PE employs additional ruses to maximize returns, including reimagining its own configuration, broadening investment areas and types of deals, and listing its firms on public exchanges. As I make clear, PE's eye is always on the end game, and the clock is ticking for the shop to exit its portfolio businesses at strong valuations. However, not a few are relinquished through bankruptcy. I also explain the catch-22 faced by pension fund managers; the enticements for founding owners to sell their places; the other professionals within the PE ambit who share pieces of the financial bonanza; and the tax havens that render the entire exploit possible. I end by briefly discussing who gains and who loses from what the industry has sown.

In chapter 2 I provide historical background to the private equity alternative market. I first examine the emergence and dramatic growth of leveraged buyout shops during the 1980s, as well as their use of junk bonds, financial engineering, and sharp cost-cutting strategies to bring in huge earnings for themselves. I provide examples of the profiteering and greed of the era that contributed to the downfall of companies such as Anchor Hocking in Lancaster, Ohio, and RJR Nabisco, led by the infamous KKR of *Barbarians at the Gate*. I describe the rollercoaster years of the 1990s, when the cyclical nature of the economy exposed the volatility of PE leveraged buyouts. I argue that GPs were able to adapt to changing conditions as they continued to generate great fortunes with which to line their pockets, if not those of the portfolio companies.

I next address the free flow of covenant-lite loans just prior to the Great Recession,[27] which was abetted by large commercial banks, and the subsequent stream of Chapter 11 filings when the economy crashed in 2008. I then detail the flourishing of the PE industry as it recovered: the nation witnessed more shops, funds, and transactions; surging investment capital; larger vehicles, including mega-funds; and high valuations, concomitant with greater debt. I detail a few of the high-profile bankruptcies (Toys "R" Us, Gymboree, Necco—of Sweetheart candy fame—Claire's, and Bumble Bee tuna) and warn that there will be more to come.

The final section in this chapter highlights the revolving door between PE players and top government officials, which guarantees the industry a friendly political climate. I note that these direct relationships are buttressed by healthy lobbying and campaign contributions. The chapter ends with the mounting criticism against PE practices, the congressional hearing titled "America for Sale?," the Stop Wall Street Looting Act proposed by Senator Elizabeth Warren and other Democratic senators, and the politically thorny bipartisan efforts to stop "surprise" medical bills.

In chapter 3 I first investigate the exploding growth of PE investments in health, especially middle-market companies. After exploring some of the factors propelling this development, including high returns on investments, resilience to business cycles, reliable revenue sources, and advantageous government policies, I discuss the malfunctioning US health system, rising costs, and the shift from nonprofit to commercial enterprises. I argue that the situation has worsened with the entrance of PE into the sector.

I then consider PE's consolidation of health industries, the ongoing quest for greater market share through add-ons and mergers, and the high valuations of acquisitions. I note that despite PE claims of greater efficiency and cost-effectiveness, limited competition has led to lean and inadequate services, worse patient outcomes, less transparency, fewer choices for consumers, and higher medical fees. Overleveraged companies can also face precarious financial conditions and end up in bankruptcy. I analyze two health cases where the PE shops filed for Chapter 11 but still came out on top. I go on to examine a few health mega-deals, both past and present, including Surgery Partners, Envision, LifePoint Health, Kindred Healthcare, and Health Corporation of America. The final section outlines the large scope of health-related

PE investments, ranging from core services and niche businesses to animal health and products, health food alternatives, and nutritional supplements. I conclude that the PE industry is reshaping the US health care system but not for the better.

In chapter 4 I begin by critically evaluating how private equity firms are quietly and steadily purchasing specialized physician practices. I explore the lure for the PE shops, especially the sector's steady revenue flow even during an economic downturn, increasing demand for services, and ultimately the potential for a strong return on investments. I review the currently high valuations of doctor offices and the sometimes-detrimental strategies to boost sale prices when offloading them to a subsequent buyer. I also address the enticements for doctors who accept PE offers, such as the financial windfall and the promise—often misleading—that they can relinquish their burdensome nonmedical office functions and spend more time practicing medicine. I then turn to the structuring of the PE buyouts through management services organizations that sidestep prohibitions against the corporate ownership of medical practices or employment of doctors. I end with an assessment of the troubling effects on patient care and society at large.

The next sections probe, in turn, selected specialties that are receiving heightened PE attention: dermatology, ophthalmology, orthopedics, gastroenterology, urology, dialysis facilities, fertility clinics, urgent care centers, and medical staff outsourcing. For each niche, I address issues pertaining to market conditions, motivations for PE firms, incentives for physicians, deal-making and financing details, PE strategies, and the real-life consequences of leveraged buyouts. I point out the main portfolio companies and platforms acquired by PE shops, along with their ongoing acquisitions, mergers, and consolidations.[28] Wherever possible, I have interviewed experts in the various fields as well as physician-owners and report their firsthand accounts.

In chapter 5 I scrutinize PE ownership of dental service organizations (DSOs), one of the first health care sectors to inspire PE investments. I explore the history of the early buyouts and expose the adverse effect on patients, such as providing needless procedures and substandard treatments. I argue that the Medicaid-funded care of children became a major target for PE, creating profit for the financial buyers at the expense of low-income kids. At the same time, a number of these highly leveraged chains declared bankruptcy, leaving young dentists, their assistants, and patients to fend for themselves.

I next tackle the PE toolbox for extracting windfall profits from dental practices and the ongoing ill effects on patients and the larger community. I also address the reasons that dentists sell their practices to PE firms and the subsequent consequences. I discuss the extent of PE engagement in the profession and delineate the ownership trajectory of several chains. I home in on the misdeeds of specific DSOs, many of which are still acquiring and scaling dental practices today.

In chapter 6, which first centers on homecare agencies, I explore the reasons for their rapid expansion, the recent appeal to GPs, and the financial bonanza for PE. I argue that the progressive takeover of the sector by PE firms and their large-scale consolidations have detrimental effects on frail elders and children, who are dependent on these services for their well-being; it leads to higher charges for families and taxpayers as well. I next take up the PACE program, which has now been opened to commercial players. Intended to keep elders at home, the government-funded initiative portends a financialized approach to all-inclusive care for the needy older population it serves. I then tackle hospice establishments, which PE firms are increasingly targeting for their portfolios. I explore the extent to which for-profit owners exploit the Medicare-supported benefit that is intended to allow the terminally ill to die as peacefully as possible.

I next zoom in on certain homecare and hospice enterprises that have undergone a succession of PE takeovers, including mega-mergers of long-standing places and a gold rush in platform purchases. I explore the impact of these investments and consolidations both financially and on the populations they serve. I also examine publicly traded chains and PE influence over them; social impact investing; and two newly converted nonprofit entities in the domain.

In chapter 7 I scrutinize addictions, beginning with substance abuse. I take up the ongoing role of private equity firms in amalgamating the rehabilitation industry, which is increasingly supported through tax-payer dollars. I also speak to the jarring disparity between evidence-based treatment and how the PE-owned chains actually provide services. I then deal with companies that were purchased by PE shops in the early twenty-first century and their history of unsavory practices, quick turnovers, extreme debt, and elevated returns. I then investigate a few of the places launched later, which are taking advantage of the opioid crisis and enhanced federal funding to combat it.

The final section of this chapter focuses on eating disorders (EDs) and why the PE industry has recently moved into the area, including more free-flowing money, limited government oversight, and over-sized returns. I then investigate specialized ED businesses, followed by chains that have acquired ED treatment centers as part of their larger enterprises. Throughout I show how PE firms have reaped financial gain at the expense of their food-challenged, largely female patients.

In chapter 8 I survey PE buyouts of autism spectrum disorders (ASD) treatment facilities. I first portray the ASD landscape, including symptoms of the disorder, its incidence, types of treatment, the comparatively recent flow of dollars from the government and commercial insurance, and the scarcity of services relative to need. I then turn to the lure for PE firms, especially the strong and quick rates of return and the sector's plethora of "mom-and-pop" shops, as well as the appeal to founder-owners who stand to gain a fortune from the elevated valuations of their businesses. I describe the large disparity between the gains of PE owners and the adverse impacts on the children with ASD they serve. I contend that autism services suit the PE model because there is a lack of clinical standardization and political oversight, allowing GPs to grow and impose "efficiency" measures that foster exceptional rates of return on the backs of their young clients.

I then paint a picture of several PE-owned chains that led the charge, beginning in 2004, in demonstrating the enormous value of the autism market. I lay bare, for each one, its acquisition and consolidation activities, mounting debt, cost-cutting tactics, and general lack of advantages—and, often, increase in disadvantages—for the people the businesses serve. I also highlight the misdeeds that abound in many of these enterprises. The final part of the chapter portrays the dizzying whirl of more recent PE buyouts, which have taken their cue from the earlier evidence of massive rates of return. These, too, have their share of malfeasance.

In chapter 9 I provide evidence for, as a 2016 *New York Times* headline outlined, what happens "when you dial 911 and Wall Street answers." I start by describing the ground ambulance terrain, its history, and appeal to GPs. I sketch the human costs of PE ownership, including worse response times, fewer supplies on hand, and more aggressive billing practices than other private or government providers. I then take on the air medical transportation industry and its monopoly control by PE firms; lax federal regulation that has permitted exorbitant fees, including surprise medical bills; and a lack of sufficient safety measures. I disentangle the transaction histories of the main PE-owned medical transport chains and the bankruptcy of several of them. I did find one family-held air transport company that is not for sale.

In the concluding chapter, I recap the secrecy of the PE industry and its lack of accountability to any public agency or, for that matter, anyone else. Nevertheless, my goal in this book is to part the curtains sufficiently to gain insights into PE's penetration of the health care sector and a host of legal and illegal harms it has perpetrated. I show that the PE firms' appetite for outsized earnings and the toolkit used to obtain them enrich the shops but do not serve the needs of clients in their medical and health portfolio companies. Drug addicts, alcoholics, children with autism disorders, girls and women with eating disorders, and elders at the end of life are mere commodities to be bought and sold for financial gain.

In the conclusion I summarize the parties that are complicit in PE's hijacking of US health care entities: public pension funds, founder-owners, insurance companies, and big banks. But none have aided and abetted PE expansion in health care more than government policies, which also fail to control any misdeeds. I argue that the PE industry has been moving full steam ahead with its highly lucrative investments, including more transactions, a growth in deal size, and ever-increasing capital commitments by public pension funds.

I then visit the sudden emergence of the COVID-19 pandemic and its concomitant financial turmoil. I contend that though the heavily leveraged PE chains are experiencing precarious circumstances, GPs are creative and flexible: they are capitalizing on the economic downturn and have even grabbed a share of the federal relief funds meant to assist small businesses. I end by calling for the federal and state governments to curb the spread of the PE industry in health care through such means as placing stringent regulations on its practices, removing tax havens that enable its maneuvers, and providing more social services instead of subsidizing those offered by financiers. Unless political leaders stop them, PE firms have no intention of curtailing their ever-growing consolidation of US health and medical services.

1

Who Even Are They?

Private Equity from Soup to Nuts

PRIVATE EQUITY is an integral part of the deepening financialization of the United States, a transformation that has attempted to monetize everything regardless of the consequences. Once an alternative, shadow sector of the US economy, PE is becoming more mainstream, participating in a larger share of the nation's wealth, and, in many ways, reshaping various segments of the market itself.[1] The industry promotes itself as creating value for companies that are acquired, but in actuality the PE firms generate wealth mostly for themselves and, to a lesser extent, their limited partners (LPs). Pension funds, endowments, and wealthy individuals finance the largest percentage of a fund's deals, but they are purely passive investors, with no decision-making authority. PE firms take over businesses using other people's money, plunder what they can, and spit out the remains.

Great-quality products, innovative designs, craftsmanship, and enhanced services to meet human needs all take second place to accumulating profits. As *New York Times* reporters Danielle Ivory, Ben Protess, and Kitty Bennett argue, "Unlike other for-profit companies, which often have years of experience making a product or offering a service, private equity is primarily skilled in making money."[2] PE managers also tend to be disengaged not only from the local communities in which their companies operate, but often from moral integrity itself.

The initial process begins with general partners (GPs) raising a pool of capital from potential donors for a new fund, which typically has a life cycle of ten to twelve years. These investment pools vary in size through self-imposed limits, with maximums depending on the PE shop's clout, inclination, capabilities, specific specialty or domain, and size, though nearly all of these funds are getting larger across the board.[3] Since 2008, GPs have become more inclined to surpass their hard caps. The interval between vintages also has shortened, averaging less than three years.[4]

Per the PE playbook, GPs have up to six years to deploy the money, generally by acquiring stakes in ten to fifteen businesses, which then become part of their overall portfolio. Subsequently, they unload the companies, usually within five years, and reimburse the LPs with their share of the profits.[5] The main intent is to cash out at a far greater valuation multiple (market price) than they had initially paid for the business. This is the mother lode of the buyout: the LPs receive their cash payouts and, if they surpass the hurdle rate, the PE collects 20 percent of the net profits (carried interest).[6] Of course, the higher the selling price, the more robust the rewards for everyone, except the company that has been sold and its employees.

At times, two or more PE firms will pool capital in what is categorized as a club deal. These arrangements allow smaller shops to acquire companies that they could not own otherwise. In other big-ticket deals, a PE house may just not want to invest too much of its fund in one asset.

Targets include publicly traded establishments, which GPs can then take private, though they often have to offer a 20–30 percent premium on the stock to entice the target firm's management and stockholders.[7] Other options are to acquire a private corporation, a division of one that is no longer wanted, a small or medium-size business, or real estate. As I discuss below, financial buyers are increasingly just purchasing from each other. Regardless, during the five to six years after purchase—or sooner—they sell off their portfolio companies and return a portion of the cash to the LPs. The GPs are now ready to start a fresh fund, though they can (and do) raise money for the next vehicle while simultaneously deploying capital for or jettisoning assets from the earlier one.

PE players take an opportunistic approach to purchasing companies.[8] Within their preferred industry sectors, they deploy capital for any target that will deliver elevated returns, regardless of product or service. They predominantly seek viable, healthy companies with strong, predictable cash flows that can service loads of debt but can also be used as collateral for add-ons and other expenses. Most attractive are relatively mature businesses with proven performance histories, low capital or research and development (R&D) needs, and a first-rate management team already at hand. Other attributes may include places with expendable assets, which can be sold to immediately pay down part of the debt or declare a dividend recapitalization (recap); firms with considerable growth potential; and companies with opportunities for cutting costs and raising revenues.[9]

The Magic Elixir: Leveraged Buyouts

The main strategy to achieving outsized profits is the leveraged buyout (LBO). Acquired firms are largely financed through debt, which in 2019 averaged roughly 70 percent of the purchase price, and sometimes more.[10] Debt, of course, is the not-so-secret sauce that makes these purchases exceedingly profitable. The bold use of debt includes financial engineering tactics like high-risk borrowing, or junk bonds, that can pile on hefty high-interest loans as part of the financing structure.[11] Even better for the PE firms, the monetary obligations are placed on the investee establishments, which are then solely liable for repaying them. Servicing the debt is crucial in order for buyout shops to realize huge returns on their investments. Thus, GPs use their portfolio companies to repay loans—and as quickly as possible. As targets pay off what is owed, the equity value for PE firms climbs. In consequence, however, the cash-strapped businesses may have insufficient funds for their labor force, equipment modernization, technical innovations, R&D, and other essential needs.

It is an exceedingly lucrative business with only limited risks for the PE shops. The business model has been painstakingly constructed so as to maximize returns from each of their portfolio companies while minimizing the GPs' exposure to loss. Sebastien Canderle observes, "Leverage . . . is firmly entrenched as a way for fund managers to make money with minimum personal risk but maximum reward."[12]

PE partners obtain still greater profits by driving up the value of the company itself through other means. A basic premise of the LBO is that the business will be sold at a far greater enterprise value (EV) than the initial purchase price—and in a relatively brief period of time. What's more, GPs milk their investee corporations by charging them a myriad of fees. For instance, expenses for due diligence—analyzing a business prior to purchase—are borne by the target, as are banking, accounting, legal, and advisory costs for the transaction. The acquired businesses assume comparable costs when sold. These extra charges for buying and selling a company generally amount to roughly 2–5 percent of the initial purchase price. There are also relatively large monitoring and directors' payments for overseeing the enterprise. Similarly, GPs can charge commissions when their portfolio companies take on acquisitions. Some, but not all, of these additional proceeds are shared with their LPs.

Managing directors regard the individual business itself merely as an asset to be bought and sold. They are not particularly concerned about what their target actually produces, its quality, or its long-term performance, as long as they can extract sizable investment returns from it. And the faster, the better. Nothing is viewed as too sacred to achieve this goal, not even hospice services, alcohol and drug treatments, fertility therapies, or emergency care.

Notwithstanding Mitt Romney's disingenuous claim during his presidential campaign that Bain Capital—and presumably PE generally—salvages failing companies and creates jobs, only a small percentage of PE shops take on this type of investing. And even when they do, the financial buyers are solely concerned with extracting value from the troubled enterprises. They are like vultures, scavenging for businesses that are on the brink of bankruptcy (or that already have filed for Chapter 11) and then buying up their debt at a fraction of the cost. As creditors, they now take control of either restructuring the company for sale or liquidating it. As usual, the future viability of the establishment is not on their radar screen.

The entrepreneurs are highly adaptable in their pursuit of monetary gain and use any number of strategies, depending on the condition of the target, the overall economic environment, and their own specific approach to financial wizardry. They are skilled at wringing money out of their portfolio companies through a strikingly resourceful array of tactics. The sizable and flexible PE toolkit includes, in addition to LBOs, strengthening cash flow, boosting revenues, slicing costs, divestitures, add-ons, enhancing operational performance, reorganization, dividend recaps, and sale-leaseback agreements.

All the same, many business leaders contend that cash flow is the most important aspect of the undertaking, even more than profits. By generating strong, positive cash flow, GPs can pay off their portfolio company's debt and borrow more money for acquisitions and even dividend recaps. To be sure, "the more cash a business produces, the more leverage it can bear, hence the numerous refinancing[s] in recent years."[13] Such ploys enhance the resale value of the enterprise, thereby enriching the PE firm with little effort on its part; nonetheless, these tactics divert resources from investment in the internal requirements of the business and can harm its long-term well-being.

Growth Equity Investing

Growth equity is a relatively recent but now flourishing type of PE investing; it represents 24 percent of all funds that closed in 2019, the highest percentage to date.[14] These non-buyout vehicles, which do not rely on extensive debt, generally are a cross between venture capital and LBOs. In this category, GPs inject money into an established, fast-growing company with solid management, a proven track record, and prospects for significantly greater expansion. Such establishments typically have insufficient working capital to bolster their ongoing development, an inability to service much debt, and a lack of access to investment banks and public markets. Unlike leveraged buyouts, the capital structure is not augmented immediately with new debt.

Success for shops specializing in this approach entails driving returns through substantial operational improvements, transformational changes, and generating far greater revenue than previously. Indeed, without high leverage, the PE firm and its management team must promote remarkable structural alterations, whether organic or inorganic. Depending on the circumstances, tactics range from national and international expansion, development of new product lines, and enlargement of existing facilities to scaling and consolidating scores of acquisitions, optimizing cash flow, and improving governance.

Still more challenging for GPs tackling growth investing is that they almost always take a minority stake in the business—contrary to their usual majority share. That means giving up full control, including the right to hire and fire top management, which is anathema to their traditional approach. Nonetheless, because the PE space is extremely competitive today, and more founding owners and families are insisting on retaining majority rights, certain PE outfits have found it expedient to move in this direction.[15]

Growth investing is particularly attractive when there is a shortage of viable LBO targets. Peggy Koenig, chair of Abry Partners, acknowledged that there were companies that she would have liked to buy, but they were not for sale. Thus, her PE firm initiated a strategy in which it would provide growth capital through senior equity financing.[16]

Voracious Appetites: Add-Ons

In the early 1980s, PE players utilized a buy-and-bust scheme whereby they bought large conglomerates through leveraged buyouts and sold off the pieces; they were adept at knowing when the parts were more valuable than the whole. New tax laws in the late 1980s rendered it less profitable to sell off divisions, and they moved on to other means of exploiting companies, such as multiple arbitrage or, as one reporter puts it, "quick-hit growth."[17]

Since 2009, add-ons have become an increasingly prominent weapon in the PE arsenal, primarily in the middle market.[18] The focus tends to be on sectors that are largely fragmented. The PE shop acquires or pieces together a company as its platform, and then seeks lower-cost but complementary acquisitions. Vertical consolidation also has become progressively more popular. It works like this: "As the platform grows, its value increases in tandem with each add-on. When sold it will have a higher exit multiple because there is a premium paid for a larger organization."[19]

Some knowledgeable observers argue that "the buy-and-build strategy has morphed from a common tactic into a cornerstone of PE value creation."[20] In large part, it is the flip side of the earlier buy-and-split approach. It can serve as a means for leveling today's exorbitant price valuations in certain industries, such as health care.[21] Rolling up small-scale businesses into larger ones, moreover, can serve to create leading regional or national enterprises. Such standing allows the corporation not only to dominate a particular market but also to control prices. At the same time, fund managers assume that consolidation will boost earnings through greater efficiency. In some cases PE firms are like the invasive multiflora rose, overpowering everything in their way.

But merger and acquisition techniques are precarious because integrating an assortment of companies complicates the scaling process, and it doesn't always pan out. Thus, the economies of scale that are expected may actually bring about financial turmoil for the acquired companies. Furthermore, though the original platform achieves immediate top-line growth with each additional purchase, its debt burden rises commensurately, necessitating tough cost controls. Consequently, while acquisitions and add-ons continue to burgeon, boosting ultimate returns for the PE firm, the portfolio companies do not always fare as well. In addition, Kosman points out that by progressively removing small and medium-size businesses from the economy, the country loses much of its entrepreneurial character.[22]

LBO Redux: Secondary Buyouts

Secondary buyouts (SBOs) are when GPs acquire companies directly from other PE firms, for example, if Abry Partners buys an enterprise and four years later sells it to Blue Wolf Capital. Although they were not prevalent in prior eras, by 2018 SBOs accounted for more than one-fourth of all non-add-on deals, up from 15 percent in 2008.[23] Clearly, the industry is facing fewer targets that have never been PE-backed and a vastly reduced number of publicly traded companies to take private.[24] SBOs are also a relatively easy means for deploying dry powder.[25] The number of tertiary and quaternary acquisitions of the same company, referred to as "echo buyouts," has been rising steadily as well. Correspondingly, quinary (fifth) and even senary (sixth) buyouts are occurring. The buy-and-build strategy, in particular, allows a PE shop to market a company within its expected time frame, thereby offering the subsequent PE owner some room for additional growth. In fact, tertiary buyouts often have a greater number of add-ons than the earlier SBOs.[26]

Many experts regard these trends as inescapable since "ideal" targets, snatched by PE houses over the decades, have steadily diminished. It is a vicious cycle: GPs that secure a business through an SBO are likely to take an equivalent exit route and hold their acquisitions for shorter periods in each round. Companies tossed around like a football, often with quick flips, may be advantageous for PE firms, but the target businesses can suffer severe consequences. For example, these multiple buyouts are unduly dependent on continual add-ons and mergers, with the companies commonly confronting ongoing piles of debt to the detriment of any operational improvements. They undergo more frequent recapitalizations (including dividend recaps), which also impose greater debt, thereby sucking out even more cash for interest payments that otherwise could have been plowed back into the establishment. The company is viewed, in effect, as a cash cow awaiting a new owner to milk it.[27]

The Unfettered Toolbox

Though a leveraged buyout is the foremost PE strategy and the core of the industry, GPs will engage in other ruses to line their pockets. The financiers branch out by adding to their tactics, specializing in specific domains, broadening into new investment areas, and diversifying their overall business. As David Carey and John Morris explain, there is "a truth about private equity that is seldom observed by those outside the financial world: It is defined more by opportunism than by conventional LBO."[28] Regardless of approach, the end game is always to squeeze as much money as possible out of a portfolio company in the shortest amount of time possible and then sell it for a sizable profit. One GP put it succinctly: "PE likes returns." The strategy is irrelevant. They will go wherever they can to put their assets to work as long as they can maximize returns.[29]

Given the competition today over top-tier investment opportunities, some PE firms—including larger ones—are turning their attention to middle- and lower-middle-market businesses, a number of which are family-owned. For these deals, GP managers market themselves as bringing considerably more to the table than just capital: they promote their financial acumen, restructuring and administrative skills, comprehensive networks of established relationships, and other know-how that supplements the field-specific experience of existing owners and management teams. It is not always an easy sell to already successful proprietors—and they are precisely whom PE is seeking.

The industry also has become increasingly specialized: more buyout shops are sector-specific or focus on a limited number of areas. A partner at a leading firm explains that although his shop is a generalist, it too is now structured by domains.[30] In truth, as a partner at another top buyout outfit makes clear, GPs are not operations people—they are financiers.[31] Therefore, they are bringing subject-knowledgeable professionals in-house or, more commonly, building an external network of go-to experts in various fields and with specific operational skill sets. Such individuals are hired as consultants or even placed in key management positions within a portfolio company. These segment-specific experts are attentive to building value so as to make the portfolio companies more attractive to buyers, not necessarily to achieve long-term growth and development. With an eye squarely on exit, they can handpick appropriate add-ons and new product lines; oversee integration, pricing, and revenues; select suitable innovations; and provide strategic direction overall.

A common refrain among GPs today is that they are paying more attention to organic growth, aimed at the top line. For example, in addition to LBOs, acquisitions, and add-ons, they rely on large-scale performance improvements as a key driver of value creation. These include increasing market share through advertising and better brand recognition, expanding sales, developing new products and services, enlarging output, and investing in capital equipment. Yet despite paying lip service to such enhancements, it appears that they are not actually allocating substantial resources to the internal requirements of their portfolio businesses. In its Tenth Annual Private Equity Perspective Survey in 2019, advisory firm BDO found that only 17 percent of the PE respondents were investing in operational improvements. Moreover, when asked where their firm would direct the most capital in the next twelve months, they replied that only 1 percent would go to "funding portfolio working capital needs."[32]

Certain PE firms also are engaging in direct lending, competing with banks to finance loans, especially for midsize companies.[33] Their transactions are completely hidden from the public and are entirely unregulated. Driven by both excess cash and a lack of government standards, direct lending has become a thriving PE business. The lending opportunities they offer are especially expedient for smaller companies that don't meet banks' criteria. Recipients also are other PE houses that are seeking loans for their acquisitions.[34] These direct-lending funds, which tend to be more borrower-friendly than banks are, customarily offer covenant-lite loans. Consequently, they broaden the potential for overborrowing and defaults. W. Blake Holden, a partner at Warburg Pincus, divulged that in one deal he was turned down by several banks but had offers from three PE places, and they all gave him a better deal.[35]

Newfangled Configurations of Themselves

A far-reaching transformation of the industry has been the public listing of certain PE firms, most of them long-standing establishments.[36] Senior PE directors have availed themselves of the opportunity to cash in on some of the stake in their business, while in most cases still maintaining control. For example, of the $6.6 billion raised by Blackstone's initial public offering (IPO), the partners collected fully $4.6 billion. The conversion also allows the buyout shops to back their acquisitions with stock, giving them greater financial flexibility. Nowadays, these publicly traded entities are steadily shifting from a partnership to a corporate tax structure (C corporation), thus benefiting from the reduced tax rate enacted under the federal Tax Cuts and Jobs Act of 2017. The revised arrangement renders stock available to index and mutual funds as well, a further financial advantage. To free greater liquid assets, especially for GPs near retirement, some enterprising places are even selling pieces of themselves to outside investors, raising roughly $14 billion in 2019.[37]

Fortunately for the rest of us, the IPOs have pierced the veil of secrecy to a certain extent: according to SEC regulations, corporations traded on the stock markets must make more information available to the general population. In the past, for example, investigators could not obtain accurate figures on PE earnings or executive income. We now know that the heads of the six main listed PE firms are the topmost earners in the United States, even compared to other leading corporations. According to a joint study by the *New York Times* and Equilar, they took home on average $211 million in 2015, or "nearly 10 times what the average bank chief executive earned."[38] Stephen Schwarzman, cofounder of Blackstone Group, was paid the most, $786.5 million in 2018; in previous years his annual income ranged from $425 million to $734 million.[39] Salaries, of course, do not convey overall wealth; many PE founders have become billionaires. Schwarzman's fortune, for instance, is estimated at $18 billion, while Henry Kravis (KKR) and Leon Black (Apollo Global Management) have a net worth of $6 billion and $8.5 billion, respectively.[40]

Feathering Their Nest: Dividend Recapitalizations and Sale-Leasebacks

PE outfits generally are not content with just the initial round of debt through an LBO and often engage in intermittent refinancing or recapitalization of their portfolio companies, which can capture exceptional returns. Secondary buyouts tend to be more at risk for recapitalizations since, arguably, they are another way of sucking more money out of a company that has already been squeezed.[41]

In the twenty-first century, there has been more aggressive use of dividend recaps. As Jason Kelly starkly states, "PE firms can use some of the companies they own as virtual ATMs."[42] In this ploy, GPs award themselves (and their LPs) bonuses by placing additional debt on their portfolio companies, often through junk bonds.[43] In 2018, PE shops helped themselves to more money than ever before; according to one expert, roughly one-third of them used debt for dividend recaps that year.[44] A few have even taken debt-financed dividends from the companies they acquired shortly after the sale. The recaps can generate impressive earnings, allowing GPs to amplify their proceeds, especially in the face of elevated valuations for their purchases.

A 2019 BDO board survey of PE players found that 84 percent of them were planning to leverage up their portfolio companies. When they were questioned as to what they intended to do with the proceeds, fully 30 percent said that they would finance dividend recaps.[45] To be sure, many partners have regained much of their original share of equity through these returns. It also moves them toward the hurdle rate, whereby they will grab the brass ring: 20 percent of the profits.

In the case of Staples, a multinational office supply business, Sycamore Partners refinanced the company shortly after taking it private in 2017. The financial buyers gave themselves a $1 billion dividend that drove Staples's overall debt to more than $5.3 billion. Even prior to exiting the chain, they had recovered almost two-thirds of their initial $1.6 billion cash investment.[46]

Similarly, CVC Capital Partners and Leonard Green & Partners bought publicly traded BJ's Wholesale Club in 2011 and, after privatizing it, completed numerous dividend recaps that paid them nearly $1.8 billion, or 64 percent of their initial outlay. When BJ's was returned to the public market in 2018, the club shouldered $2 billion in debt.[47]

The arts-and-crafts retailer Michaels is yet another typical example of GPs seeking to enrich themselves via loans, at the expense of their investee companies. Through a dividend recap, Michaels reimbursed Blackstone and Bain Capital nearly half of the $1.7 billion they had paid to purchase the chain. The PE shops then went on to accrue more than twice their money in a 2014 IPO.

Leonard Green & Partners also wrings millions from portfolio companies. In 2014, the PE firm bought Mister Car Wash for $8.2 billion in equity, with the remainder in loans. Two years later it grabbed a $213 million dividend recap from the auto-cleaning service, and in 2019 took another for $215 million, all financed through debt. Leonard Green recaptured nearly all of its initial investment. The leverage multiple for these dividend recaps, however, became so extreme that the company was downgraded to "speculative" by Moody's.[48]

Dividend recaps divert cash flow from companies to their PE owners. It is especially egregious when a business is experiencing financial stress and can be pushed into bankruptcy. Moreover, as John Puchalla, a senior vice president at Moody's, asserts, "It limits their flexibility to ride through the economic cycles."[49]

Similarly, PE houses can engage in sale-leaseback arrangements, another attractive maneuver when valuations are elevated. Through this tactic, GPs formally separate the enterprise from its real estate (land and buildings), sell the property, and then lease it back. They then use the proceeds to recoup part or all of their initial equity investment while also returning cash to their LPs, thereby enhancing internal rates of return. The portfolio company itself, on the other hand, is now burdened with paying rent on land it had once owned. Such asset stripping amounts to legalized theft. In just one example, Sun Capital Partners acquired Shopko Stores for $1.1 billion in 2005, immediately sold the valuable real estate for $800 million, and leased it back to the stores. With the company now saddled with immense rent, additional revenues were sucked out of the already debt-laden chain, and by 2019 Shopko was forced into bankruptcy.[50]

Seizing the Gold: Exiting Portfolio Companies

PE titans are not known for their sentimentality; rather, as soon as they acquire a company, they position it for their successful exit. And the sooner the better. The clock begins ticking immediately after the firm purchases a business. Though the holding period generally ranges from three to six years, quicker exits tend to yield higher returns.[51] At the same time, quick flips are more likely to generate financial stress for both the workers and the company without adding much of value for them.

There are essentially three means of disposing of a portfolio company: sell it to a private company in a related industry (generally, a strategic buyer); sell it to another PE shop (financial buyer); or put it on the public market through an IPO. In some cases, the PE firm might retain shares in the public company beyond what is required by law and off-load them periodically as stock prices rise.[52] In the right circumstances, an IPO can offer an immense payday. However, there have been far fewer IPOs since 2010.[53]

To a great extent, secondary buyouts have become the exit of choice, especially for middle-market companies. SBOs reached 54 percent of the total in 2018 as compared to 43 percent for corporate acquisitions. One of the most vital concerns for PE shops in the aftermath of the Great Recession was to locate lucrative exits for their portfolio companies, many of which they had been forced to retain well beyond their customary holding time. GPs were eager to garner the carried interest for themselves, and LPs were anxious for their cash. SBOs are less bureaucratically complex, less costly, and less time-consuming than preparing for an IPO. As with corporate purchasers, SBOs deliver full liquidity earlier.

Relapse buyouts, where a PE firm sells an asset and after a short time repurchases it, have cropped up more frequently as well. A case in point is the TPG / Leonard Green & Partners buyout of J. Crew from its founding family in 1997 for $500 million. After an IPO nine years later, the GPs in 2011 again took it private in a $3 billion leveraged buyout.[54]

From Bedrock to Bankrupt

PE firms are adept at piling debt on their investee companies, siphoning cash from them, and when necessary using the US bankruptcy laws to protect their interests. They shrewdly insulate themselves from any debts or other financial obligations of their acquisitions. Every fund is created as a separate partnership, and each business within it is a legally distinct entity, responsible for its own financial well-being. The partners do not have to shore up any of their stressed assets, and in the case of bankruptcy, they are liable only for their initial equity stake in the business. Their other portfolio holdings are not only sheltered but any actual financial losses may have been recouped through earlier returns, such as dividend recaps and the multitude of management fees.[55] The evidence suggests that they often exit their insolvent companies either with limited consequences or, at times, sound profits.[56] In addition, they can use bankruptcy to slash a company's unsustainable debt, revoke contracts with unions, jettison pension commitments, and discount the company's obligations to suppliers.[57]

Overly indebted portfolio companies and subsequent filings for Chapter 11 protection have been endemic in PE over the decades. Retail has been hit the most, especially in the early years, but any industry with untenable debt is susceptible to default. The situation is even more precarious if a company encounters a market disruption, for example, new state-of-the-art technologies where it should spend extra cash on catching up rather than servicing debt. Other factors, such as a change in consumer preferences, intensified competition, or a rise in interest rates, could make it difficult to sustain large financial liabilities. Furthermore, it is challenging enough to run a company encumbered with huge loans during advantageous economic times. It is even more demanding when conditions worsen or the economy descends into a recession. Under these circumstances, as we have witnessed during the COVID-19 pandemic, there are countless bankruptcies and insolvencies. A significant number of PE executives continue to fail to provide a buffer against future upheavals.

In 2019, Moody's Investors Service warned, "The number of low-rated companies deemed highly vulnerable to default may jump 'dramatically' in the next downturn, possibly exceeding levels seen in the financial crisis, as a result of private equity activity." According to the investor rating service, PE owns nearly 80 percent of North American enterprises shouldering B3 ratings (five levels below investment grade) and 68 percent of those rated Caa (speculative grade). Its report notes, "A burdensome debt load and an overly aggressive acquisition strategy and integration challenges can push viable businesses into the Caa category."[58] The upshot was that ninety-nine PE-owned companies received a distressed credit rating in 2019, up 29 percent from 2018.[59]

The Funders: Limited Partners

As mentioned above, PE firms draw predominantly on other people's money for their transactions and personal accrual of wealth. Limited partners are the lifeblood of ready cash in the industry's playbook; they are expected to provide nearly all the equity capital for investments. For the most part, GPs have contributed only 1–2 percent of total acquisition costs. Since the 2008 financial crisis, however, LPs have been demanding more "skin in the game," especially as fund sizes have climbed. In 2019, the expected share was closer to 2.9 percent, or slightly more in certain cases.[60]

LPs pour vast amounts of cash into PE coffers—trillions of dollars—despite the problematic nature of the industry.[61] It is the money of workers and retirees, nonprofit foundations, university endowments, insurance companies, high-net-worth families, and to a lesser extent, sovereign wealth funds (i.e., Norway, China). By the end of the 1990s, state and local pension plans had emerged as the foremost source of PE financing.[62] Today, nearly half of PE investment capital comes from public and private pension funds worldwide.

Seeking huge windfalls, these funds have steadily enlarged their allocations to the asset class as compared to other investment options. One source observes that in earlier times, "LPs contributed 4–5 percent of their total resources; now they are in double digits."[63] Analysts expect institutional investors to dole out even more in the coming years, even though survey results for 2020 indicated that they are concerned about a potential recession or whether their PE shop will actually deliver the expected high returns.[64] Concomitantly, the investor base overall has grown enormously, with more state and local pension funds committing money. Not even the COVID-19 pandemic slowed these trends down.

Institutional sponsors are willing to risk their capital and relinquish liquidity for the lifetime of the fund (generally ten years) in order to garner far greater returns relative to traditional markets.[65] Public pension plans, in particular, tend to be desperate for high-yield investments because a significant percentage of them are underfunded and have been for years. The flood of baby boomer retirements as well as longer life-spans have exacerbated the situation. It is estimated that the shortfall in promised state and local government benefits has reached $5 trillion today, or just under 75 percent of what they need to meet obligations.[66] Funded ratios (assets divided by liabilities) average only 66 percent and, according to one source, would have been 50 percent or less if they had invested fully in risk-free securities.[67] Pew Charitable Trusts data indicate that only twelve states are sufficiently funded while the rest are vulnerable, in dangerous condition, or experiencing critical financial health with the prospect of insolvency.[68] And these deficits are rising.

Presumably, pension fund managers are attempting to compensate for the inability or unwillingness of state and local authorities to allocate sufficient resources to meet accruing and burdensome pension obligations. Otherwise, they might have to drastically cut promised retirement benefits. Most of these institutional investors plan to increase their PE investments. Seduced by the extra-large returns promised by savvy PE marketers, especially during periods of low interest rates such as today, they are ready to disregard the moral ramifications. For example, in addition to serious risk, some of these pension investments may be at odds with the health and well-being of the workers and taxpayers who contribute to the systems and the retirees who depend on them.

There is also the question of fiduciary duty: trustees of pensions, endowments, and other types of capital reserves generally have a legal (and ethical) responsibility to act in the best interest of their beneficiaries. Yet once they commit assets to a PE fund, they relinquish all control over the money to the GPs.[69] One PE executive explained that investors execute due diligence on a PE's track record but then let it "run the show without interference." Another says, "You make a contract with LPs and then they give you a blank check."[70] Though LPs would appreciate greater transparency, they mostly accept the loss of command over their money and being kept in the dark about transaction details.

Nevertheless, they are concerned about management fees, which is one of the more contentious issues between LPs and their PE partners. GPs fill their coffers by extracting cash from the investors to the tune of 1.3–2.5 percent annually on committed capital during the life of the fund, irrespective of how well the investments perform. In a 2020 LP Perspectives Survey of 146 institutional investors, 73 percent agreed that the rising fees charged by private equity funds are difficult to justify internally.[71] These charges, which can amount to nearly 20 percent of the overall fund assets, are a significant and valued portion of earnings for PE partners.[72]

The financial buyers are fully aware that unless they keep their LPs happy, the well could run dry. And the paramount means for satisfying them is through internal rates of return (IRR) that are far greater than safer investments, especially those that have more liquidity.[73] As stated by Jeff Aronson, founder and chair of Centerbridge Partners,

IRR is the most important criterion for LPs in choosing a PE partner. Evidently, they expect, as a minimum, yields in the mid- to high teens.[74] If a shop is struggling with an exit for any of its portfolio companies, thereby threatening to lessen the fund's overall IRR, it will turn to other means to up the indicator, such as dividend recaps. Nowadays, however, even the indicator itself is being questioned.

Institutional investors are not always passive bystanders. A few are demanding lower management and other fees as well as co-investment opportunities, which usually have lower charges and higher returns. They have also asked for more PE equity on investments. Further, they can pressure GPs on issues of importance to them; in one case, when a firm appealed to a potential LP group for funding, several members expressed concern about the limited number of women it employed.[75] In another instance, LPs (among other parties) leaned on Bain Capital and KKR to pay severance to the displaced workers of their bankrupt Toys "R" Us chain. Of course, LPs could do far more to protect labor, communities, and the beneficiaries of their pension plans.

But to the contrary, they tend to gloss over the noxious underpinnings of the PE industry. Rather than confront GPs over ethical violations, LPs tend to be more concerned with maintaining elevated profits. For instance, in a survey of 62 institutional investors by Eaton Partners, 63 percent were troubled by how present-day political and media attacks on PE will affect their earnings. Similarly, according to a Coller Capital study of 113 LPs worldwide, the Global Private Equity Barometer, more than 75 percent of them would prefer that PE associations, such as the American Investment Council, stand up for the industry more forcefully.[76]

Top Management: Supervising the Enterprise

Small and medium-size businesses, including founders, have gotten into the act as well. In prior decades, GPs targeted mostly larger corporations, at times in hostile takeovers. As Carey and Morris find, high-level managers were presented with stakes in the organization "that potentially could make them richer than they could ever hope to become collecting stock options in a public company. 'Sign me up!' CEOs said."[77] Today, smaller businesses are either invited in by owners or wooed by the GPs who, again, offer irresistible financial incentives. Besides, because of bank consolidations since the 1980s and the ensuing loss of community and independent commercial banks, less sizable enterprises find it challenging to obtain financing elsewhere.

PE houses typically exert rigid control over their portfolio company's strategic goals, which mainly are the servicing of debt and attaining strong earnings. They establish the business plan, timetables, and labor guidelines; closely monitor the enterprise; and approve budgets and capital outlays. GPs tend to dominate the board of directors; normally, one or more of their representatives sit on it for as long as they own the company. Particularly noteworthy is that they hold full power to hire and fire CEOs and other high-level executives, including the founders of the companies they have bought.

Despite that, top-tier managers are highly valued for the day-to-day governance of the acquired company. A common refrain among the founders I interviewed was that "as long as you bring in the money," the PE shop leaves you alone—unless a matter entails substantial financial expenditures. GPs understand that good management is central to a portfolio company's success. They strive to retain existing directors post-acquisition, but where senior executives are viewed as inadequate, they will appoint their own team. Perhaps 50 percent of PE transactions entail a leadership change.[78]

Of course, effective management for a PE firm is viewed as alignment with its short-term interests. To ensure or strengthen similar aspirations, the senior executive team—or founder-owner—usually is granted or expected to hold on to an equity stake in the business. Typically, they end up with 5–20 percent of the entity. By becoming part owners in the buyout, senior executives are incentivized to concentrate on attaining huge, quick earnings. They may also receive bonuses if they meet periodic targets.

Additional Feeders at the Trough

It's an open secret that investment banks cash in on the private equity industry. They receive sizable fees for underwriting debt, financing bridge loans, arranging deals, marketing a company to potential buyers, and arranging IPOs. As Burrough and Helyar write, in mergers and acquisitions—win, lose, or draw—they secure fees for advising, divesting, piecing together, and lending money.[79] During the 2003–2007 buyout boom, banks derived about 20 percent of their profits from PE business. In 2007 alone, the large shops paid them an estimated $16.3 billion in fees.[80] Certain banks dedicate entire divisions to the highly profitable LBO space.

The PE industry is surrounded by other professionals who also feast at the table. A plethora of accountants, lawyers, insurance agents, brokers, consultants, tax advisors, and more partake in its deals. In some cases, there can be eight or more lawyers and bankers working on a single acquisition. Each takes a bite out of the assets for every transaction, including the sourcing, purchase, additions, marketing, and sale. In the 2018 buyout of the publicly traded Kindred Healthcare, a homecare and hospice provider, the PE firms had the assistance of thirty-four advisors and twenty-seven lenders.

Sprinkling Fairy Dust: The Federal Tax Haven

An essential aspect of the PE industry is the highly advantageous tax breaks, especially for debt, that allow GPs to attain their enormous wealth. Kosman asserts that it was these loopholes that launched the industry in the first place.[81] Not only does heavy debt magnify the PE industry's gains, but the interest it pays on the loans is tax deductible. Reduced taxes because of leverage alone may well represent up to 20 percent of a company's worth. Kelly calls this the "mother's milk" of the PE buyout.[82] Just as advantageous, when earnings from carried interest are distributed to the partners, the money is taxed as capital gains rather than at the much higher ordinary income rate. Such taxpayer subsidies augment the value of portfolio companies for their PE owners without benefiting the businesses themselves or "creating new wealth for the economy."[83] The federal government has lost billions of dollars over the decades from these and other tax avoidance schemes.

Despite some politicians' threats of harsh revisions to the existing code, the Tax Cuts and Jobs Act of 2017 did not alter the carried interest loophole. The measure did cap the deduction of interest from loans at 30 percent of the total, potentially encouraging PE partners to place slightly less debt on their acquisitions or, alternatively, encouraging them to put down more equity.[84] Nevertheless, the evidence suggests that GPs have not chosen either of these options, which would have lowered their earnings considerably. In addition, PE is now required to keep its portfolio companies for at least three years, up from the previous mandate of twelve months; businesses flipped sooner are taxed at the higher short-term capital gains rate. This stipulation, however, would have affected less than 17 percent of exits in 2017.[85] It could in the future slightly cramp the GPs' style in their roll-up strategy because they might have to time their portfolio companies' add-ons with greater precision.

The Tax Cuts and Jobs Act decreased the corporate tax rate from 35 percent to 21 percent, which has had mixed implications for the PE firms. On the one hand, the places that they own benefit from higher cash flow, allowing them to pay off debt easier and quicker. On the other, publicly traded corporations have more capital for acquisitions, thus enabling them to compete more effectively with the PE shops and thereby driving up valuations for everyone.

Many experts believe that overall the 2017 tax act has not been unduly burdensome for PE firms, and certainly it was far more favorable than it could have been. For example, lower corporate taxes appear to be compensating for the limits on interest deductibility, especially since GPs have not reduced leverage on their buyouts. Regardless, they are skilled at tax arbitrage and have been restructuring their firms, debt, and deals to circumvent any of the negative effects.[86] Besides, the industry received a reprieve through the Coronavirus Aid, Relief, and Economic Security (CARES) Act of 2020: the bill temporarily raised the allowed percentage on deductions of interest from loans.

Concluding Remarks

A foremost mantra among GPs is that they create value for the businesses they purchase, even as they extract outsized earnings for themselves and their LPs. But there can be considerable adverse social and economic aftereffects associated with a leveraged buyout and its hefty profits. Who exactly bears these costs? As noted earlier, buyout shops disregard all concerns other than maximizing financial gain; they have flourished at the expense of workers, communities, and in the case of bankruptcies, the businesses themselves. As Kosman puts it, "the private equity industry is not about, and never has been about, building strong, healthy companies."[87]

PE-owned enterprises employ a significant and expanding percentage of the US labor force. With fewer than 5 million Americans on their payrolls from 1980 to 1999, nowadays more than 11 million people (nearly 9 percent of private-sector workers) are at the mercy of GPs and their firms.[88] Though the financial buyers may value effective top management, the rest of the labor force is viewed merely as a liability on their accounts. Given the secrecy of the industry, it is challenging to uncover precise data on the effects of private equity on workers, but in the main, its business model engenders severe repercussions for them. Greater productivity and "efficiency," whether in retail, services, or health care, translate into economizing on operating costs, sometimes ruthlessly. For labor, this implies streamlining personnel, intensifying workloads, limiting training, lowering wages, and slashing benefits with the aim of reducing spending and repaying heavily leveraged loans. Up to half a million more workers than in comparable non-PE-owned enterprises were let go between 2000 and 2008.[89] A 2019 study, "Private Equity: How Wall Street Firms are Pillaging American Retail," reveals that while PE-controlled retailers employ more than a million workers today, they were responsible for more than 1.3 million job losses since 2009.[90] Terminated staff lose health insurance, vacation benefits, sick days, and severance pay, unlike CEOs and other high-level executives who can secure golden parachute packages worth millions.

GPs tend to use any positive cash flow to service debt and for dividends, mergers, and acquisitions. Because the partners are not interested in the long-term prospects of the businesses they hold, there are few resources available for research and development. Supplies and equipment are accorded short shrift as are customer services and capital spending. They can raise prices on products where they have gained monopoly status. They will do anything to enhance the bottom line, at least for the short term, and to ready their acquisitions for sale at vastly improved prices. It takes a certain financial acumen—and ruthlessness—to extract everything you can from a company and simultaneously build its market worth for resale. But how much "value" are the PE owners actually adding to the business versus what they take out? One observer acidly remarks: "Overnight, a financially healthy company becomes one that is living on the edge—not for any benefit for employees or customers, but solely for the financial benefit of the PE firm that bought it."[91]

Are PE firms adding value to the society at large, or are they just takers? A number of state and local pension funds are beneficiaries of the industry to an extent; their executive managers certainly seem to think so, given their ongoing and growing financial backing of PE. Then again, because of the industry's tax gambits, federal, state, and local governments are deprived of millions, perhaps billions, in revenues. Consumers often lose as small companies get rolled up into regional or national monopolies: prices rise, and choices are restricted. Bankruptcies engender a loss to everyone, although PE partners mostly take their equity out beforehand. Communities can experience acute damage, as numerous insolvencies over the decades have shown. GPs are like an elephant stampede, crushing everything underfoot.

2 |

The Emergence of the Alternative Asset Class

FIRST KNOWN as leveraged buyout (LBO) shops, private equity emerged in the 1960s and 1970s. These PE firms were largely two- or three-person partnerships engaged in relatively small transactions, generally well under $30 million.[1] LBOs began flourishing in the 1980s. According to Eileen Appelbaum and Rosemary Batt, there was a proliferation of leveraged acquisitions, more than 2,500 during that period, including a number of hostile takeovers that rapidly marked the firms as corporate raiders.[2] The LBOs then exploded into billion-dollar deals or more, which soon became the norm for many of them. Total leveraged buyouts swelled to $74 billion by the end of the decade, up from $3 billion in 1981.[3]

The energetic pursuit of bigger and bigger ventures was abetted by deregulation and tax policies, which LBO shops exploited to the fullest extent. In addition, investment banks, including First Boston, Morgan Stanley, Salomon Brothers, Merrill Lynch, and Goldman Sachs, became an integral part of their operations; they found the massive financing and advisory fees irresistible.

By the mid-1980s, the scale of LBOs accelerated and the business became more convoluted, particularly because of the introduction of junk bonds, which allowed for even grander purchases and greater debt. Spearheaded by Michael Milken through his firm Drexel Burnham Lambert, these risky, high-interest financial instruments released huge amounts of unsecured debt for outsized takeovers.[4] Drexel raised long-term, relatively covenant-free capital that was not accessible to midsize companies anywhere else, especially those firms below investment grade.[5] Bryan Burrough and John Helyar contend that Milken and his company "almost single-handedly transformed the takeover business in the mid-1980s."[6]

For the most part, LBO shops bought private companies or divisions of those that were publicly traded; a substantial number of conglomerates, which had increased their size and diversity of products during the previous two decades, were now shedding assets unrelated to their primary business. Several of the larger LBO firms took entire public establishments private with the aim of dismembering them: the various sectors were worth more than the whole. These shops would acquire a company, sell off enough parts to pay the purchase price, and keep the core business at nearly no expense. Their targets generally had sufficient positive cash flow to pay down the high debts that were incurred in the leveraged takeovers.

In conjunction with the heavy use of junk bonds, financial engineering, and sharp cost-cutting strategies, the PE partners extracted as much money as possible for themselves. The unrestrained profiteering of the era enabled the accumulation of considerable personal wealth, which could be realized expeditiously and without significant outlays of the recipient's own capital. The multibillion-dollar leveraged buyout industry embodied excessive greed and predatory behavior; it offered lavish lifestyles for the newly minted millionaire partners and often hefty monetary rewards for top management and stockholders, while contributing to the collapse of companies, decent jobs, and once viable communities.[7]

One example is the disquieting story of a thriving Fortune 500 company, Anchor Hocking, which was based in a flourishing small town in Ohio. Brian Alexander in Glass House recounts how a series of leveraged buyouts, beginning in 1986, systematically destroyed both the company and Lancaster's community.[8] The first of these new owners,

Daniel Ferguson, CEO of Newell Corporation, immediately fired staff, sold off parts of the business, and instituted a number of other "efficiencies" that enhanced profits while sabotaging the workers. In 2004, Anchor (along with two other businesses) was sold to Cerberus Capital Management in another heavily leveraged purchase.[9] Although still profitable, the now seriously indebted company was forced to pay millions in interest, along with dividend recaps and "advising" fees to Cerberus. At the same time, the firm neglected to contribute its share into the employees' 401(k) pension fund and to maintain equipment, leading to continual breakdowns. By 2006, loaded with more than $400 million in debt, Anchor was driven into bankruptcy.

Monomoy Capital Partners, the next owner, sounded the death knell for Anchor after buying it out of Chapter 11 in 2007. The LBO shop continued the practice of increasing value only for itself by laying off more workers, charging high "monitoring" and "consulting" fees, borrowing money for dividend recaps, pocketing 1 percent of the value of all transactions, and engineering a sale-leaseback for the real estate that Anchor owned. According to Alexander, by 2012, Monomoy had received $54 million in known dividends and fees; the total corporate debt was roughly $181 million more than when the PE firm had bought it.[10]

The following year, Monomoy took the company public, retaining two-thirds of the stock.[11] The GPs received $90 million in cash from the transaction, piled up $265 million more in liabilities, and demanded additional givebacks from the workforce. Nevertheless, with more than $400 million in debt and only $100 million in total assets, Anchor—now named EveryWare—in 2015 filed for Chapter 11 again. Previously a successful business with a great deal of potential, it was now a beaten-down company in a downtrodden, drug-plagued town. Newell Corporation, Cerberus, and Monomoy continue to thrive.

There were a substantial number of other disastrous buyouts during the 1980s that ended in bankruptcy or the breakup of viable corporations. Of the twenty-five enterprises between 1985 through 1989 that relied on junk bonds for LBOs, companies worth in total more than $1 billion (slightly more than half) entered into bankruptcy.[12] Kosman asserts: "Still, the LBO kings, who had long ago been paid their fees, consistently [made] money on these deals, and lots of it."[13]

As the most prolific and voracious PE outfit of the era, Kohlberg Kravis Roberts (KKR) acquired quite a few giant establishments, including RJR Nabisco, Duracell, Stop & Shop, Safeway, Motel 6, and Beatrice Companies. At the time, KKR controlled roughly one-third of the nearly $20 billion in capital held by buyout firms. Its second largest acquisition, Beatrice (1986), cost $8.7 billion, most of it in debt. KKR promptly began selling off subsidiaries, such as Avis Car Rental and Tropicana, until it nearly liquidated the corporation. From the initial deal alone, KKR netted $45 million in fees while lawyers and bankers collected $250 million. Additionally, the original six top corporate officials were granted golden parachutes amounting to more than $22 million for agreeing to the deal. After less than four years, KKR had extracted $2 billion for breaking up the conglomerate; the LPs garnered an average of nearly 50 percent annually from their $407 million investment.[14] As usual, thousands of people lost their jobs.

The $4.2 billion buyout in 1986 of Safeway—the largest supermarket chain in the world at the time—was even more lucrative for KKR, its LPs, top management, stockholders, bankers, and lawyers—and just as devastating for employees and localities. Entire divisions and individual "underperforming" stores were swiftly closed down; some were sold for their valuable real estate. KKR, which controlled two-thirds of the board of directors, particularly aimed its ax at supermarkets employing union workers enjoying relatively decent wages. All told, Safeway shed 53 percent of its shops.[15] Susan C. Faludi, in her Pulitzer Prize–winning article, "Safeway LBO Yields Vast Profits but Exacts a Heavy Toll," observes, "But while much has been written about the putative benefits of LBOs, little has been said about the hundreds of thousands of people directly affected by the decade's buy-out binge: employees of the bought-out corporations. In the case of Safeway, a two-month investigation of the buy-out reveals enormous human costs and unintended side effects."[16]

More than 55,000 people, many of whom had worked for Safeway for years, lost their jobs; those who managed to find employment elsewhere faced drastic wage cuts, sometimes up to 30 percent, or were forced into part-time work. KKR drove the remaining labor force hard by imposing punishing quota systems for managers. Unlike the liquidation of Beatrice, the leaner and meaner Safeway soon engendered enhanced productivity and rising profits. In due course, Safeway was placed on the public market again. By the time it fully cashed out, KKR had turned its initial $129 million equity investment (only 3 percent of the buyout) into $72 billion, pocketing fifty-six times its money in thirteen years. Investment bankers, advisors, accountants, and others derived $292 million in fees and expenses related to the deal. Several decades later (2014), Safeway was subjected to another take-private LBO, this time by Cerberus Capital Management, which paid $8 billion for the company.[17]

Without a doubt, the greed and excesses of the era are epitomized by KKR's well-publicized takeover of RJR Nabisco, the tobacco and food giant, in 1989.[18] As chronicled by Burrough and Helyar in *Barbarians at the Gate*, a ferocious bidding war had taken place involving management, several LBO firms, investment bankers, and other Wall Street contenders. KKR triumphed. At $25 billion, the purchase was by far the largest LBO in history, a record it held for nearly twenty years. It was also the most highly leveraged: the LBO shop borrowed fully 90 percent of the total amount of the acquisition, much of it in Drexel junk bonds. Interest payments alone were $1 billion annually.[19]

KKR maintained a firm grip on the company even after taking it public in 1991; eight of its executives sat on RJR Nabisco's fifteen-member board.[20] In order to meet the crippling debt, its new management team was forced to sell off pieces of the business, raise prices, and steadily lay off workers. On the other hand, the previous top managers ran off with golden parachutes worth millions of dollars. Investment banks, the junk-bond peddler Michael Milken, and other investors did equally well in fees for the deal.[21] KKR collected $75 million in payments from its LPs alone and millions more in other fees.[22]

The Roller Coaster 1990s

The cyclical nature of the economy exposed the volatility of the asset class: the LBO slump in early 1990, expansion later in the decade, downslide in 2001, prosperity a few years later, and standstill during the Great Recession of 2008. The age of exceptionally high-debt LBOs temporarily petered out toward the end of the 1980s. Two factors were the scandals and the subsequent public condemnation of buyout practices. The ignominy of the RJR Nabisco fiasco had solidified the public's view of the entire buyout industry as voracious plunderers, and for a while it was considered Wall Street's bête noire.

Declining economic conditions toward the end of the 1980s took a significant toll as well. The US economy deteriorated, and along with slow recovery, a large number of earlier acquisitions floundered. Many filed for bankruptcy, fully exposing the vulnerability of unduly leveraged companies. Investment banks and regulators became concerned and, at least for the moment, ramped up their scrutiny of the buyout shops.[23] At the same time, the junk-bond market collapsed, and Drexel was liquidated, thus drastically reducing the size of potential deals. The period of easy access to credit for outsized buyouts, excessive leverage, and hostile takeovers was abruptly curtailed.[24]

Several years later, however, a mixture of circumstances spurred the revitalization of LBO activities. The US economy not only perked up but experienced a high-technology, internet, and telecommunications boom. Interest rates were now at historically low levels, credit became widely available again, and more pension funds and other institutional investors began pouring money into "alternative investments."[25] To take better advantage of such favorable tailwinds, the LBO shops rebranded themselves as private equity firms; junk bonds were renamed high-yield bonds.

The PE firms also broadened their strategies due to negative popular opinion about splitting up companies, the fact that there were fewer of them available to dismantle profitably, and a modification of the tax law in 1987: under the revised rules, new corporate owners would be taxed on the sale of any of a purchased company's divisions.

According to Kosman, this slowed down the "buy-and-bust strategy" of the 1980s, unless the transaction involved real estate or selling pieces of a company at a loss.[26] Consequently, the financial buyers began to concentrate on enhancing the EV of their purchases. According to Carey and Morris, " 'value creation' would be the new mantra": this meant pursuing higher-margin goods and services; growing businesses both organically and through acquisitions; and extending companies' geographic reach both nationally and internationally.[27]

The sheer amount of money accumulated by PE burgeoned, as did the number of acquisitions. For example, in the late 1990s, KKR and Blackstone amassed record-breaking buyout funds, totaling $5.7 billion and $4 billion, respectively.[28] Again, GPs generated great fortunes for themselves. As Kosman found in his investigation of the ten largest LBOs during the 1990s, although the ultimate financial situation of these companies differed considerably, they all shared one aspect as a result of their takeovers: the PE partners raked in millions of dollars.[29]

PE in Jeopardy? The Great Recession of 2008

Although PE firms were riding high, in the early twenty-first century they again succumbed briefly to a sudden downturn in the economy. With the crash of the dotcom bubble in 2000, more PE-owned companies were forced into bankruptcy: sixty-two prominent establishments became insolvent during 2001, and forty-six more collapsed in the next six months.[30] Buyout activity also slowed down notably.

As the economy began recovering in 2003, free-flowing, low-interest loans became available once more, jump-starting the buyout industry. Large banks, eager again for hefty transaction fees, not only provided abundant capital but attached few restrictions on the loans.[31] Institutional investors, too, were willing to hand over more money than ever before; PE shops were finally cashing out the companies that they owned, realizing large returns from them.[32] With mounting millions (and, for some, billions) in their funds, GPs engaged in frenzied dealmaking at increasingly elevated sums and with heavier leverages. At the end of 2007, debt on some buyouts had reached 70 percent or more of the purchase price.[33] Because of the magnitude of certain ventures, PE turned to club deals, where two or more firms partner to finance them.[34]

During this boom period, PE shops bought nearly a thousand businesses listed on the stock exchanges, totaling almost a trillion dollars, which nearly doubled the number previously owned. As usual, after the purchases they would cut back customer services, raise prices, and drastically reduce any reinvestment in the establishment; the improved cash flow, along with inexpensive interest rates, would then allow them to regularly load more debt on their portfolio companies so they could pay themselves dividend recaps. Kosman notes that this was the case for nearly 40 percent of the establishments owned by fourteen of the largest PE houses between 2002 and mid-2006. He adds, "Private-equity firms are often reckless when they have their companies declare dividends."[35]

And then the economy collapsed, this time to a far greater extent, setting in motion the most challenging time for the industry. The Great Recession and its aftermath rendered countless portfolio businesses incapable of paying the hefty interest on the debt that had been laid on them. Appelbaum and Batt report, "In all, 260 PE-owned companies entered bankruptcy during the 2008 to 2011 period."[36] One such corporation was the 133-year-old mattress manufacturer Simmons Bedding, which various PE houses had bought and sold seven times over two decades. In 2009, its last owner, Thomas H. Lee Partners, filed for Chapter 11 bankruptcy protection. According to the *Financial Times*, 25 percent of the workforce was laid off, whereas Thomas H. Lee earned $77 million, including dividends, over its six years of ownership. Overall, the several PE firms that had controlled Simmons walked off with an astounding $750 million.[37]

At the same time, since credit had frozen in the summer of 2007, GPs could not invest the roughly half trillion dollars of capital that they had accrued from their LPs during the boom years.[38] Nor could they offer an IPO for the companies they held or find buyers for them; ultimately, they were forced to keep them far longer than they had intended.

Resilience: PE Rearing Its Head Again

The world of private equity did not stagnate in the aftermath of the Great Recession. As conditions gradually improved, especially by 2013, the shops yet again resumed their self-enrichment activities, albeit in innovative ways. According to some observers, the business model had evolved, and PE started relying less on the creation of value through financial engineering and highly leveraged buyouts.[39] However, shortly thereafter PE firms slipped back to elevated debt once more, abetted by low interest rates and expanding target valuations. The PE industry continues to transform as it adapts to changing social, political, and economic circumstances.

The alternative investment space by 2020 had emerged out of the shadows: not only had it turned mainstream, but it was flourishing. The United States and the world have witnessed a spiraling number of PE funds in what has become nearly a $4 trillion industry. The number of shops also has exploded: in 2019 there were 3,749 PE firms, and they owned roughly 8,000 companies valued at $5 trillion, up from fewer than 2,000 at the turn of the twenty-first century.[40]

GPs are wheeling and dealing with an escalating pool of capital as well, enabling them to arrange ever-larger transactions. PE increasingly appeals to financially hungry pension funds and the like and has attracted a larger number of LPs willing to commit capital and at higher percentages of their total investable assets. Since 2016, there has been a fundraising bonanza, with a flood of money pouring into vehicles of all sizes and reaching record numbers: the firms accumulated nearly $442 billion in capital for new funds during 2016 and 2017 and amassed another $166.4 billion in 2018.[41]

Certain houses, especially the most established, have shown a strong appetite for mega-funds that are larger than some of the precrisis ones.[42] Despite backing off from supersized vehicles in the wake of the Great Recession, by 2017 the GPs were at it again. PitchBook analysts note that CVC Capital Partners, KKR, Silver Lake, and Vista Equity Partners, among others, raised funds of $10 billion or more that year; far more shops closed mega-funds during 2019 and 2020. Clearly, these prodigious vehicles reap commensurately greater management fees for the GPs.

The funds could have been even bigger, but the buyout shops have been forced to cap them; otherwise, there could be too long a lag in investing the money, leading to a lower internal rate of return (IRR), which would seriously trouble LPs.[43] As it is, their money-raising success has produced a swelling amount of dry powder, reaching record levels by 2020. It was estimated that PE firms had $1.45 trillion in committed capital at their disposal worldwide, generating pressure to spend it within the industry's stipulated time frame.[44] According to one LBO shop titan, "PEs are shoveling money out the door as fast as possible."[45] In 2020, they had nearly $4.5 trillion in assets under management.

Deal-making has abounded, with robust investments everywhere. In 2018, GPs engaged in a record-breaking number of transactions, estimated at 4,828 with a total value of $713 billion.[46] Mega-buyouts have materialized as well, similar to some purchases between 2004 and 2007. Deals of more than $1 billion and several of more than $5 billion accounted for nearly one-third of overall investment by 2018.[47]

Investment banks bolstered ongoing trends by offering easy access to credit and with relaxed terms. Anxious to resume their lucrative relationship with the industry and flush with cash, banks began feeding risky leveraged buyouts again, including junk bonds. The evidence indicates that more than $356 billion of loans (75 percent of the leveraged institutional market) in the first half of 2018 were covenant-lite, with little or no lender protection. Concurrently, competition in every aspect of the alternative investment space—from LP capital to choice acquisitions—was at an all-time high, though long-standing PE firms continue to have a distinct advantage.[48] It seems that GPs are pulling out all the stops for top-tier companies.

The mixture of massive fundraising and dry powder, freely flowing low-interest loans, and enhanced rivalry has driven up valuations. Purchase prices had steadily risen to a median multiple of 11.6 times EBITDA (earnings before interest, taxes, depreciation, and amortization) by the end of 2018, up from 8.4 times in 2013.[49] As James

Christopoulos of CVC Capital Partners put it, "We are living in a world of high multiples."[50] Another PE titan noted that except for energy, "the multiples are breathtaking."[51] Obviously, the industry is not daunted by these excessive valuations.

Despite initial caution after the Great Recession, the leverage on buyouts has escalated. Equity contributions in 2018 averaged only 39.6 percent, close to the 30.9 percent in 2007.[52] Leverage guidelines were issued in 2013 by several US agencies, but they were only recommendations; in any case, the Trump administration withdrew them. The Federal Reserve reports that a number of PE-owned companies today have liabilities exceeding those in 2007.[53] The elevated debt is quite risky, especially given the generally covenant-lite terms of the loans, raising troublesome questions about the future viability of US businesses.

The precarious condition of many PE-owned enterprises has been compounded by the stepped-up practice of extracting extravagant dividend recaps from them. GPs go full force in leveraging their portfolio businesses in order to take big bites out of them. Sycamore Partners, for example, gorged itself on Staples, taking out fully $1 billion in a leveraged recap that added to the office supply company's already bloated liabilities of $5.3 billion. By doing so, Sycamore recaptured almost two-thirds of its purchase price. CVC Capital Partners and Leonard Green seized $1.8 billion in dividends (65 percent of the buyout cost) from BJ's Wholesale Club before placing it on the public market in 2018. In another case, Silver Lake, the Singapore sovereign wealth fund GIC, and other members of an ownership syndicate in 2019 took nearly a billion dollars from their portfolio company Ancestry, which they had purchased for $2.6 billion four years earlier; a similar sum had been taken by its previous PE owners.[54]

There have been a multitude of PE-led bankruptcies of late. One source finds that 40 percent of retail and supermarket chains that filed for Chapter 11 from 2015 to 2017 were controlled by PE firms.[55] Likewise, an analysis by FTI Consulting concludes that in 2016–2017, two-thirds of insolvent retailers were PE-owned, accounting for 61 percent of the job losses in the industry.[56] Though not all bankruptcies end up in liquidation, a significant number of workers and suppliers, along with their communities, may be devastated nevertheless.

In 2017, weighed down with debt, high-profile failures included Toys "R" Us, Payless ShoeSource, and Gymboree. The following year, additional notable companies collapsed, such as New England Confectionery Company (Necco), Claire's, and David's Bridal. Eighty-eight other PE-owned businesses in 2018 were graded as financially distressed.[57] A few of these companies have confronted insolvency twice, mainly because of the unmanageable debt PE shops have placed on them. Payless ShoeSource's 2017 bankruptcy primarily stemmed from its overwhelming $840 million liability at purchase in 2012, along with subsequent dividend recaps. Its owners, Blum Capital and Golden Gate Capital, had helped themselves to more than $350 million in 2013–2014. Though Alden Global Capital bought Payless four months after its filing for Chapter 11, 400 stores had already been shut down. In February 2019, Payless was in bankruptcy once more, losing 2,500 more outlets and 16,000 jobs.[58]

Likewise, in 2017 Gymboree and its Crazy 8 shops collapsed under the weight of liabilities. Bain Capital had bought the children's clothing company in 2010 for $1.8 billion, borrowing $1.3 billion of the total. Seven years later, after it added a host of new outlets that raised interest payments to an unsustainable level, its lenders seized the chain. They could not cope with the lighter but lingering debt, and Gymboree filed for bankruptcy protection again in 2019.[59] It finally liquidated its stores, with losses of hundreds of jobs.[60]

The nation is feeling the effects of earlier deals as well, such as in the case of Toys "R" Us, an iconic seventy-year-old company. Acquired in 2005 in a $6.6 billion LBO by Bain Capital, KKR, and Vornado Realty Trust, it went into Chapter 11 protection in 2017 and was liquidated the following year.[61] Although the three owners maintained that the problem entailed factors beyond their control, knowledgeable observers argue that the company was just too heavily loaded with debt. For instance, in a 2018 *Bloomberg Businessweek* article, the reporters write that despite real competition from Amazon, the chain could have been turned around, especially given how much children and families adored the stores. They lay the blame squarely on the overwhelming liabilities that accumulated over time: Toys "R" Us had to pay roughly $400 million in interest annually for more than a decade. According to these authors, that was nearly half of the chain's operating profit, even during its better years; others argue that the percentage was actually higher.[62]

As usual, workers paid a huge price for the takeover. Stores were shut and positions cut right from the start, and there were vastly lowered wages for the residual workers. At the time of liquidation, more than 33,000 additional people suddenly lost their jobs—with no advance warning—and they did not receive any severance payments, estimated at $75 million. In many places, the employees also lost vacation and sick pay owed to them. Vendors, too, experienced hardship; losses for them totaled $350 million. For example, Toys "R" Us had been Mattel's second largest customer, and the manufacturer ended up laying off personnel as well. In addition, the financial health of the New Jersey community where the business had been based suffered: it lost millions in tax dollars.[63]

But the investors, lawyers, bankers, and advisors managed to extract close to a billion dollars in fees and other payments for their efforts in the bankruptcy and liquidation proceedings. The prebuyout CEO of Toys "R" Us had received a $65 million golden parachute.[64] According to Bryce Covert, a writer for the *Atlantic*, fees for the two PE shops over the years "more than covered the firms' losses in the deal."[65]

Facing a strong lobbying effort by the laid-off workers aimed at LPs, congressional Democrats, and the public, the GPs capitulated, at least in part. Bain Capital and KKR agreed to contribute $10 million each toward severance money—a pittance given the $75 million owed to the workers and the millions collected by the financiers. The lenders that had forced the liquidation appropriated the brand name and sold it to Tru Kids, Inc., in January 2019. Along with software retailer b8ta, Tru Kids opened two upgraded stores in 2019 but shut them less than two years later.[66]

Another pre–Great Recession LBO, Necco, defaulted on its loans. The manufacturer of Sweethearts, Necco wafers, and other well-known candy brands had been in business for 150 years prior to its acquisition by PE.[67] American Capital bought the corporation in 2007 for $57 million and before long reduced expenses sharply, including by limiting sanitation services. In due course, the plant developed a rat infestation. In 2017, Ares Capital Corporation took control of Necco and sold its real estate to a real estate investment trust (REIT), which in turn charged the candy maker a devastating $2.5 million in rent annually. As a result, Necco was forced into bankruptcy and in April 2018 was auctioned off to Round Hill Investments for $17 million. After receiving a warning letter from the US Food and Drug Administration about the rats, Round Hill shut the factory down. In September 2018, Necco was sold to Spangler Candy, which relaunched the manufacture of the candy hearts in 2020.[68]

Claire's is also a victim of a prerecession LBO. Taken private in 2007 by Apollo Global Management, the operator of teen-oriented ear-piercing and jewelry stores crashed in March 2018, burdened with $2.1 billion in debt.[69] Analogous to other bankruptcies, Claire's has off-loaded its debt, leaving others to bear the consequences.

Bumble Bee seafood, which filed for Chapter 11 in November 2019, was drowning in debt. It had been seriously enervated by a long series of LBOs, at least five since the company emerged from its first bankruptcy in 1997. During Bumble Bee's financial whirl over the years, each of the PE firms along the way soaked up its share of profits and then threw the assets to the next predator. The last owners, Lion Capital and Carson Private Capital—which bought Bumble Bee for $980 million in 2010—incurred a $25 million fine from the federal government for price-fixing. Almost immediately after Bumble Bee was declared insolvent nine years later, it was bought by FCF Fishery for $926 million in another highly leveraged buyout—with nearly 70 percent in debt financing.

Even prior to the COVID-19 pandemic, it was clear that bankruptcies were looming for many more PE-owned businesses. Moody's Investors Service had rated a mounting percentage of them with unsatisfactory credit scores, noting that the problem had reached an "alarming level." The credit agency emphasized that the situation would become particularly troublesome if economic conditions deteriorated.[70] Alex Lykken, a PitchBook analyst, suggested: "And should another significant correction be lurking around the corner, it may be the middle market that absorbs most of the pain the next time around."[71]

The year 2019 was the tenth year of the bull market run. PE executives were convinced that an extended long downturn in the economy would occur in the near future. According to advisory firm BDO's survey, 89 percent of respondents had expected a long-term slump by 2020 or 2021.[72] Christopoulos of CVC Capital Partners said: "We all know that a recession is coming sooner or later."[73] At the Wharton conference I attended in 2019, a number of panelists were questioned about how they were positioning themselves for a potential slowdown in the economy. One GP snapped, "We're paid to invest through all cycles."[74] Obviously, despite the looming economic crisis, PE shops had not been dissuaded from heaping more debt on their investee businesses, nor had investment banks and PE direct-lending funds refrained from doling out the money. But beginning in March 2020, the pandemic and its financial ramifications began to put the PE industry to the test.

PE Goes to Washington—and Back

The rapacious behavior of PE partners, the often crippling debt placed on businesses, and the harmful effects on society only occur because our political leaders allow it and, indeed, buoy up the practices. It is not only on Wall Street that the asset class has emerged from the darkness but also in the political realm, where PE has become a powerful player. GPs regularly populate all levels of government, whether as electoral candidates or as high-profile appointees. Such infiltration is both purposeful and effective. It allows the industry to convey the issues that it thinks are important directly to top officials. Individual shops also bring prestigious public officials on board to take advantage of their influence and to enhance the firm's overall standing. In turn, politicians cash in on their contacts by accepting these highly compensated positions. There is an intricate web of connections through which people weave back and forth between government and business.

Carlyle Group has had a roster of Washington insiders. The Center for Public Integrity cautions, "Critics have long denounced Carlyle's practice of recruiting former high-ranking government officials at the same time as it invests in companies regulated by their former agencies," dubbing it "access capitalism." It has been like this from the beginning. A cofounder of Carlyle, David Rubenstein, served as deputy assistant for domestic policy under President Jimmy Carter. Even former president George H. W. Bush became a senior member of the firm's Asia advisory board.[75]

Carlyle has particularly profited from access to the US Department of Defense. In 1992, former defense secretary Frank Carlucci joined Carlyle, and subsequently the buyout shop "became a major player among defense contractors." For example, about $42 million (42 percent) of its first fund in the early 1990s was in aerospace and defense companies; it parlayed that into $372 million overall at exit. Six PE firms received a total of $14 billion in defense contracts between 1998 and 2003, and twelve Carlyle-owned establishments received slightly more than 66 percent of the total.[76]

Carlyle also hired James Baker in 1993, following his stint as secretary of state under George H. W. Bush; he was able to use his networks to help the firm expand into international markets, especially in Asia and the Middle East.[77] Later, while he was still a partner at Carlyle, Baker assisted George W. Bush as a special presidential envoy to negotiate for Kuwait in attaining money that Iraq owed the country. According to the Nation, "Carlyle has sought to secure an extraordinary $1 billion investment from the Kuwaiti government, with Baker's influence as debt envoy being used as a crucial lever."[78] And he apparently had been a key player earlier, as secretary of state, in requiring payment of the huge arrears in the first place.

Other examples include William E. Kennard, Bill Clinton's Federal Communications Commission (FCC) chair, who became a managing director of Carlyle's global telecommunications and media group, "directing the firm's business investments in companies he regulated."[79] Similarly, shortly after Julius Genachowski left his position as FCC chair in 2013, he also teamed up with the shop. As a Reuters reporter makes clear, Carlyle "has deployed more than $18 billion of equity in investments in the technology, media and telecom sectors globally since its founding in 1987."[80]

Blackstone Group, too, has signed up its share of former government officials as executives and advisors, including Paul O'Neill, secretary of the treasury under George W. Bush; and Wesley Clark, a four-star general and NATO supreme allied commander in Europe. Pete Peterson, cofounder of the firm, had been secretary of commerce under Richard Nixon. Ironically, through a foundation he later formed, Peterson strove to oppose the growing federal budget deficit even though his PE house has always depended on extensive debt for its outsized earnings. Similarly, Mitt Romney, who cofounded Bain Capital, lectured about fiscal austerity and balancing the budget during his 2012 presidential campaign while reaping millions from Bain's highly leveraged buyouts.

Other PE firms, of course, have recruited Washington powerhouses as well. Forstmann Little, for instance, took on Henry Kissinger, Donald Rumsfeld, George Shultz, Colin Powell, and Newt Gingrich, who later moved on to JAM Capital Partners.[81] In 2013, Warburg Pincus hired Timothy Geithner as its president; earlier, he had facilitated the passage of the Dodd-Frank bill that culminated in negligible oversight over the PE industry.[82] In March 2021, Jay Clayton, the Securities and Exchange Commission chair from 2017 to 2020, became the lead independent director on the board of Apollo Global Management. The list is endless, guaranteeing that the industry is working in the friendliest political climate.[83]

President Joe Biden seems to be upholding this questionable tradition. Shortly after his election, Pine Island Capital Partners (founded in 2016) and WestExec Advisors (founded in 2017) were recruiting grounds for early key appointments. These included two Pine Island partners: Antony Blinken (secretary of state) and General Lloyd Austin (secretary of defense). Richard A. Gephardt (former House majority leader), Tom Daschle (former Senate majority leader), and Don Nickles (former chair of the Senate Budget Committee), among others, are also affiliated with the PE firm. Pine Island specializes in government-funded aerospace and defense contractors; near the end of 2020, it raised a $218 million fund specifically for that sector. Biden also named Avril Haines from WestExec as his director of national intelligence, and he enlisted a number of other people from the consultancy firm for his transition team. Its clients are companies that profit from millions of dollars in defense contracts; thus far WestExec has been able to shield itself from scrutiny because of nondisclosure agreements.[84]

Given the alternative market's enormous wealth, it is not surprising that its political donations and lobbying are not only abundant but escalating. The Center for Responsive Politics shows that from 2005 to 2015, PE tripled its outlays for lobbying, and campaign contributions rose sixfold. In 2018, five shops alone spent slightly more than $14 million on political campaigns and $4.5 million on lobbying. Particularly noteworthy, between 56 percent and 84 percent of PE's lobbyists had previously held government positions.[85]

Both Democrats and Republicans are recipients of PE money, ensuring its ongoing political impact regardless of election results. For example, in 2016 KKR was the third largest funder for Max Baucus (D), chair of the Senate Finance Committee; he was one of the most influential members of Congress on the question of taxes. As Ryan Donmoyer of *Bloomberg News* notes, Baucus jettisoned provisions of the Tax Cuts and Jobs Act of 2017 that would have increased rates on carried interest, the bread and butter of the PE industry.[86] By the same token, as a candidate, Donald Trump (R) pledged to eliminate the carried interest loophole, but after he assumed the presidency he backpedaled on the issue. Leaders from KKR and Blackstone Group had met with key political players in Congress and federal department officials, such as treasury secretary Steven Mnuchin. Steve Schwarzman, cofounder and CEO of Blackstone, met directly with the president; Schwarzman was a fundraiser for and unstinting donor to Trump's campaigns.[87]

The Trump White House was jam-packed with PE representatives, who often proposed self-serving policies. One case in point was the appointment of Schwarzman to chair the President's Strategic and Policy Forum. Nicholas Confessore of the *New York Times* notes that

Schwarzman's ties to Trump were instrumental in achieving a Blackstone deal for $20 billion from Saudi Arabia. In another instance, John F. Kelly, secretary of Homeland Security, previously had been an advisor to DynCorp, Cerberus Capital Management's portfolio company that is dependent on Defense Department contracts.[88]

GPs increasingly have been attempting to sway lawmakers at the state and local levels as well. An investigation by the *New York Times* in 2016 found that they engage in "sophisticated political maneuvering—including winning government contracts, shaping public policy, and deploying former public officials to press their case."[89] In certain states they have particularly advantageous relationships, although much of the influence is indirect, generally exerted through the companies they own.

However, criticism of the PE shops has gained traction: the good ol' boys are facing mounting scrutiny. This was kicked off by the bankruptcy of Toys "R" Us and, shortly thereafter, transgressions related to private prisons and surprise medical bills, mostly by hospital staffing and emergency medical transport companies. Introduced by Democratic presidential contender Elizabeth Warren and her fellow senators Kirsten Gillibrand and Tammy Baldwin in mid-2019, the bold Stop Wall Street Looting Act would, if enacted as is, upend the industry. Among other stark and, in my view, indispensable PE-related provisions, the legislation would render GPs partly liable for the debt placed on their portfolio companies; curb dividend recaps within a year of an LBO; fully tax the monitoring and transaction fees; sharply limit the deductibility of interest payments; assist workers in capturing their back pay, severance, and pensions in cases of bankruptcy while restraining executive payoffs; tax carried interest as personal income; and require more extensive disclosure to the Securities and Exchange Commission.[90]

At the end of 2019, those three Democratic senators and other critics set up a special congressional hearing, "America for Sale? An Examination of the Practices of Private Funds," through the US House Financial Services Committee. Representative Maxine Waters, committee chair, made clear that she was particularly troubled about PE ownership of places that operate essential social services,[91] concerns that I address in subsequent chapters. The point of the hearing was to deliver a litany of PE wrongdoings, which Chris Witkowsky of *Buyouts Insider* had earlier observed would be a "public flogging." Instead "the hearing became a lovefest of sorts, with Congressional representatives from across the country expounding on the benefits that private equity investments brought to their districts." Witkowsky says that such support is based on the benefits that PE brings to communities nationwide.[92] The evidence suggests that it is more likely due to the intense PE lobbying, the campaign money pouring in, and the current placement and future opportunities in the industry for political officials.

PE's foremost pressure group, the American Investment Council (AIC), which had earlier helped curtail any serious tampering with PE's flagrant tax loopholes, has been decidedly active in railing against the Stop Wall Street Looting Act. Not unexpectedly, its main approach has been to categorize the alternative market as "an engine of growth and innovation," touting its ostensible job creation successes and reminding everyone that public pension retirees are reliant on the industry. The president and CEO of AIC, Drew Maloney, was the assistant secretary for legislative affairs at the Department of the Treasury from mid-2017 to mid-2018.[93]

During the 2020 presidential primary season, Senator Warren became a persona non grata in PE-land. The stream of industry-related opposition emails on my computer was a telltale sign, and there was palpable fear of her possible ascendancy to the presidency. It seems that GPs' hackles go up when their lucrative livelihoods are being threatened. In response, the financial entrepreneurs flooded the campaign coffers of friendly candidates on both sides of the aisle. According to the Center for Responsive Politics, GPs spent $170 million on the 2020 election, slightly favoring Democrats.[94]

Concluding Remarks

Private equity firms and their leveraged buyouts flourished in the 1980s, mostly through junk bonds. Many of these deals ended in the breakup of previously viable public companies, and some of them were driven into bankruptcy. Regardless, PE titans gained considerable personal wealth.

The 1990s exposed the vulnerability of PE buyouts to economic conditions and interest rates. Leveraged buyouts were on a roller coaster of fluctuating levels of deal-making throughout the decade, and GPs continued to enrich themselves.

The 2008 Great Recession and its aftermath gave momentary pause to PE activities. Until roughly 2013, GPs were forced to hold on to their companies longer than usual, and LBO deal-making and exits slowed down considerably, as did the amount of capital invested. PE firms accumulated high levels of dry powder they couldn't deploy. Concomitantly, the extreme debt on their portfolio businesses engendered financial distress and a substantial number of bankruptcies. As usual, business owners, workers, and communities—rather than the PE firms—paid the price.

In the third decade of the twenty-first century, PE is again flourishing, with ever-increasing firms, funds, capital, deals, and companies owned; mega-funds are increasingly common. Investment banks provide easy access to credit and at covenant-lite terms. At the same time, valuations, leverage on buyouts, and dividend recapitalizations are at an all-time high, along with a new spate of bankruptcies.

National policies have buttressed much of the financial engineering and outsized profits pursued by the shops. Such support is buoyed by the revolving door between the industry and government: GPs populate government positions, and prominent political officials are invited to join PE firms. The titans also donate generously to congressional and presidential campaigns and aim intensive lobbying at both political parties.

Beginning in 2019, a few Democrats began to scrutinize the consequences of private equity leveraged buyouts. These efforts could gain traction now that the Democrats have gained the presidency and both houses of Congress. Needless to say, the American Investment Council is fighting back with its huge array of resources.

3

Consolidating Health Care

THE BARBARIANS are now at the gate to hijack our medical needs and personal well-being.[1] Though health care has experienced much profiteering for decades, the private equity exploitation of our medical requirements has hit full throttle. General partners have moved into health care with purpose and doggedness. A motivating factor is that large conglomerates in retail and other industries, where GPs had previously carved out pieces for huge gains, provide far more limited opportunities today. For all practical purposes, a significant number of the most valuable corporations have already been picked over—and a few more than once. As I suggested above, the vast amount of dry powder, over $1.5 trillion globally, also has been instrumental in the current surge in health investments.

PE buyouts overall have exploded in recent years, and health care, along with information technology (IT), have been driving forces. Benjamin Edmands, a partner at Consonance Capital Partners, asserted, "Twenty years ago there were only a handful of funds that would invest in healthcare. Now everyone has a healthcare team. Everyone wants more in healthcare."[2] In 2017 the number and volume of US deals in the sector "broke records," reaching 440 transactions valued at $52 billion. The following year, deal-making was even more robust—531 deals amounting to $65 billion—and the numbers are still rising.[3] Presently, the domain represents nearly 15 percent of all PE acquisitions.

Although PE portfolios are generally not centered on any one market sector, quite a few are gradually zooming in on health care industries. In 2018, eighty-four specialized health funds reached their hard cap, totaling $22 billion overall.[4] Since then, there are even more niche investment firms focusing solely on health-related companies. PE shops are also expanding their in-house expertise in certain industries, notably health, whereas a decade ago they employed mostly generalists.[5]

The present-day foray into health-related businesses has precedent in earlier eras, although the number of transactions was far more circumscribed. By and large, GPs had been wary of health services because of their inordinate complexity, especially the multitude of players and an unpredictable regulatory environment.[6] Nonetheless, by the early 2000s the number of leveraged buyouts expanded, and several of the largest PE firms plunged into a few massive deals.[7]

In 2006, for example, the $33 billion take-private purchase of Health Corporation of America (HCA) by Bain Capital, KKR, and Merrill Lynch Global Private Equity was the largest LBO ever at the time. Prior to placing the assets back on the public market in 2010, the PE firms helped themselves to $4.25 billion in three separate dividend recaps, financing them partly through junk bonds. The GPs, of course, netted millions in various fees that they charged HCA. After the IPO, each of the investors sold $500 million in stock, recovering their initial investments. In 2012, Bain and KKR, which still had a 40 percent stake in the hospital chain (valued at $4.8 billion), received another $360 million in dividends.[8]

These windfall profits apparently prompted PE firms to take over at least thirty-five more hospital chains over the next several years.[9] If HCA is to serve as an example, PE ownership could come at a huge price for the institutions, communities, and patients. A 2012 investigation of HCA by the New York Times, which included hospital records, lawsuits, regulatory probes, and interviews with physicians, nurses, and administrators, found severe irregularities that jeopardized patients, providers, and payers. Among other issues of concern, HCA manipulated billing codes in the emergency room (ER); it turned away individuals who presumably had nonthreatening ailments unless they paid in advance; and the staff sometimes missed serious conditions. Moreover, doctors and nurses told interviewers that after the PE buyout, they often felt pressured to focus on profit at the expense of essential services. The *New York Times* also found a number of unnecessary but lucrative Medicare-funded cardiac procedures and dangerous understaffing, which led to bedsores and other adverse conditions.[10] In addition, HCA financed far fewer capital improvements than comparable hospitals, presumably to enable the GPs to pocket the massive dividends.[11]

"PE Loves Healthcare"

In health industries, PE houses tend to concentrate on middle-market targets—and at times, the lower middle market—especially in certain subsectors. The services area has been particularly vigorous, characterized by health care reporter Harris Meyer as a "hot market," but life sciences and IT have also aroused considerable interest.[12] PE titans expect such deals to intensify in the coming years. Justin Sunshine, now with General Atlantic, explained that although his previous firm, Blackstone Group, is capable of sizable transactions, those in health tend to be on a smaller scale.[13]

Medical products and services, in various forms, have become ubiquitous in the PE world. In the words of Chris Witkowsky, editor of PE *Hub*, "PE loves healthcare."[14] In addition to the factors of overflowing dry powder and more limited prime retail and industrial opportunities, the health sector conforms to key criteria of the PE business model, affording great prospects for GPs to enrich themselves. Health-related concerns tend to be associated with some of the more stable businesses in the United States, earning impressive rates of return. Several knowledgeable observers find that health care has been among the three foremost areas for returning large PE profits since 2011.[15] Another source showed that, compared to other industries, in 2017–2018 a significant number of health subsectors had the greatest rates of return.[16]

Health care's substantial growth over the years has been relatively resilient to business cycles, even coping well throughout the 2008 Great Recession, though less so in some niches during the coronavirus pandemic. Despite the vicissitudes of the economy, health platforms tend to have ongoing sources of revenue through Medicare, Medicaid, and other public health programs. In 2018, Medicare expenditures were $582 billion (14 percent of the federal budget); Medicaid and the Children's Health Insurance Program (CHIP) comprised roughly $400 billion (9.7 percent). States spent another $236 billion that year, averaging 20 percent of their general funds.[17]

With an aging population—along with the rising prevalence of chronic diseases—the customer base for health services is progressively increasing. In tandem with a greater number of elders, especially the increasing number of the oldest-old, is a mounting demand for medical attention, devices, and supplies; prescription drugs; and especially post-acute rehabilitation services and long-term care. Just as important, government policies have been propelling a movement from institutional care toward "alternative sites," most of them funded by taxpayers. GPs are taking advantage of this steady transformation and the increased flow of Medicare and Medicaid dollars into home health, hospice, urgent care, and ambulatory surgical centers. The Affordable Care Act, which expanded health insurance coverage appreciably, has been a bonanza for the PE industry as well by adding even more abundant revenue streams.

The Monopoly Game

In the past, as I discussed above, PE houses would acquire a conglomerate and carve it up, selling off each division: the parts were worth more than the whole. Nowadays, they unify their new acquisitions: the whole is worth more than the parts. There is an ongoing tendency in certain health sectors for PE shops to source businesses from founder-owners; as baby boomers continue to retire, the availability of such places has been increasing.[18] The PE industry is devouring small to medium-size health enterprises at a rapid pace, and there seemingly is no end in sight. It is like a relay race as they amalgamate various niches through a series of LBOs and then pass the larger company to the next financial player, which concentrates the enterprise even more.

As with its other types of investment, the PE industry acquires health care targets that have proven track records. Since health markets are still largely fragmented, a PE shop can take a particularly strong company as a platform and then roll up numerous similar businesses to achieve scale and expand its geographic reach. Since 2011, add-ons and mergers have become the modus operandi in certain health-related sectors, especially provider services. During 2018, for example, add-ons accounted for 64 percent of all US buyouts, up from 54 percent in 2015. As they achieve greater market share, whether local, regional, or national, the consolidated enterprises are capable of boosting prices, cash flow, and earnings. In turn, they often attach complementary businesses and products to foster multiple revenue streams and to protect against cost controls, regulations, and emergent competitors.[19]

This flourishing buy-and-build model enhances a platform's financial value. It also helps GPs to contend with the pricy health care marketplace. Intense competition from both other financiers and public corporations, which have far more disposable cash since the Trump administration's tax cuts, has forced procurement price tags upward.[20] Benjamin Edmands at Consonance Capital Partners stressed that in some niches the purchase multiples are way beyond anything he's ever seen.[21] PE partners justify the exorbitant valuations by using smaller, less expensive add-ons to blend down the overall price.

Who Wins? Who Loses?

Financial players maintain that consolidation provides countless benefits for health care, especially by rendering delivery systems more cost-effective and efficient through economies of scale. For instance, according to a 2018 *Bain Report*, integrating small health clinics into chains "unlocks" a portfolio company's value at both the top and bottom lines through amplified volume, pricing, and productivity.[22] The PE industry also argues that scale allows it to take advantage of technological developments in software and hardware as well as digital health, thereby providing consumers with the latest advances. Nevertheless, the main beneficiaries seem to be the GPs: costs are lowered and earnings increased, but at the same time, consumer prices rise, access to decent care often deteriorates, and choice diminishes.

PE partners, whose only goal is to magnify short-term profit, keep their eye on the only ball that matters: return on investment. From their standpoint, health care is just another industry to exploit. But compared to other PE sectors, the stakes are higher: they are dealing directly with people's lives, safety, and medical well-being. In this arena, financial players are preying, for example, on youngsters and their parents who are desperately in need of services for autism spectrum disorders, or on people dealing with eating disorders or substance abuse. By the third buyout, common in these realms, the GPs have already skimmed most of the cream, leaving lean, frequently inadequate services. Greedy value creation on the financial side too often seems to be accompanied by value destruction in quality of care.

In 2018, the American Medical Association (AMA) initiated a yearlong inquiry to evaluate the effect of venture capital and private equity on medical services. Marni Jameson Carey, executive director of the Association of Independent Doctors, scoffed: "We know that when corporate medicine takes over the practice of independent medicine, costs go up, quality goes down, and patients and doctors lose. . . . We don't need a study for any of this. We just need common sense to prevail."[23]

According to one research report, among other problems, "less competition can lead to worse patient outcomes, especially when prices are set by regulators, as in the Medicare program."[24] Further, in order to generate extreme returns the newly consolidated company may be forced to enhance productivity by speeding up the flow of patients. Physicians, for example, sometimes receive daily quotas on how many people they must attend to or how long they can spend with each one; they also might be pushed to encourage more expensive treatments. Another strategy is to substitute lower-level employees for higher-paid, better-trained professionals, at times without ample supervision. These and other tactics, including the elimination of critical but low-profit procedures, all adversely affect the quality and safety of medical services.[25]

Eileen Appelbaum has found that with less competition, hospitals tend to deliver "lower health outcomes for patients and greater variability in the quality of care." In her study of PE-held hospitals, she notes that because of the short time frame, the temporary owners generally fail "to invest in technology, workers' skills, and quality improvements, all of which require a longer time frame to pay off."[26] To make matters worse, to pay off massive debt, the facilities must cut expenses, such as reducing staff and shutting down less lucrative divisions. And in highly concentrated localities, a particular hospital system may be the only game in town.

It is also challenging for consumers to obtain accurate information on the quality of provider services, whether from physicians, dentists, hospitals, or nursing homes. Therefore, patients need to trust them and assume that their welfare is first and foremost. GPs tend to keep their ownership of health-related businesses under cover. Certainly, it would be disconcerting for the family of an elder receiving hospice care to find out that the company's top priorities are maximizing profits and quickly building value for a sale.

Despite industry claims to the contrary, economists have warned that the rising concentration in various health subsectors contributes to higher prices. William Galston writes in the *Wall Street Journal*, "Companies in concentrated sectors can engage in 'exclusionary' conduct that keeps new competitors from entering a market and 'exploitive' conduct that allows dominant companies to take advantage of their market power such as predatory pricing."[27] These businesses can achieve bargaining leverage to press payers for larger fees and medical suppliers for lower charges. PE-owned enterprises are more likely to apply any gains to their bottom line rather than pass them on to consumers.

Hospitals are a prime example of how consolidation adversely affects fees. Although monopolization had been occurring before PE entered the picture, the shops are now a dynamic force in merging facilities. In 2018, for example, GPs spent $10.4 billion on hospitals and clinics, up from $250 million in 2009.[28] Appelbaum argues that even if hospital concentration results in lower overall costs, consumers do not reap the economic benefits; to the contrary, supersizing allows a facility sufficient clout to bargain for higher reimbursements from commercial insurers and patients alike.[29] The evidence suggests that hospitals that have achieved monopoly status in a region charge roughly 16 percent more than those with four or more competitors.[30]

Customers thus tend to have less choice as PE firms monopolize health markets. In certain situations, especially medical emergencies, patients may be forced to pay exorbitant rates. Such is the case with air and ground ambulance transportation, where providers often have a lock on services. There also is negligible price transparency when a PE portfolio company is in control. Patients are more exposed to balance billing (surprise bills for out-of-network services) under such conditions. Emergency room visits are particularly susceptible to this shady practice, which is regularly carried out by PE-owned Envision and other such companies. Inflated fees also are typical of hospital-affiliated specialty physicians, particularly radiologists and anesthesiologists, many of whom are being acquired and consolidated by GPs.

Further, consolidation is not always beneficial for the enterprises themselves. Of particular concern is the expanded debt that accompanies each new acquisition. According to Fitch Ratings, the improved revenues and efficiencies that have been anticipated by PE players are not completely compensating for the swelling liabilities.[31] Overleveraged—and overpriced—businesses are highly risky. They are notably precarious in today's environment of covenant-lite loans and unstable markets. Uncertainties regarding national and state government health policies and Medicare and Medicaid reimbursement rates further threaten the viability of companies sunk in debt. Peggy Koenig, chair of Abry Partners, noted that a few of her firm's former portfolio companies had to file for bankruptcy because of altered public policies.[32] There are definitely winners and losers.

It is evident that the buy-and-build strategy doesn't always pan out. Several PE partners, including Edmands, have cautioned that many of the consolidated health investments, such as physician practices, just won't make it.[33] Avinash Amin, managing director at Madryn Asset Management, added that such health LBOs have been tried many times before—and they ended badly.[34] The aggregation of independent doctors' offices by physician practice management companies (PPMCs) in the 1990s failed miserably, forcing "many practices to the brink of financial disaster."[35]

Bankruptcies: Two Cases in Contrast

Hahnemann University Hospital and St. Christopher's Hospital for Children, PE-owned medical facilities, filed for bankruptcy in June 2019 and were shut down two months later.[36] The 171-year-old Hahnemann, located in the center of Philadelphia, had served low-income families, two-thirds of them on Medicaid or other public aid. The venerable institution had been through two earlier takeovers, the last by for-profit Tenet Healthcare Corporation, which had bought it out of bankruptcy from the Allegheny Health, Education, and Research Foundation in 1998. Not known for tender loving care of its facilities and patients, Tenet claimed that Hahnemann was losing money and cast it off (along with St. Christopher's Hospital for Children) in January 2018. In a $170 million LBO, the buyer, American Academic Health System—through Paladin Healthcare Capital—placed a heavy debt on the already struggling hospital.[37] Joel Freedman, American Academic's founder, chair, and president, also had started Paladin.

According to numerous sources, the failing Hahnemann would have required an injection of capital for upgrading equipment and IT, along with the acquisition of smaller facilities—such as urgent care— to offset its relatively lower reimbursements from public programs. Instead, Freedman used any positive cash flow to pay off the hospital's hefty liabilities. He did very little to improve the facility's financial viability; in fact, Freedman starved Hahnemann of basic supplies, laid off 175 staff members, and failed to pay into the employees' pension, health, and training fund, depriving it of $2 million.[38]

Ominously, although not uncharacteristically, Freedman had separated the hospital's operations from its real estate, including a few associated medical office buildings and a parking garage. All along there was speculation that he had bought the hospital with the intention of redeveloping the valuable land as luxury condos and not to save a low-income community's hospital. Appelbaum says, "It's the first time I know for a hospital being bought by a private equity company in what appears to be a pure real estate play."[39] Because of the bankruptcy, slightly more than 2,500 employees were laid off, medical students lost their residency placement, and the community was deprived of its main safety-net hospital.[40] Freedman, his PE firm, and perhaps the PE debt holders were the winners.

+ + +

In the second bankruptcy case, 21st Century Oncology (the largest integrated cancer care network in the United States) eventually survived. After being placed on NASDAQ in 2004 by its founder, the company (then named Radiation Therapy Services) was taken private again four years later by Vestar Capital Partners in a $1.1 leveraged buyout. Over the next nine years, at least eight PE firms invested in the chain as it piled up debt from everywhere. It soon had 124 radiation oncology treatment centers and 170 clinical offices. After a failed IPO in 2016, presumably because of its excessive liabilities 21st Century filed for Chapter 11 the following year.[41]

The oncology company emerged from bankruptcy in January 2018, $500 million lighter in liabilities but loaded with new capital (and liabilities) from Beach Point Capital Management (its major debt holder), Oaktree Capital Management, and others.[42] GenesisCare, an Australian provider of cancer and heart disease services, picked up the pieces by acquiring the company in May 2020 for $1.5 million.[43] In this instance, the company was saved; the winners were an array of PE firms. The losers, as usual, were communities and their residents in need of treatment for cancer. For example, in Naples, Florida, Genesis has monopoly ownership of the only four radiation centers in the city.[44]

Middle Market to Mega-Market

Despite the prevalence of middle-market transactions in the health realm, mega-deals are also flourishing, mostly because GPs are taking over targets that the PE industry has been rolling up for more than a decade. In 2017, there were a dozen transactions worth $1 billion or more.[45] One prominent leveraged buyout that year was Bain Capital's $3 billion takeover of Surgery Partners, a company that had been placed on the NASDAQ by H. I. G. Capital in 2015 after nearly six years of ownership; H. I. G. had pocketed $271 million in the IPO and retained majority shareholder control. A subsequent Bain transaction involved the acquisition of National Surgical Healthcare and its merger with Surgery Partners, its rival.[46] Together, the two chains operated 125 surgical facilities across thirty-two states.

The year 2018 witnessed more hefty health deals, with PE outfits continuing to buy already amalgamated companies that serve the nation's vital medical needs. For example, the largest physician staffing company, Envision Healthcare, was taken private by KKR for $9.9 billion after a long history of add-ons, mergers, IPOs, and LBOs.[47] Envision's partial consolidation of the physician outsourcing industry occurred in 2016 when it joined another large staffing and ambulatory surgical center, Amsurg. There are few major competitors now providing hospitals with medical personnel for ERs, radiology, anesthesiology, neonatology, pathology, and other departments.[48] Yet the enterprise has been mired in complaints about its egregious surprise out-of-network billing practices and in multiple lawsuits. Ellie Kincaid, writing for Forbes, states, "Critics say the company, which outsources doctors to hospitals, represents U.S. healthcare at its ugliest."[49] Indeed, it was one of the instigations for the Stop Wall Street Looting Act.

LifePoint Health was another enormous LBO deal in 2019; it offers essential rural services, including hospitals, physician practices, and regional health systems. Apollo Global Management took the enterprise private for $5.6 billion, merging LifePoint with another portfolio company it owned, RCCH HealthCare Partners.[50] Apollo apparently intends to wring outsized profits out of one of the few health systems operating in underserved rural communities and small towns. According to the LifePoint website, "It is the sole community healthcare provider in the majority of the non-urban communities it serves."[51]

After a series of mergers and acquisitions, Kindred Healthcare emerged as the largest home health company and second biggest hospice provider.[52] Seizing on the opportunity to capitalize on the needs of frail and dying elderly people, TPG Capital, Welsh, Carson, Anderson and Stowe (WCAS), and health insurance provider Humana bought the then-public company for $4.1 billion. After separating the enterprise into two divisions,[53] the consortium immediately expanded the at-home branch. Six months later, it purchased Curo Health Services, a hospice chain that had already been tossed around among several PE houses, for roughly $1.4 billion. As a result, Kindred became the leading hospice operator in the United States (see chapter 6).[54]

Concluding Remarks

The health industry is quite expansive, encompassing a diverse range of concerns. At the core is direct patient care and the ancillary services that people rely on for safeguarding their quality of life, treating ailments, and maintaining overall physical and mental fitness. PE firms are snapping up assorted places that deliver essential assistance for behavioral health (i.e., substance abuse, eating disorders, autism spectrum disorders); dialysis; dentistry; homecare and hospice; fertility issues; physical and occupational therapy; specialty physician practices; diagnostic labs and imaging centers; hospital health systems; urgent care and ambulatory surgery facilities; pharmaceutical companies; and medical device businesses, which reach into every vital aspect of medicine, from pacemakers and surgical devices to artificial joints and catheters.[55]

Nibbling along the edges of health care, PE houses are also attracted to businesses that serve the industry overall: IT and software (telemedicine, remote monitoring), life sciences, diagnostic imaging, biopharmaceuticals, insurance and managed care, patient scheduling, health care credentialing, medical supplies, medical scribes, and more. Scores of financiers continue to make inroads into these niches.[56]

Every health-related nook and cranny is being explored for potential windfall profits. Since pet ownership is spreading, as is a commitment to animals' health and comfort, GPs are in hot pursuit of places catering to these demands.[57] They are particularly appealing because there is even less regulatory oversight of pet facilities and products than those for people. Concurrently, a greater awareness of and interest in healthy food alternatives and vitamins among the US population is serving as an invitation for PE shops to probe for financial advantages. They are already invested in all-natural nutritional supplements and remedies, meat alternatives, organic groceries, and gluten-free fare.[58]

Expert Ludovic Phalippou, author of the textbook *Private Equity Laid Bare*, questions whether private equity's playbook is appropriate in every type of business.[59] Undoubtedly, health care is an unsuitable industry for PE. These are essential human services. Can we really afford, as a nation, to have newly consolidated dental, physician, therapy, homecare, and autism chains collapse, similar to Toys "R" Us?

Clearly, PE firms have emerged as a significant participant in the reshaping of health care in the United States. One of their most influential effects has been to compel other types of owners to engage in more bottom-line-focused care. As I show in the next chapters, the industry's foray into US health care has not improved access to affordable services and safer procedures. Nor has it delivered better health outcomes. To the contrary, the PE business model, which is centered on elevated, relatively quick profits, is ravaging our already broken health care system. It contributes to higher public program expenditures (Medicare and Medicaid); more burdensome medical bills; rapid, assembly-line treatments; less credentialed practitioners; and other deleterious effects on the payment for and delivery of services and products for our health.

4

It's between Me and My Doctor?

AMERICANS TREASURE the autonomy of our physicians, eschewing the notion that government or commercial enterprises should interfere with medical decisions. Nonetheless, we have the most corporatized health care system in the industrialized world, where community-based practitioners have increasingly become employees. Indeed, fewer doctors than ever own their practices: only 47 percent in 2018, compared to 76 percent in 1983 and 53 percent in 2012. They tend to be affiliated with groups, but only one-third of these entities are still independent.[1]

Since the turn of the twenty-first century, physicians and physician groups have been increasingly bought out by nonprofit hospital health systems that aim to curb competition, ensure referrals, and provide all-inclusive medical networks. About one-third of doctors work in hospital-owned medical practices, although some sources put it as high as 48 percent.[2] Research suggests that this growing vertical consolidation has led to higher prices and greater health spending overall.[3]

Currently there is an even more troubling phenomenon: an increase in the control of medical care by non–medically trained owners. Seeking to curb inroads into their profits, a few commercial insurance companies have entered the market, but thus far they have hired only 2 percent of doctors.[4] More alarming is the aggressive acquisition of single and group practices by PE firms. One reporter writes, "In a growing and powerful trend, private-equity and venture-capital groups have been swooping in with ever larger offers for all kinds of specialty practices."[5] In 2018, GPs announced more than 120 such transactions.[6]

PE shops were initially drawn to dermatology and dentistry, mostly because their services are generally paid out-of-pocket or, in the case of surgical procedures, have dependable, reoccurring insurance reimbursements. Orthopedic surgery and ophthalmology, too, have captured their attention owing to high surgical volumes and profitable ambulatory surgery centers. Nowadays, investments in other specialties—gastroenterology, optometry, women's health, urology, primary care—are burgeoning as well, along with hospital-based fields, such as anesthesiology, radiology, hospitalists, and ER doctors.

Enticements for PE

As usual, for PE firms there is no interest in a particular physician sector other than what it can provide in returns on investment. And the earnings have been strong in recent years. The purchase of specialty offices represents yet another opportunity to scale established businesses into regional or national brands: PE is mainly interested in practices that are already successful.[7]

Retail health services are highly fragmented and offer high-margin prospects and ample cost-cutting potential. Just as important, by positioning itself strategically, a PE-backed physician conglomerate has greater clout to bargain for higher reimbursement rates from insurance companies and other payers. One health care strategist suggests, "It's a war of who can get big enough in any area to get payers to treat you with respect."[8]

Medical practices also ensure a steady revenue flow, often regardless of economic conditions. After all, even in a recession, families cannot forgo emergency care, treatment for cancerous lesions, nonelective surgery, and other interventions. Greater insurance coverage since the Affordable Care Act has rendered services more prevalent as has population aging and older people's guaranteed coverage through Medicare.[9]

PE transactions for specialty practices are rising not only in quantity but also in purchasing costs. These elevated prices since roughly 2014 are due to the extraordinary levels of dry powder, which the shops must deploy as quickly as possible, and greater competition for these coveted entities. Forbes reports, "While retail health businesses with fewer than ten outlets have been commanding multiples of around four to seven times EBITDA, those with 10 to 50 clinics are selling for seven to nine times, and some marquee assets with more than 50 clinics are trading in the low teens."[10] For some places that are well managed and productive, multiples have been as high as ten to twelve times EBITDA or more.[11] In lay terms, the higher the multiple, the greater the value of a company, and nowadays PE firms are paying premium prices for these specialty offices.

Obviously, with such extreme valuations along with substantial debt, GPs must enhance the worth of their physician portfolio companies through stark measures. For instance, as Robert Aprill of Provident Healthcare Partners points out, they engage in "multiple arbitrage" by acquiring a large number of groups locally, regionally, and nationally: "As the platform organization grows, its value increases in tandem with each additional acquisition."[12] Therefore, the more add-ons, the greater the exit value of the enlarged platform. Together with the buy-and-build strategy, the PE-backed physician groups may engage in organic growth by expanding the number of offices in each locality with de novo facilities. They also must enhance cash flow significantly to manage the concomitant rise in debt.

Luring the Doctors

Typically, the physicians are paid up front with cash through a leveraged buyout, along with equity in the PE-backed management platform they have joined.[13] After the sale, they generally receive a reduced salary (up to 30 percent) and often a productivity-based bonus; they also surrender valuable assets to the new owner.[14] The financial bonanza occurs when the practice is sold several years down the road, when they cash in on their equity stake.

According to one GP, the vast majority of deals in the area are based on proactive initiatives: the PE firm approaches the physicians.[15] Understandably, the doctors often are tempted by the millions in bids for their practices. This is particularly attractive for those intending to retire in the near future or who desire to leave medicine as a career. Studies show the mounting burnout, low morale, loss of control, and low job satisfaction among physicians. They are especially frustrated with the expensive, poorly designed electronic health records systems imposed on them and the myriad other complex bureaucratic hurdles they increasingly face.[16] Physicians also may seek to enlarge and centralize their practices so as to have more leverage in negotiations with health insurers and to raise capital for their administrative, technological, and specialized equipment expenses.

In its pitch to doctors, GPs contend that their "investment facilitates larger, better capitalized groups with sophisticated technology and management that can provide higher-quality and more efficient care."[17] They insist that they won't interfere with the doctor-patient relationship but will solely carry out back office functions, such as record maintenance, accounting, regulatory compliance, patient scheduling, marketing, and IT services. "We let doctors practice medicine," a chief refrain among PE managers, is quite appealing. Many physicians who are satisfied with their chosen profession accede to a buyout with the intention (and relief) of handing over nonmedical functions to others. Nevertheless, as I show below, the PE shops generally seize tight control over all aspects of their acquired practices, including the physicians, if predetermined financial targets are not met.

Structuring the Practices

Unlike other health care subsectors, there are unique regulatory concerns for PE firms acquiring physician practices. In particular, they must consider the corporate practice of medicine (CPOM) doctrine, the federal Anti-Kickback Statute, and the Stark Law. Violation of the latter, which prohibits doctors from referring Medicare recipients to any health-related entity in which they have a "financial interest," engenders civil penalties. The Anti-Kickback Statute relates to all national health care programs, and noncompliance potentially results in both civil and criminal consequences.

The most challenging for PE ownership is the CPOM doctrine, originating from the AMA in 1847. The policy was an attempt to prevent the commercialization of medicine: its overarching mandate prohibits corporations from practicing medicine or employing a physician to provide professional medical services. Though states have their own interpretations, regulations, and exceptions to the rules, the general intention is to keep businesses from controlling patient care. As Dr. Liz Epprecht asserts, commercial firms and medicine have vastly different goals and, accordingly, "a corporation might be tempted to involve itself in physicians' medical decisions, which could endanger patients and the medical practice as a whole."[18] Given the outsized financial performance expected by the PE industry, there is even more danger from its intervention.

GPs painstakingly attempt to circumvent CPOM policies by legal maneuvers and a reconfiguration of ownership. They initially form a PPMC, which then becomes the purchasing vehicle for the medical practices.[19] The PE portfolio company thus is constructed in such a manner that it has, as Yves Smith explains, "all of the economic and control benefits of owning a practice. Nominally, the doctors 'own' the practices when they file with state authorities."[20]

The Fallout

PE investments in certain physician specialties, structured through practice management platforms, first emerged in the 1990s. For the most part, they were disastrous, with the companies failing, and everyone—including the physicians—experiencing considerable losses.[21] Now, they are engaging in similar buyouts but even more expansively both in size and types of specialties. Vast additional capital is going to be required to service these ongoing LBOs.

Physicians are the lifeblood of the US medical delivery system, responsible for much of the health and well-being of families. There already are serious doctor shortages in many parts of the country.[22] Are we placing thousands of doctors, along with their newly debt-laden practices, in jeopardy? Government rules and regulations could change; reimbursement rates could shrink; and the economy could stall or fall into a recession. Any combination of dire—or even less extreme—circumstances could challenge the ability of the PE-owned physician chains to meet their financial obligations.

There is more than potential financial collapse at stake when physicians come under the umbrella of PE. Once the financiers gain control of the business, they take over far more than back office functions: in the end, they are seeking efficiencies in all aspects of the business. After the LBO, doctors typically are no longer in full charge of their practices or any ancillary businesses. Quality of care can easily suffer under PE control. For example, the new owners can substitute paraprofessionals for more expensive MDs to a greater extent than before. The employment of nonphysician providers, such as nurse practitioners and physician assistants, is shown to augment productivity and profits. However, when one skimps on employee costs by placing lesser-trained practitioners in positions for which they are not qualified, patients are at serious risk.[23]

Physicians working in PE-owned firms encounter troubling demands that can have an impact on the quality of care as well. They may have to work different and longer hours than before, rush through patients, rotate to different satellite sites, and operate an electronic medical record system they didn't choose and are not comfortable with.[24] As Smith remarks, although physicians themselves were stepping up the pace of patient care and the number of appointments per day, "PEs are speeding up these negative trends."[25]

In some places, doctors are under duress to upcode insurance bills, hard-sell products and treatments (some of which may be unnecessary), and be parsimonious with medical and other supplies. Trust in doctors and perhaps the whole health care system is undermined when profits trump medical needs. Health considerations should be the only measure when suggesting particular courses of treatment to patients who rely on the physician's expertise. PE-owned practices also tend to be less tolerant of individuals who need to pay for their services in installments, and even previous, long-term customers may be turned away.[26]

In the long run, PE's increasing takeover of physician practices not only is negatively affecting care, but is driving up US medical expenditures for the government and everyone else. Consolidation has been intensifying, and as in other PE-owned health sectors the loss of competition raises prices.[27] As PE titans pocket their massive rates of return on physician acquisitions and kick the practices to the next buyer to chew on, Americans are paying for it with their health, well-being, taxes, and paychecks.

Are the consequences of the PE takeover of physician practices worse than the results when the purchase is by a hospital system? Marni Jameson Carey, executive director of the Association of Independent Doctors, adamantly maintains that the adverse effects of PE-owned and hospital-owned physician practices are the same. Among other arguments, Carey told me that they have equally negative impacts on health, the US health care system, and physicians: they both lessen competition, drive up costs, mandate that doctors meet certain quotas, reduce patient access (independent doctors, then, have difficulty in getting referrals), and shift physicians' allegiance from the patient to the new owner. Carey also noted that in the case of hospitals, they add steep nonprofessional facility fees.[28]

The larger issues, of course, are the regrettable loss of physician independence and of the ability to keep patient needs first and foremost in the practice of medicine. Shawn Morris, CEO of Privia Health, asserts that despite the obstacles in today's medical environment, research indicates that "independent doctors are happier practitioners than their employed colleagues and less likely to burn out. . . . The bottom line is independent physicians are crucial to an effective healthcare marketplace."[29]

Nevertheless, it seems to me that at least hospital systems are concerned with and knowledgeable about medical care, and profits are not their exclusive goal. In the cases of university-based and nonprofit facilities, they can foster research, subsidize care for indigent people and underserved communities, offer residencies, and address community needs more generally, benefits that are antithetical to the PE playbook.

Skin in the Game: Dermatology

Despite the merger and acquisition movement by hospital health systems beginning in the first decade of the twenty-first century, dermatologists mostly continued to practice alone (35 percent) or in independent, single-specialty groups (41 percent).[30] But since 2014, their practices have increasingly piqued the interest of private equity firms. Dermatology management groups have become a leading target for PE. A JAMA *Dermatology* investigation by Harvard researchers found that seventeen private equity–backed dermatology management groups acquired 184 practices from 2012 to 2018, accounting for 381 clinics in thirty states. In 2018, there were thirty-six dermatology deals, nearly all by PE firms.[31]

Dermatology is a large, thriving, and relatively lucrative market, amounting to about $16 billion annually. With more than 11,000 practices and the three largest representing just 3 percent of the total, the market is still wide open for mergers and consolidations. Among other inducements, dermatology benefits from an aging population, a shortage of specialists relative to demand, a rise in biopsies and detection of skin cancers, diverse product lines, and potential expansion of internal pathology labs and other ancillary services. One of the most alluring aspects of the specialty is cosmetic surgery and beauty products, where a significant percentage of the population, especially women, is willing to pay out-of-pocket.[32]

Exceptional valuations have drawn the attention of owner-MDs as well. Such deals range from three to five times EBITDA for a single practice, five to seven times for a small group, and up to thirteen times for a larger, multisite organization.[33] Given these numbers, the PE shops must up the company's worth commensurately, preparing for future sale. In addition to developing more sites and rolling up the business through acquisitions, the financiers commonly place inordinate pressure on the management teams to implement various "efficiencies," such as hiring lower-wage practitioners. The expectation is to ultimately generate from two to five times the initial capital they invested in the practice.[34] The original owners, who usually retain a minority equity stake in the business, eventually profit once more.

Dr. Clifford Perlis, a dermatologist in Philadelphia, attests that private equity investment in dermatology "adds value to practices, creates more practice options, enhances advocacy, and better manages the complexity of practices."[35] Similarly, other professionals maintain that PE improves the infrastructure of the business, brings in financial and operational expertise, and establishes governing boards (usually with representatives of the new PE owner).

A few dermatologists who have affiliated with PE-backed groups, such as Dr. Betsy Wernli, president of Forefront Dermatology, lament the overwhelming regulatory burdens that forced her and her colleagues to abandon their solo practices. Another, Dr. Manfred Rothstein, makes clear: "I love dermatology. . . . But the non-dermatology part was getting more onerous, cumbersome, time-consuming, and frustrating." Dr. Risa Jampel sold her practice to PE-owned Anne Arundel Dermatology in March 2016, and Dr. Colby Evans sold his to Abry Partners's portfolio company U.S. Dermatology Partners for similar reasons. Evans states, "Personally, it has made my life easier."[36] The advantages of PE ownership, then, are spread all around. But what is wrong with this rosy picture?

Trouble in Paradise

One of the foremost critics of dermatology practice consolidation is Dr. Jack S. Resnick, professor of dermatology at the University of California's College of Medicine. His overarching concern is with the commoditization of skin diseases and their treatment: patients' well-being and physicians' know-how tend to take second place to the chase for return on investments.[37] In an interview with the *Dermatology Times*, he notes that colleagues who sold their practices to PE were reporting pressures "from private equity owners to change the way they practiced medicine to maximize financial returns for investors." The lure of big money and back-room assistance must be weighed against some devastating drawbacks. Resnick elaborates on the downsides: PE firms divert vital practice revenues to pocket fees and carried interest (perhaps as much as 20 percent); are more interested in the short term than in the long-term sustainability of the practice; buy at inflated price tags that carry the potential of bankruptcies; broaden the employment of unsupervised physician assistants, who may work in separate allied sites; place control over where specimens are analyzed, regardless of a patient's needs; and may encourage unnecessary procedures.[38]

In response to continuing uneasiness about the future of the specialty, several dermatologists formed the Group for Research of Corporatization and Private Equity in Dermatology. Dr. Sailesh Konda, an assistant clinical professor of dermatology at the University of Florida's College of Medicine; Dr. Joseph Francis, a licensed dermatologist and adjunct clinical assistant professor at the University of Florida's Department of Dermatology; and others have put forward several issues, many of them concurring with Resnick's view. They point out that under PE ownership, nonphysician managers may have significant authority over doctors, with the latter losing their autonomy even over medical decisions. The organization is apprehensive about insolvencies and the overuse of inadequately trained and improperly supervised assistants. In the end, the members conclude, "It is difficult to mix PE and optimal, ethical patient care as the goals of each are inherently conflicted."[39]

In October 2018, the group (with lead author Konda) wrote a paper highly critical of PE ownership of dermatology practices, which was published online by the *Journal of the American Academy of Dermatology* (JAAD).[40] In a particularly disturbing incident, the journal's editor soon withdrew it, citing factual errors, an assertion adamantly denied by the writers. It is quite unusual to take down a paper from JAAD's website once it has been positively peer-reviewed. In this case, there had been objections to the article by PE titans and a few dermatologists who had sold their practices to them.[41] After a stormy exchange of emails, the piece was reposted the following month.

In 2017, the *New York Times* investigated PE firms with dermatology portfolios and their employment of nonphysician practitioners. Predictably, the reporters uncovered an upsurge in physician assistants, mainly unsupervised, carrying out dermatological procedures. The researchers found large numbers of unnecessary procedures by these assistants and missed diagnoses.[42] The following year, Emma Court, a reporter for *Market Watch*, interviewed dermatologists who had sold their practices to PE firms. Most of their comments were off the record since they had signed nondisclosure agreements and feared lawsuits. Nevertheless, their critiques are disturbing:

> [They were] pushed to refer patients to specialists within their organizations and have lab tests processed in-house, even if they thought another specialist or lab technician was better suited for a patient or a condition.

> [There is] pressure to sell products and procedures. . . . Her practice treats her more like a salesperson than a doctor.

> [The midlevel practitioners] misdiagnosed and mismanaged medical conditions on a daily basis . . . , diagnosing a skin cancer as eczema and missing skin cancers, Lupus and genetic syndromes.

> [There was] systematic upcoding by the practice when it came to billing for common procedures like biopsies.

> [There was] cost cutting on medical supplies.

> [There were] pressures to meet production numbers for procedures; sell products like acne creams, anti-aging products, and sunblock; and refer patients to in-house estheticians for chemical peels, extractions, and microdermabrasion.[43]

Overall, the dermatologists interviewed by Court confirmed that because of the stress on ramping up profits, corners were cut, and patient care deteriorated. They highlighted the dangers of lesser-trained practitioners providing treatments for which they are not qualified and the subsequent risk to patients. In addition, the evidence indicates that these health workers performed more biopsies in diagnosing skin cancer; one dermatologist dubbed such providers as biopsy "factories."[44]

Dr. Arash Mostaghimi, a dermatologist and researcher at Brigham and Women's Hospital in Boston, provides a nuanced view of the situation. In an interview with me, he spoke of the positive potential of PE buyouts, such as eliminating waste, economies of scale (sharing records, availability of human resources staff, use of common labs and surgeons), and enhanced leverage for negotiating rates with insurers. However, he was concerned about the potential impact of PE buyouts on patients as well as on the health care system overall. He notes that the addition of financial considerations for a practice is not necessarily harmful, but there are lines that need to be drawn. Although stressing efficiency, one must be vigilant that physicians are not overcrowding their schedules, delivering unnecessary procedures, providing shoddy treatments, or using an overabundance of midlevel assistants for techniques they are not qualified for. He also worries about the pressure to ready a practice financially for the next buyer.[45]

Nevertheless, he is insistent that "we don't have the data yet" to know what will happen to patients being treated in practices under PE ownership. He agrees that "at best it's a high risk," and there's "a high potential to get burned," but at this point "emotions have outpaced the available data."[46] I strongly disagree. Though this physician does not want to rush to judgment on the more recent buyouts, the evidence is already available on dermatology practices that have been in PE hands for several years, and it does not paint a pretty picture.

Harris Meyer, a writer for *Modern Healthcare*, points out, "Some early studies already have raised concerns about private equity ownership of dermatology groups leading to a loss of physician autonomy, conflicts of interest, increased utilization of high-cost services and inadequate supervision of midlevel clinicians."[47] There is enough apprehension that an editorial in *JAMA Dermatology* coauthored by Dr. Joshua Sharfstein, vice dean for public health practice at Johns Hopkins University, called for a halt to all acquisitions until more information is available on quality of care and costs for patients and insurers. Sharfstein argues that "policymakers and medical leaders can't afford to wait for more data."[48]

Critics are also troubled by the impact of PE acquisitions on the future of the profession and young practitioners. Resnick, for example, says, "The consolidation and commoditization of dermatology practices and their services is rapidly changing the specialty and the choices of practice venues for future dermatologists."[49] Others agree that it is dividing generations; there are fewer opportunities and options for early and mid-career dermatologists. And the possibilities that remain may be undesirable, especially for newly minted doctors with a passion for practicing dermatology.

Dermatologists who have sold their practice characteristically argue that they carefully sorted through many proposals and chose the one that best fit them. Nonetheless, even if they are initially satisfied with their selection—which few are—they have no power over the next LBO, only a few years away, or other flips that will follow.

In my interview with Mostaghimi, I asked about the dermatologists who give up ownership of their practices. He viewed that as a reasonable exit strategy since, unlike in prior decades, it is difficult to find young practitioners to buy them. The newcomers to the profession can't afford to do so, and they also are concerned about market uncertainties, such as the unpredictability of insurance rates. The dermatologists who have turned over their offices to PE firms do not view it as hurting anyone, Mostaghimi said. But they have been subjected to moral outrage, including from some in the dermatology community.[50]

It is challenging to get prior owners to discuss their actual experiences post-sale. One person agreed to provide information to me on the condition of anonymity. This interviewee had a sound practice and wanted assistance with regulatory requirements and other back office issues. He and his co-owners sought to grow the practice, but they did not have sufficient resources to do so. This dermatologist envisioned a buyout as a win-win situation for everyone. He had conversed with quite a few PE shops before choosing the current one and had felt confident about the ultimate selection.[51]

Unfortunately, my interviewee contended, he had not fully understood the ramifications of the deal. "I was naïve. . . . I've lost control over my business," he said. "I wanted to maintain our culture, but I'm not sure if I do anymore." The PE firm has contributed some benefits to the practice, including infrastructure, additional clinics, modernized offices, technology, and marketing. On the other hand, some days he "feels regret": the company had been better off under his leadership. The dermatologist lamented that the PE firm aggressively goes after patients for their payment balances; puts pressure on managers; skimps on supplies; short-staffs clinics; overworks personnel; and triggers high staff turnover. When these concerns were brought to the attention of the PE-installed CEO, "he didn't care," the dermatologist added.

This doctor also provided an example of a particularly concerning event. He had a special needs patient who required laser surgery that his insurance would not cover. The dermatologist wanted to do it without pay, but the chief operating officer refused. He had to persuade the CEO in order to proceed with this case.

Now that the portfolio company is shaping up for a sale, the PE is squeezing pennies even further to "sweeten the pot," the dermatologist told me. The financiers are keeping an even tighter check on resources. The dermatologist said that he is nervous about the next PE buyout because the practice is heading into the unknown; nevertheless, he "is happy that the current leadership will go." He further offered that the PE-selected managers do not understand what dermatology is about and are not even interested in finding out. He would prefer a long-term, silent partner in the future.

PE investment in dermatology management groups and the subsequent scaling with add-ons is prospering and at high valuations. Nonetheless, there is disquiet among a number of practitioners about what is happening to the profession, particularly the loss of control by physicians, rising costs, and the effects on quality of care. In the next section I explore selected PE leveraged buyouts and some of the consequences.

The Players

With the acquisition of Texas-based U.S. Dermatology Medical Management, Vicente Capital Partners apparently was the first PE shop to purchase a dermatology management group. The company became insolvent and sold its practices to independent dermatologists at the end of 2011. Since 2015, dermatology has become all the rage in PE-land.

Advanced Dermatology and Cosmetic Surgery

The largest player in the nation in both size and deal price is Advanced Dermatology and Cosmetic Surgery, founded by Dr. Matt Leavitt in 1989. ADCS was first purchased in 2012 as a platform by Audax Group, which shortly thereafter engaged in a forceful buy-and-build strategy. Four years later, ADCS was passed on to Harvest Partners in an SBO for $600 million; the company was valued at fifteen times its $40 million in earnings and was left with $324 million in liabilities at the time.[52] Since then ADCS has accumulated consistent debt and has paid multiple fees to its PE firm for purchases of forty-five dermatology groups and labs across the nation.[53]

ADCS has created a strong brand name, and all of its acquisitions display the official sign on office doors and buildings. The headquarters in Maitland, Florida, as described by Katie Hafner and Griffin Palmer in a New York Times article, is elaborate. The company is tightly organized from afar, with a central call center answering questions and scheduling appointments. According to the reporters, ADCS has a large number of physician assistants performing skin checks, which can be problematic; research suggests that they tend to perform more unnecessary biopsies than more highly trained physicians do and have missed potentially cancerous lesions.[54]

Bedside Dermatology, owned by ADCS through Harvest Partners, mostly employs physician extenders.[55] The company deploys mobile clinics, sending them out to nearly seventy-two Michigan nursing homes, and charges Medicare and Medicaid for the services. Its mid-level staff performs cryosurgeries and other minor surgery, and also injects steroids, all presumably without direct physician supervision. The evidence reveals that 75 percent of its patients, nearly all at the end of life, had some form of dementia and that the removed lesions most likely were harmless. Even worse, some of the procedures likely had adverse side effects, given the frailty of the patients.[56]

Forefront Dermatology (rebranded from Dermatology Associates of Wisconsin)

The second largest dermatology practice in the United States, Forefront Dermatology began its rapid expansion subsequent to its first LBO by Varsity Healthcare Partners in 2014.[57] It was flipped after only eighteen months, creating a bonanza of $450 million for Varsity, more than thirteen times Forefront's annual revenues.[58] Through an SBO, Forefront's next PE owner, OMERS Private Equity, stepped up the geographic reach, and by mid-2019 Forefront had locations in seventeen states.[59] Since its takeover by private equity, Forefront has accumulated at least $400 million in loans, thus enduring heavy debt loads and continuous refinancing.

As it gobbled up and consolidated Wisconsin dermatology practices (thirty-eight by 2019), Forefront was rewarded with up to $850,000 in state tax credits over three years, depending on how many jobs it ultimately created through its corporate expansion in Manitowoc. Taxpayers, as usual, are paying the bill.[60]

It is risky to make conclusions based on limited employee and patient reviews of a conglomerate such as Forefront, but I was struck by the harsh tone of most of them on indeed.com. Here are four typical comments by ex-employees (based on ninety-six reviews):

> All this place is about is the Executives, Investors, and doctors making money. They don't care about the patients, they do everything they can to squeeze every penny out of anyone who comes in for care, every employee is just a number and they only like the ones that are making them money.

> Never work for a company with a high turnover rate. Accept a position with this company at your own risk. I repeat, stay away at all costs.

> Forefront bought out our previously known private practice—the switch to private to corporate was a hard adjustment. . . . I felt like once the contracts were signed we were out of sight out of mind. They were more

focused on how many practices they could buy as soon as possible. Fee schedule was too high for our area.

The pace is fast to the point breaks cannot be taken, almost daily. Schedules are overbooked on a routine basis which leads to much longer days, and an environment that could easily lead to errors—in turn compromising patient and employee safety.[61]

I also sorted through twenty customer reviews on Yelp. They painted a picture of a company that gorges on fees and rushes patients through appointments like they're on an assembly line. Some typical caustic remarks: "You need to avoid this place like the plague"; "They are ripping people off and need to be stopped"; "They only think about how much money they can make but no patient care or concern. Rushed appointments and reluctant to take time answering questions"; "I would not recommend this group to anyone"; "I will never do business with Forefront and advise strongly that everyone take heed to this warning"; and "I smell a scam."[62]

U.S. Dermatology Partners (rebranded from Dermatology Associates)

The third largest dermatology company in the nation, Dallas-based U.S. Dermatology Partners (founded in 1996), has been owned by three PE shops since its first LBO in 2013 by Candescent Partners. The company was flipped in merely seventeen months to Spring Capital Partners in an SBO in 2014.[63] Only two years later, U.S. Dermatology was pitched to Abry Partners in a tertiary LBO, with the previous PE owners dividing $322.5 million from the sale. Spring Capital Partners's main contribution to the company appears to have been financing its leveraged add-ons and mergers. When Abry took over, it continued the prowl for acquisitions; the company rolled up more practices and ever more debt.[64] Fourteen doctors and staff departed and sued, claiming that US Dermatology interfered with medical decisions and hired frontline workers with no training in dermatology, putting patients at risk.

Schweiger Dermatology Group

Launched in 2010 by Dr. Eric Schweiger as Clear Clinic, SDG has experienced a long history of debt financing, venture capital, and minority PE investments. Similar to ADCS, the company has been guided by its founder-CEO. Nonetheless, at least two of the minority investors, LLR Partners and SV Health Investors, have representatives on the board of directors, presumably to ensure that the ship's finances are steered according to the PE business model.

With a goal of de novo expansions and acquisitions, SDG's initial financial sponsors provided $14 million in 2013 and 2014. Schweiger raised millions more during the following years; in 2015 SV Health Investors and in 2016 LLR Partners and others supplied at least another $35 million in debt capital for the company's ongoing growth. The money continued to roll in as SDG consolidated dermatology practices in the New York metropolitan area. In 2018, LNK Partners and Zenyth Partners joined, eager for a piece of the action. SDG is now the leading dermatology practice in the tristate area and the fourth largest in the nation. With more leveraged buyouts in 2019 and 2020, not even the COVID-19 pandemic halted the company's ravenous appetite for add-ons and their concomitant debt financing.

Dermatology Solutions Group (rebranded from Gulf Coast Dermatology)

Started in 2006 by two doctors and based in Brentwood, Tennessee, DSG has an unusual history. It faced its first PE investment in September 2013, when Cressey & Company recapitalized the company and provided $58 million in development money. According to its then-CEO, Christopher Brooks, the PE firm supported aggressive growth of the enterprise. However, the original owners—who still held significant equity in DSG—did not agree with Cressey's mission and vision for the place. The PE firm did not have health care expertise, training, or experience. "It was a mismatch," Brooks told me. According to him, everything unraveled, and roughly eighteen months later (May 2015) the doctors bought most of their business back.[65] DSG operates twenty-five locations in four southeastern states.

Despite the negative experience, Brooks said that at some point the dermatologist-owners might approach another PE firm. They have done some financing on their own, but without private equity assistance they could not raise sufficient capital for a substantial acquisition. They would be more careful next time, he noted, and look for more congruency of goals rather than take the highest bidder.

Brooks asserted that a practice must get larger to compete and survive. The insurance companies and other payers are always seeking to reimburse providers as little as possible, and only sizable places can obtain adequate rates. But it is unfortunate, he said. The independent physician, who has more ability to operate as he would like, generally provides better-quality care as opposed to PE's cookie-cutter approach to treatments.

Meanwhile, Cressey wiped DSG off the "prior holdings" list on its website. But it kept the company's mid-Atlantic assets, and just under a year after separating from DSG, the PE firm invested, along with Apple Tree Partners, in QualDerm Partners (QDP).[66] Cressey is now doggedly growing QDP, and since 2017 has acquired at least four more dermatology practices, each with several locations.[67]

Anne Arundel Dermatology

One of the largest brands in Tennessee, Maryland, Virginia, and later North Carolina, Anne Arundel Dermatology was purchased from its founders in September 2015 by New Mainstream Capital in a management LBO.[68] Since that time, AAD acquired in rapid succession twenty practices; it now has fifty-five clinic locations. It also brought in a minority investor, Pantheon Ventures, in 2018.

Again, I was disturbed with the overall tenor of the reviews by AAD employees on the website indeed.com. Below are a few typical comments (out of twenty-five) in 2018:

Front desk receptionist, Columbia, Maryland: "The company is the worst company I have worked for and I only have been working for 5 months. I'm already looking for a new job."

Former medical assistant and phlebotomist: "This is the worst place I have ever worked. We were a small practice that everyone was family and once AAD bought our practice things changed for the worse! This place has gone downhill since AAD took over!"

Former front desk clerk, Knoxville Tennessee: "After working for my company for over 10 years we were recently bought out by AAD. The family atmosphere was gone quickly, and the corporate feel set in. You are expected to do a pretty impossible amount of work, especially at the check in position, with no raise in sight. . . . The days are longer and the lunch breaks are shorter. . . . I would never recommend working for this company to anyone."

Former working supervisor, Maryland: "AAD is all about the money and how many patients they can see, not patient care. We had a family environment that changed once AAD took over to one where everybody is just trying to survive the drama."

Former medical assistant: "My experience at AAD was horrific. . . . The word to describe AAD is greed. The company as a whole is pathetic. They lack patient care and ethics."

Current manager at Severna Park, Maryland: "They are so busy trying to buy new practices and expand that they offer no support to existing practices. . . . Horrible environment."

Current medical assistant, Glen Burnie, Maryland: "Anne Arundel Dermatology is a complete joke. Horribly understaffed . . . unrealistic expectations, no formal training whatsoever. Management DOES NOT care about their employees AT ALL!!!"

Current medical assistant, Annapolis, Maryland: "Poor patient care—Depending on the doctor, usually she/he will be double and triple booked throughout the day seeing 2–3 patients every 15 minutes, cramming in too many patients. . . . Hands down worst company I have worked for."[69]

Ultimately, New Mainstream did not have to be concerned with the deteriorating quality of care or the staffing issues. In the fall of 2020, it offloaded Anne Arundel Dermatology to Ridgemont Equity Partners and pocketed its outsized earnings.

DermOne

One company that did not survive, though the reasons are still not public, is DermOne, owned by Westwind Investors. Acquired by the PE firm in 2012, the company went defunct in 2018. It had been one of the nation's fastest growing networks of dermatologists; in just a few years it had acquired forty practices in five states. The sudden collapse of DermOne is intriguing since Westwind has no limited partners and finances its acquisitions for the long term. In any case, Schweiger Dermatology in an SBO snatched the nine bankrupt New Jersey locations, most likely at a bargain basement price, and then continued DermOne's acquisition and consolidation journey.[70]

+ + +

By 2017 the dermatology market had taken off, and some initial LBOs had already turned to secondary ones; it is most likely that many will flip again in due time. Each PE hungrily pushes ever more acquisitions, actively recruiting and enticing physician-owners and groups to join its portfolio platform company. As one of the most lucrative specialties, dermatologist practices are in high demand and command inviting buyout prices, but those come with rising debt and myriad fees paid to the PE houses. GPs are on the move in this sector, with no end in sight.[71]

More than Meets the Eye: Optometry and Ophthalmology

Eye care, including treatment of cataracts, corneal disease, and glaucoma; refractive, oculoplastic, and laser surgery; medical optometry; dry eye management; and optical services, was first discovered by PE firms in the mid-1990s. At the time, as is true today, a preponderance of ophthalmologists practiced in single-physician or relatively small, private multiphysician offices. GPs began piecing together a number of these independent offices through PPMCs and then taking them public.[72]

Before long, due to poor decisions based on the PE playbook in conjunction with a national economic decline, most of these investments failed, resulting in disaster for everyone involved—except perhaps the PE shops. In their haste to purchase ophthalmology practices, the financiers had neglected to develop sufficient infrastructure.[73] According to John Pinto, practice management editor of Ocular Surgery News, "The history of that wave of commercial experiments was pretty dreadful. . . . Virtually all of the firms that were developed went away. Along the way a lot of doctors were financially harmed, and even those who weren't financially harmed had to undergo a lot of frustration."[74]

By 2012, PE firms were displaying renewed attention to the specialty. According to a study of ophthalmology and optometry acquisitions between 2012 and 2019, GPs bought 228 practices, comprising 1,466 sites, through twenty-nine platform companies; fully 82 percent of the LBOs were during the last two years of the study. The researchers found that multispecialty, retina, and optometry practices were 56 percent, 40 percent, and 4 percent, respectively, of the total takeovers.[75]

Dr. Paul Koch was the first to take the plunge into PE's world with the LBO and recapitalization of his company in 2012. With Koch Eye Associates (a chain of eye care centers in Rhode Island) as its platform, Candescent Partners formed Claris Vision.[76] In turn, backed by a plethora of PE houses, Koch acquired a series of eye care companies, including Seacoast Eye Associates (Rhode Island) and Eye Health Vision Centers (Massachusetts). Six years later, after priming the company for a high-value resale, Candescent sold Claris Vision to Eli Global; unlike PE firms, Eli Global keeps its independent portfolio businesses for the long term.[77] Koch encouraged and applauded this decision since he believes that this non-PE alternative is best for physician practices, young doctors, and patients.

Koch, who served as chief medical editor of *Ophthalmology Management*, became disillusioned with the PE business model. He writes: "The younger doctors in the practice got nothing out of the original deal, and they were stuck in a situation where long-term planning was discouraged. Requests for equipment and facilities that would enhance the practice over the long term stalled."[78] He also laments that the PE firm had zero interest in continuing his long-standing sponsorship of the local community, such as Little League teams.

Nonetheless, the latest iteration of PE investments in eye care continues. Climbing from four PPMC acquisitions in 2013, nine each in 2014 and 2015, and thirteen in 2016, the overall PE movement into eye care accelerated rapidly thereafter; there were more than eighty-seven investments during 2017 and 2018, many of them newly developed platforms. Some observers suggest that there may be fifty PE firms or more drawn to the sector.[79] The rate of PE acquisitions in the ophthalmology space is expected to quicken even further in coming years. One source drolly writes:

> The Annual Meeting of the American Academy of Ophthalmology is the marquee event for ophthalmology, with presentation of landmark research, unveiling of innovative technology, hundreds of educational symposia, and updates on the dynamic ophthalmology marketplace. What was the hottest topic at AAO 2017? I'm not referring to the topic with the largest symposium audience, or the topic covered by the trade journals or media outlets. I'm referring to the topic most discussed among colleagues at the bar, whispered among friends between meetings, or nervously researched by anxious ophthalmologists seeking answers. So, what was this hot topic? The return of private equity to ophthalmology.[80]

Why has there been such renewed interest in this previously failed enterprise? As I mentioned above, PE firms have so much dry powder (capital) to invest that they keep searching for more opportunities in health care. Ophthalmology, in particular, has a number of attractions for them. It offers the prospect of complementary revenue streams, always a welcome addition to pay off debt. Ambulatory surgery centers, for example, are increasingly profitable since, according to the

American Academy of Ophthalmology, more than 24 million Americans over age forty have cataracts, a number that is expected to grow dramatically. Laser surgery also is experiencing rising demand as more people opt to forgo their contacts or glasses.[81] Other means for augmenting cash flow include retailing eye wear. In addition, PE shops can take advantage of intensifying diabetes and obesity among the population and the associated incidence of eye disorders.

Notwithstanding earlier consolidations, the specialty is still sufficiently fragmented to allow for regional and national branding: in 2018, there were 23,000 independent optometrists and 18,000 ophthalmologists in private practice (nearly 70 percent of the total).[82] Will high valuations for eye care practices, driven by intense competition, entice practitioners to relinquish ownership? One knowledgeable observer comments that as with other specialties, the price tag for buying out a retiring ophthalmologist is generally more than a newly minted doctor can afford. Previously, the cost was one or two times the physician's previous annual earnings; now, PE firms are paying far, far more.[83]

Like physicians in other specialties, ophthalmologists usually lose control over their practice, something many of them do not foresee. At times, they have been completely squeezed out of their practice with few viable alternatives.[84] During a roundtable discussion of private equity in ophthalmology, one doctor warned practitioners who were entertaining a sale: "Be prepared to lose financial control over your organization and to live with that. Decisions will be made in cooperation with the financial interests of the organization and may not be what you have traditionally done."[85] The prior doctor-owners get a dose of reality when they realize that taking management responsibilities off their backs is not why PE shops invest in their practice. Pinto advises: GPs are "about making a profit for their investors, not helping doctors manage their practices." He adds that taking non-patient-oriented chores from ophthalmologists is a selling point, but PE associates tell him that, in fact, they do not really think about that part very much. Their own income and bonuses depend on the number of deals they make and the amount of earnings they bring into the firm.

"They're not going to be rewarded by whether this or that practice is running more smoothly," says Pinto.[86]

The Surging Crowd in Vision Care

EyeCare Services Partners (ESP), based in Dallas, and Eyecare Partners, located in St. Louis, are two of the more prominent ophthalmology companies created expressly as platforms by PE firms prior to 2017. Founded in 2014 by Varsity Healthcare Partners, ESP experienced its second LBO and recapitalization three years later by Harvest Partners. During that short time, the business had acquired twenty locations in California, Colorado, Delaware, Illinois, and Maryland; Katzen Eye Group, through a management buyout, was the first and most significant of its acquisitions. Along the way, of course, ESP accumulated millions in debt and engaged in at least one refinancing, but the PE shop had earned enough to pull out early. Piggybacking on Varsity's purchases, Harvest Partners then took its turn to increase the value of ESP for itself. It went on a tear, buying one eye care company after another; by mid-2019 it had fifty locations and seven ambulatory surgical centers under thirty-two brand names.

Eyecare Partners, created as a platform by FFL Partners in April 2015, also swiftly expanded to embrace multiple optometry, ophthalmology, and ambulatory surgical centers. By the end of 2018, it had bought more than 275 eye care locations across twelve states in the Midwest, Southeast, and Mid-Atlantic, with seemingly no end in sight.—And then FFL dumped it in early 2020 for an astounding $2.2 billion. Indubitably, its new owner, Partners Group, will continue to devour practices in an ongoing consolidation of the chain. Eyecare Partners, too, kept individual brand names, in this case twenty of them. Are these examples of stealth branding, where customers do not know they are actually seeking vision services from PE-owned firms?[87]

By 2017, the PE shops were on a roll, with acquisitions, mergers, and consolidations mimicking the earlier and ultimately disastrous trend in dermatology.[88] The 2017 crop included Shore Capital Partners, whose overall portfolio focuses on health care companies that range from urgent care to autism. Their eye care platform, EyeSouth Partners, created with Georgia Eye Partners, has more than thirty-eight offices in Georgia, Florida, and North Carolina and is seeking to expand throughout the US Southeast. Another was Waud Capital Partners, which formed Unifeye Vision Partners as a platform in conjunction with Minnesota Eye Consultants. Waud seems to be tightly controlling the enterprise: it has three of six members on Unifeye's board of directors. Also in 2017, Chesapeake Eye Care Company and Whitten Laser Eye were acquired and merged by Centre Partners, creating the platform Vision Innovation Partners. With millions of dollars in debt financing, Centre Partners's Chesapeake Eye is still buying practices in the mid-Atlantic states, where it hopes to be a regional force for insurers to reckon with. The 2017 list of PE newcomers in this domain seems boundless.[89]

The rapacious buying spree continued into 2018 as more PE shops dived into eye care platforms at a rapid pace; they were awash in debt financing.[90] In 2019, the specialty witnessed the largest buyout yet: West Street Capital Partners acquired the holding company of MyEyeDr.—an optometry-focused enterprise—for a whopping $2.7 billion.[91] Its prior owner, Atlas Partners, which had acquired the management services company in 2015 for $775 million, earned 3.5 times its investment in only four years.

At this point, it is too early to determine how doctors, their assistants, and patients will fare, but if one takes past experiences of PE ownership of physician practices into account, there is not cause for optimism. The preponderance of these later entrants holds, in addition to their eye care acquisitions, a potpourri of portfolio companies ranging from cable, media, and food to energy, logistics, technology, and consumer products. We do know that the firms flocking into ophthalmology and optometry like swarming locusts are not seeking to improve the eye health of the US population.

Taking on the Musculoskeletal System: Orthopedics

Orthopedics is among the fastest growing health care segments in the United States, engendering more than 137 million visits to doctors, emergency rooms, and hospital outpatient clinics. Indeed, a significant number of people (approximately 60 million) experience chronic musculoskeletal distress.[92] Medicare alone pays billions of dollars for the treatment of back pain, including shoulder, back, and neck surgeries. There are also more than a million joint replacements annually.[93] These disorders are expected to continue their upward trend in coming years as the population ages. Just as important, it is likely that surgeries will increasingly take place in ambulatory centers rather than in more expensive hospital settings.

Orthopedics is one of the few specialties that has been relatively unharvested by PE firms, and it is the most fragmented; most practices consist of only a handful of orthopedists.[94] Nevertheless, PE interest has built, especially since 2017, and it is expected to continue to escalate.[95]

It is surprising that it took so long for the moneyed interests to swoop in, given the ongoing dynamics in orthopedics, which usually put a fire in their belly. First, demand is intensifying because of an aging population and because of more injuries among young and middle-aged people who are exercising to a greater extent. Sports medicine, for example, has become one of the heavy hitters in the specialty. Second, ancillary services, such as imaging, physical and occupational therapy, durable medical equipment, and pain management, are ripe for picking. H. Lee Murphy argues that orthopedics is "viewed by experts as a potential gold mine for its ties to income-producing ancillary services."[96] Third, insurers are to a greater extent demanding that procedures take place in ambulatory surgery centers, which are often owned by the orthopedic practices themselves.[97] Fourth, according to Jeff Swearingen, cofounder of Edgemont Partners, orthopedic practices tend to be "big businesses with a lot of cash flow."[98] Fifth, orthopedic procedures tend to generate substantial reimbursements from insurers, though a cut in rates may be looming.[99]

One of the first orthopedic practices to fall into the private equity orbit in 2017 was Southeastern Spine Institute, which was recapitalized by Candescent Partners.[100] Located in Mount Pleasant, South Carolina, and founded in 1990, the all-inclusive medical campus is the largest spine practice in the state. The PE firm's goal is to become a regional force by acquiring and consolidating practices in the surrounding areas. There are only a few multistate providers (for example, Centers for Advanced Orthopaedics and OrthoCarolina), and none of these are PE-owned yet.[101]

HOPCo, the management company of the Center for Orthopedic Research and Education (known as CORE Institute), is a provider of musculoskeletal care that wound up in PE hands. I spoke with Dr. David Jacofsky, one of the initial physician-owners of the practice, who is still the chair and CEO.[102] He told me that CORE affiliated with HOPCo (around 2014) because it provided growth capital, infrastructure, and software for claims analysis and tracking of outcomes, which helped them become more effective in their performance. The main goal was to transition to value-based care.[103] Jacofsky was adamant that HOPCo did not interfere with their medical procedures.

In 2017, Frazier Healthcare Partners, Lorient Capital, and Princeton Ventures moved in as investors, providing more growth capital to the company. As with Southeastern Spine Institute, the CORE Institute encompasses the whole gamut of orthopedic services. By early 2019, only two years after investing in the business, Frazier began to search for a buyer. Given that the CORE Institute was the first PE-owned orthopedic group to flip since 2017, the industry carefully watched to see what the leveraged buyout would fetch. In the summer of 2019 the enterprise was acquired by Audax Group and Linden Capital Partners for more than $400 million.

The Orthopaedic Institute was first acquired in 2017 through a management LBO and recapitalization by Varsity Healthcare Partners, which formed its holding company, Orthopedic Care Partners, at the same time. According to Dr. Andrew Rocco, the Orthopaedic Institute's chief medical officer, steering the twenty-five owner-physicians into an agreement was not easy. He suggests, "The fact that our group got to a resolution speaks to the fact that most practices are looking at their options." As of mid-2019, he and his colleagues were pleased with the uptick in patient volume the PE imposed and with the revenue growth target of 25 percent annually. Rocco says that Varsity has renegotiated all the company's managed care contracts for the better, at least for the Orthopaedic Institute and the PE house. Varsity also has lived up to its promise of maintaining a hands-off approach to treating patients, but Rocco admits that there is some uncertainty about the next PE firm, which is sure to arrive when the time is ripe.[104]

Varsity aims to expand the Orthopaedic Institute's footprint from its current north-central Florida locations to clinics throughout the state and eventually consolidate into a multistate provider. The Steadman Clinic is one of its out-of-state purchases, acquired in 2019; its Vail, Colorado, centers are perhaps the most prestigious sports medicine facilities in the world. With this acquisition, Orthopedic Care Partners almost doubled its number of surgeons—from thirty-three to sixty-one.[105]

As mentioned above, there has been growing PE interest in the specialty. For example, in 2018, Atlantic Street Capital Management took control of OrthoBethesda, which provides orthopedic services through four centers in the greater Washington, DC, area.[106] In another recapitalization and LBO that year, Bow River Capital Partners and Capital Southwest acquired Precision Spine Care, a practice with seven facilities in East Texas. Also in 2018, Midwest Orthopaedics at Rush, a large, physician-owned practice in Chicago with fifty doctors, initiated the process of seeking a buyer. Nonetheless, the PE titans will have to sweeten the pot: one investor claims that in an eventual LBO, this practice could be valued at $250 million, and each of the doctors could receive $2 million–$5 million. The physicians, of course, would forfeit a percentage of their future salaries in any deal.[107] Riding the tailwinds into 2019, Kohlberg & Company led the pack with its acquisition of Orthopaedic & Neurology Specialists, followed by Revelstoke Capital Partners's formation of a management services organization with Beacon Orthopaedics and Sports Medicine in Ohio.[108]

As with other hot physician niches, there appear to be boundless possibilities if the notoriously reluctant and highly paid orthopedists continue to assent to buyouts. Obviously, it is far too early to assess the impact of private equity on the quality of care, physicians' and physician extenders' satisfaction, and the fate of the orthopedics specialty overall. All the same, given that earnings trump all other values in the PE business model and that the industry already has its hand in the cookie jar, it is not much of a stretch to suggest that the orthopedics specialty will soon face vast consolidations and most likely deteriorating services. As I indicate throughout this chapter, PE is just not suitable for physician practices, unless the only goal is to make money for financiers and perhaps the owner-doctors.

Sitting Heavy on the Stomach: Gastroenterology

PE investment in gastroenterology—a specialty that treats diseases of the esophagus, stomach, small bowel, colon, rectum, gallbladder, pancreas, and liver—is still in its initial stages. Audax Group, through its purchase and recapitalization of Gastro Health in 2016, was the first investor in the gastrointestinal (GI) space.[109] Formed in 2006 by the merger of three groups—GI Care Center, Gastroenterology Associates, and Gastroenterology Group—the company was particularly appealing for a takeover since it had a savvy management team that was already deeply engaged in debt financing and acquisitions. By 2016 Gastro Health had sixty practices; through Audax it acquired more than forty and is still adding offices, all in Florida.

Despite its relatively late start, the gastroenterology niche is ripe and ready for harvesting, like a crop of juicy peaches. According to Eric Oliver, GI practices are on the verge of being snapped up by private equity.[110] Although gastroenterologists represent a tiny percentage of physicians (1.7 percent), the specialty is vastly fragmented: 37 percent work in single-specialty office-based practices; 16 percent in multigroup office-based practices; 15 percent in solo office-based practices; 12 percent in hospitals; 10 percent in nonhospital academic positions; 8 percent in health care organizations; and 1 percent in out-patient clinics.[111] The emergent appeal of the GI field is also due to its short supply of physicians and rising demand for services. Undoubt-edly, the aging of the population and the concomitant rise in GI-based diseases of the elderly have piqued PE interest. For example, colorec-tal cancer is the third most common cancer diagnosed in the United States, and it is predominant among individuals age fifty and over. The specialty also benefits from a need for recurrent checkups, such as colonoscopies, and from technological advances in procedures, such as endoscopic retrograde cholangiopancreatography, a means of diag-nosing and treating problems of the liver, gallbladder, bile ducts, and pancreas; and esophagogastroduodenoscopy, a means of examin-ing the lining of the esophagus, stomach, and first part of the small intestine.[112]

In a 2018 management buyout, Waud Capital Partners plunged into the GI field by acquiring the largest gastroenterology management company in the nation, Texas Digestive Disease Consultants. Waud re-named it GI Alliance, and the goal is to extend its reach so as to be-come the foremost brand in the United States.[113] In that same year, Fra-zier Healthcare Partners swooped into the relatively unplumbed specialty by establishing a new gastroenterology management plat-form, United Digestive, with Atlanta Gastroenterology Associates. The latter had all of the essential features attractive to private equity: it was already a well-run group with sixty locations and ninety-six physicians, encompassing nearly one-third of gastroenterologists in Georgia; it owned its ambulatory facilities; and it delivered all ancil-lary services, such as pathology, pharmacy, infusion, and anesthesi-ology.[114] The physician-owners had their own goals that coincided with Frazier's. According to Dr. Steven Morris, a cofounder of Atlanta Gastroenterology Associates, the group intended to aggressively build up a strong network of practices in three or four more southeastern states and required PE capital to do so. Similar to other physician practices, the doctors were seeking greater leverage to negotiate more effectively with insurers. And, as usual, they were looking for-ward to the PE firm taking the business operations and government regulations off their hands. Morris states that Frazier had no interest in interfering with patient care, but again there was anxiety about the subsequent PE: "There's always apprehension about the second owner and the second bite of the apple," he offers.[115]

Two more buyouts took place in 2019. Amulet Capital established a new management group, U.S. Digestive Health, and simultaneously merged three Pennsylvania gastroenterology practices under its ownership in a $130 million LBO; it is now the seventh largest GI group in the United States.[116] At the end of the year, Varsity Healthcare Partners bought Peak Gastroenterology Associates, the largest practice in Colorado; the group, uncharacteristically, both engages in research and participates in more than seventy clinical trials.[117] I wonder if such critical but unlucrative endeavors will slow down under PE ownership; they certainly don't fit into its playbook.

As with other physician specialties, there are deep fears about the movement toward corporate medicine. Some practitioners are also concerned that the "PE need for growth and profit may forgo opportunity to design and create a more effective independent physician practice model for the next generation of gastroenterologists."[118] Will future gastroenterologists become employees of commercial chains, with little control over treatments and lab choices? Will colonoscopies become like mass production assembly lines? Will Medicaid recipients lose access to GI care? Today, 73 percent of gastroenterologists accept Medicaid patients.[119]

Moving into the Urinary Tract and Male Reproductive System: Urology

For PE firms, there are even more uncharted territories in physician specialties to plumb; they unrelentingly seek additional mother lodes of opportunities. Because of immense competition among PE firms for practices, such as in dermatology, and their huge price tags, they are foraying into new areas. Urology has already experienced a number of mergers but mostly through hospital and health systems and physician-led amalgamations. By 2020, there were more than fifty leading regional groups. Nonetheless, of the roughly 12,000 urologists in the United States, 60 percent are in private practice (with most of them in solo or relatively small group offices and nearly all the rest in institutional settings).[120]

The first PE to gamble on the specialty was the Audax Group with a 2016 LBO of Chesapeake Urology (CU).[121] Since its founding in 2006, CU engaged in debt financing nearly every year, but Audax Group stepped up both the sum ($114.5 million in 2018) and the number of its acquisitions. In 2018 alone, in rapid succession, its LBOs included Peninsula Urology Associates (twenty-four offices and a few ambulatory centers in Maryland and Delaware); Tennessee Urology Associates (eleven offices in Tennessee); and three groups in Colorado (Advanced Urology, Alpine Urology, and Foothills Urology), which were merged at the time of the buyout.

Also in 2018, New Mainstream Capital blazed a trail into urology through its leveraged management buyout of Central Ohio Urology Group.[122] With the goal of spreading its reach throughout the United States, Central Ohio Urology already had a centralized system for its eighteen offices in Ohio. A new platform company for urology—Urology Management Associates—was also formed that year by J. W. Childs Associates in partnership with New Jersey Urology.[123]

Integrated Medical Professionals (IMP), owned by sixty-seven physicians, took the plunge at the end of 2018 and began the process of seeking a PE investor. Already the largest urology-centric multispecialty provider in the United States, these doctors, too, want to grow their footprint across the nation. The decision of the Centers for Medicare and Medicaid Services (CMS) to change the payment method for outpatient surgery to site-neutral reimbursement rates appears to have been the precipitating factor in their decision.[124] In June 2020, Lee Equity Partners won the deal, simultaneously acquired a separate independent practice, the Urology Group, and combined the two enterprises into a new management services organization named Solaris Health.[125]

As of 2019, there still were few urology clinics in PE portfolios, but the specialty is sufficiently enticing to lure the moneyed interests over the next several years. Lisette Hilton, writing in *Urology Times*, delineates the financial benefits for urologists, intimating that they will soon succumb to the temptation. But she warns, "The real impact of these partnerships on urologists, their patients, and health care in general remains unknown."[126] As more and more PE investments occur in urology, consolidating the niche, we will ultimately be forced to contend with the consequences of these financially focused deals on individual urologists, patients, and the specialty overall.

Failing Kidneys: Dialysis Clinics

I am particularly interested in kidney disease because one of my closest friends in college, Bill O'Connell, was able to live for decades with the illness only because he had Medicare funding for a few years of dialysis and eventually a successful transplant. Kidney malfunction can be lethal without dialysis; it is the ninth leading cause of death in the United States. Nearly 30.3 million people (more than 9 percent of the population) has some stage of the disease, and the number is expected to rise because of higher rates of diabetes, obesity, and hypertension, as well as earlier and improved diagnosis. Just as important for the financiers, the passage of the Social Security Amendments of 1972, which entitle individuals with the condition to Medicare coverage, spurred a for-profit dialysis industry; it is the only disorder for which the age-based program provides coverage for everyone.[127] Furthermore, the US government has incentivized the growth of stand-alone dialysis centers rather than the provision of services in hospitals.[128]

Consequently, far more people are treated for the ailment, which has spurred the construction and consolidation of ever more free-standing clinics. Dialysis is expensive, and the bulk of its funding derives from Medicare. In 2016, the treatment accounted for $34 billion of the program's overall spending.[129] And reimbursement rates are rising: in 2017, dialysis clinics received $80 million more in government payments, followed by an increase of $190 million the next year. Beneficiary copayments went up by $30 million.[130] Dialysis is a $24.7 billion industry that generates huge profits, certainly not something PE firms would overlook. In 2018, the pretax earnings of the two leading dialysis companies were nearly 20 percent annually—not a bad pay day.[131]

Of the largest dialysis companies, approximately half are private equity–owned. The top two, DaVita HealthCare Partners and Fresenius Medical Care, control nearly 75 percent of all PE-owned places.[132] DaVita, founded in 1994 and listed on the New York Stock Exchange (NYSE) the following year, has been steadily expanding across the country ever since. Fresenius has a more complicated history since the publicly traded company has bought a series of enterprises with long PE trajectories. It has been enmeshed in a convoluted web of interlocking buyouts and is now the second largest dialysis provider in the nation.[133]

The third biggest provider, U.S. Renal Care, owns 4–5 percent of all centers.[134] Founded by Chris Brengard in 2000, it has been cast from PE to PE over the years, beginning in 2005 with $30 million in funding from several venture capital firms (SV Health Investors, Salix Ventures, and Select Capital Ventures). Cressey & Company took a 25 percent stake in 2006 and paid itself and the other owners a $137.5 million dividend recap in 2011. Leonard Green & Partners bought U.S. Renal Care the following year in a management buyout, and then in 2019 sold it to Bain Capital, Summit Partners and Revelstoke Capital.[135]

The owners of publicly traded American Renal Associates, the fourth largest dialysis company in the United States, are seeking to cash out; PE firms still own 40 percent of the stock. American Renal Associates began its PE journey in 2004 when it was acquired by Pimlico Capital in a $20 million LBO. After receiving development capital from two PE shops for numerous acquisitions over six years, it was sold to Centerbridge Partners in a 2010 SBO for $450 million. Centerbridge subsequently borrowed another $200 million to pay itself a dividend recap in 2013, just before putting the chain on the NYSE in 2016; the PE firm realized $165 million and retained some stock.

Clearly, consolidation in kidney treatment brands is extreme and ongoing. Not only has the sector been a gold mine for numerous PE firms along the way, but the consolidation has raised the cost of treatments, mostly paid by taxpayers through Medicare and Medicaid. It also has limited the choices for vulnerable people living with renal failure. Without serious regulation, the industry appears to be a free-for-all even compared to nursing homes, which have notoriously appalling conditions and lax enforcement. The dialysis centers are supposed to be inspected only once every three years and even that tends to be disregarded. Sanctions are few and far between, and violations have been on the rise. Doctors are scarce at the facilities, and there is often only one registered nurse—the minimum requirement—and at times there is none.

In earlier years, the procedure had been carried out in hospitals. Since the movement to corporate, for-profit medicine, and especially private equity ownership, quality of care has become a serious problem. The United States also has one of the highest dialysis fatality rates in the industrialized world, despite the greater costs.[136] One of the major reasons is the undertrained, underpaid, and overworked technicians who are responsible for most of a patient's dialysis care. Such centers are often short-staffed, and Medicare does not have staffing level mandates. Only a few states have imposed them, and efforts to do so in other places, such as California, have been soundly defeated through industry pressure.[137]

What is more, the centers are plagued with unsanitary conditions and generally poor care. In 2010, Robin Fields did a comprehensive investigation of clinics across the country and uncovered egregious safety violations in numerous practices. In order to cut costs, she found, owners are running their clinics "like factories, turning over three shifts of patients a day, sometimes four" and expecting their technicians to monitor more individuals than safety experts recommend.[138] The more daily shifts that can be fit in, the more money the owners earn. But it means shorter sessions for patients and less time between them, adversely affecting their well-being and even life expectancy. In addition, infection-control breaches "exposed patients to hepatitis, staph, tuberculosis, and HIV."[139]

Mortality at the large profit-making enterprises tends to be more than that of nonprofits or public centers. One investigator reports a 19 percent and 24 percent greater risk of death at Fresenius and

DaVita centers, respectively, than at the nation's major nonprofit chain.[140] Research by the political comedian John Oliver finds that for-profit centers have 35 percent fewer nurses per patient than other facilities. He further comments: "Companies like DaVita will cut any corner possible to turn a profit, even if it means putting the wellbeing of its patients in jeopardy." Oliver aptly concludes, "The care of America's kidneys is way too important to be treated as a fast food experience."[141]

Even worse, a study in JAMA (September 2019) reveals that patients treated at for-profit dialysis centers, as compared to those served at nonprofit facilities, are 64 percent less likely to be placed on a transplant waiting list and 56 percent less likely to receive a transplant from a deceased donor. The investigation by a team of researchers at the Emory School of Medicine analyzed the records of more than 1.5 million patients diagnosed with renal failure from 2000 to 2016. Plainly, "the implication is that for-profit facilities may be biased toward keeping patients on dialysis."[142]

The top commercial companies have also been accused of pushing their patients onto commercial health insurance instead of publicly funded care, which pays them far less. When the Affordable Care Act was implemented in 2014, it mandated insurance coverage for people with preexisting conditions—including renal disease—and the dialysis clinics had a new, higher-paying source of revenue.[143] For instance, just months before American Renal Associates was taken public, the PE-owned company faced a lawsuit over allegations that it had persuaded Medicaid patients in Florida and Ohio to purchase United-Healthcare plans, whose premiums would be paid by the nonprofit American Kidney Fund. Unsurprisingly, this health insurance premium program (HIPP) is funded by the largest dialysis companies, presumably to capture the higher commercial reimbursement rates. Private payer fees at the time were roughly $4,000 for each treatment, compared to only $200 from Medicaid. But HIPP recipients pay a price: they are charged copays by the insurance companies and lose their Medicaid/Medicare funding for a future kidney transplant if an organ becomes available.[144]

In 2019, California attempted to curtail the practice through Assembly Bill 290, which would have prevented clinic owners from "encouraging" low-income Medicaid patients to enroll in HIPP. A federal judge blocked the legislation until a lawsuit against it—mainly brought by DaVita and Fresenius Medical Care—was resolved.[145] Shelby Livingston reports, "While in their public statements the companies focus on how the new law would affect patients, the companies are also likely worried about their bottom lines. . . . DaVita's then-CEO, Ken[t] Thiry, said that the law could reduce operating income by $24 million to $40 million."[146] As of the spring of 2021, the lawsuit had not been resolved, and the law had not taken effect.

In 2018, California had also endeavored to limit the amount of money the state's dialysis clinics could earn from commercial insurance: Proposition 8 would have capped charges at 15 percent more than the cost of treatment. It also would have mandated staffing levels, annual inspections, and other safeguards. The measure, which was supported with $18 million from the Service Employees International Union, was defeated: DaVita, Fresenius, and U.S. Renal spent $67 million, $34 million, and $8 million, respectively, to fight it.[147] DaVita and Fresenius own 72 percent of the clinics in California and collect $3 billion in profits from them. One business columnist states starkly: "More generally, the Proposition 8 campaign is a reflection of the dialysis industry's reputation for profiteering from a life-preserving procedure."[148]

In 2019, President Trump, in a supposed money-saving measure, signed an executive order that, among other provisions, is intended to move more dialysis patients away from clinics and into having treatment in their homes. CMS has proposed a pay model that would push dialysis patients toward such care, along with fostering transplant operations. Unfortunately, too many people undergoing dialysis do not have sufficient help at home to accomplish this, and the number of available kidneys is far too limited at this point in time. Nevertheless, top dialysis companies simultaneously are advocating against the initiative and are moving in step with what may come. Fresenius, for instance, is expanding its home dialysis business and altering some of its clinics into training centers for people performing homecare. DaVita is investing in technology to assist such individuals. The money-making financiers are not going away anytime soon.[149]

Et Tu, Brute? Fertility and Women's Reproductive Health

There is no physician specialty that private equity would avoid if it could make an outsized profit in a short amount of time. The relatively untouched area of fertility (and other women's health domains) is primed for exploitation, especially given that physicians in the field are thriving. More than 8 million babies have been delivered through in vitro fertilization (IVF) since the birth of Louise Brown in 1978. In the United States, there are 250,000 cycles of IVF procedures annually in nearly 500 mostly small, independent clinics.[150] Why shouldn't PE firms now consolidate them and snatch a share of the wealth for themselves?

Considerable charges for fertility treatment (averaging upward of $15,000 for each attempt) combined with restricted insurance coverage had held the PE industry back; as late as 2015 there were few investments.[151] But many shops are overcoming their reticence, and changing conditions have been part of their reconsideration. At least fifteen states have mandated coverage by insurance companies, and even a few businesses are covering their employees' IVF expenses. Since 2016, the US Department of Veterans Affairs has allowed wounded soldiers to receive such services as well. There is a confluence of other tempting factors for the PE industry: more women are having children in their thirties or later, leading to a higher incidence of infertility; the legalization of same-sex marriage and the rise of single parenthood have enlarged the number of individuals seeking services; and advancements in technology have rendered it more attractive for people who have had difficulty conceiving to pursue the option.[152]

According to several knowledgeable observers, there is apprehension that the PE focus will be on enrolling greater numbers of young, healthy women for egg freezing and other measures to enhance the bottom line at the expense of the population's actual needs (i.e., more affordable treatment options). Dr. Ravi Gada of Dallas Fort Worth Fertility Associates (co-owned by four physicians) says his clinic "has brushed off interest from private equity firms. He worries that the impromptu flexibility possible in a clinic like his—such as offering a discount for a woman coming back for a second or third IVF cycle—wouldn't be possible in a chain backed by private equity money."[153] The CEO of physician-owned Shady Grove Fertility, Mark Segal, is particularly worried that outside investors could push the clinic toward "more of a focus on just continuing to add more patients . . . without necessarily focusing on how that would impact patient care."[154]

One of the first PE platforms, Ovation Fertility, was pieced together in 2015 by PE firm WindRose Health Investors through the fusion of four IVF laboratories. It was cast to its second PE owner only four years later. In the short interim, Ovation rapidly acquired fertility labs across the United States and began offering new moneymaking services, such as egg freezing, long-term storage of embryos, donor eggs, and surrogacy services.[155] Nate Snyder, Ovation's CEO, described his experiences with the chain. He graduated from the Wharton School, he told me, and sensed great opportunity in the fertility market. A former fellow student was employed at WindRose, and using Snyder's business model, they decided to partner in the acquisition and consolidation of in vitro fertilization and genetic testing labs. According to Snyder, they were so successful that Ovation grew faster than they had anticipated, and by 2019 WindRose was ready to cash in on its investment. It was well positioned for even greater growth, Snyder added. Fully forty PE firms expressed interest in buying the business, more than any other portfolio company WindRose had ever owned; Morgan Stanley Investment Management's bid ultimately won.[156] The company does not accept either Medicaid or commercial insurance; despite its financial success, then, Ovation Fertility is only benefiting families that can pay on their own or are forced to go into debt.

In 2016, Lee Equity Partners and businessman Martin Varsavsky assembled a joint venture, Prelude Fertility, by piecing together Reproductive Biology Associates and MyEggBank North America. By 2019, they had acquired sufficient clinics to become the largest provider in the United States, with a market share of 8 percent.[157] The partners intend to continue expanding its national geographic reach, at least until sale time.

In 2017, Women's Health USA was acquired by Sverica Capital Management. The company had been founded in 1997 by attorney Robert Patricelli, who apparently had no particular interest in fertility but foresaw its financial potential. Through venture capital funding from Sprout Group, he grew the enterprise into one of the largest physician management services organizations associated with women's issues. It was ripe for the picking, and Sverica, a multisector PE investor, opted in.[158]

Also in 2017, Audax Group formed the platform Axia through a merger of Women's HealthCare Group of Pennsylvania and Regional Women's Health Group. Further consolidation began with its 2018 purchase of Abington Reproductive Medicine for $10 million; it was renamed Sincera Reproductive Medicine two years later. I spoke to Dr. Jay Schinfeld, who retired just before the buyout of his Abington practice. To say the least, he is dismayed by the consequences of the sale. He says that his previous partners, who signed the contract with Audax, were paid up front for the takeover, but everyone else has suffered. "Axia is a mess," he told me. "Everyone's miserable. The practice has had a hard time." According to him, working conditions have changed for the worse. The PE-owned company also has turned to cheaper health care insurance for its employees and imposes tighter schedules on them. Schinfeld noted that before Audax, his company had provided every worker with a free lunch and allowed an hour to enjoy it. He said, "We believed in sharing the wealth." He pointed out that such an attitude is good for everyone, including the business and patients. Not only has the practice eliminated the complimentary meals, but the break has been cut down to a half hour.[159]

A substantial number of his prior staff have quit or were fired without warning, especially the nurses. One of the embryologists, who had been with the practice for twenty-four years, was dismissed on the spot because he needed an unanticipated day off. In addition to his concern about the employees, Schinfeld is worried about the patients. Doctors are restricted in what equipment and products they can purchase, and services have deteriorated. "Axia is not interested in the quality of care." The new owners are just there to make money. The PE firm has engaged in aggressive marketing but also in hard-hitting billing practices. "Private equity is not good for medicine," Schinfeld concluded.

One of the physicians who participated in the buyout, Dr. Stephen G. Somkuti, maintained that there have been certain advantages from the takeover by Audax and its acquisitions and mergers, including improved ability to negotiate with insurers and decreased overhead costs. He insisted that the PE associates, who are all businesspeople, have no interest in micromanaging patient care. Nonetheless, he acknowledged that there have been a number of day-to-day frustrations. Everything is slow, he explained, due to the multiple levels of bureaucracy. He also allowed that the company has grown too fast and that infrastructure has not kept pace. Further, Somkuti told me that the PE shop has replaced many nurses with lesser-trained medical assistants (although he added that the nurses may have been overqualified for some of these positions). Budgets are tight as well: although equipment used to be replaced or upgraded immediately as needed, now the physicians "must make do with what they have."[160]

In 2021, now with eighty centers, the company was tossed to Partners Group at a price of $800 million.

Have people who desire to get pregnant become the latest cash cow? Will their reproductive health succumb progressively to corporate medicine in the PE style? As the financiers swell the number of deals and aggregate small businesses in this lucrative theater, what will happen to costs, affordability, quality of treatments, and types of service? Given the PE business model and the evidence thus far, it is most likely that GPs will feather their nests without putting people and their genuine fertility needs as top priority.

PE is making headway in other areas of women's health as well. According to a study of buyouts between 2010 and 2019, PE firms acquired seventeen obstetrics and gynecology practices, consisting of roughly

533 offices.[161] Because of a stable clientele, fragmentation, the potential for auxiliary services (e.g., ultrasounds), fertility, related laboratory requirements, and shortfalls in personnel, the specialty is ripe for more rapid and extensive PE takeovers in the coming years. It is projected that by 2025 there will be a dearth of nearly 5,000 employees nationally for such services.[162]

Cornering Emergencies: Urgent Care Centers

Also known as retail health clinics, freestanding urgent care centers (UCCs) have been popping up everywhere around the country. As a more than $18 billion industry—and mounting—the niche has tempted hospital health systems, insurance companies, retailers (such as Walgreens Boots Alliance), and naturally, PE shops. The latter, which own slightly more than half of all UCCs in the United States, are also participating in joint ventures with hospital systems.[163] Patients, too, are drawn to the retail clinics, given their lower cost than emergency rooms (ERs), longer available hours than primary physician offices, and convenience.[164]

PE firms began investing in UCCs beginning in 2010, and the sector remains robust. Seemingly, their main appeal is the strong potential for stepping up the pace, and therefore the volume, of patient visits. As reported in DocWire News, "The business model is easy to understand: treat many patients as quickly as possible and the money will start to add up."[165] Since, despite the "urgent care" tag, these clinics only serve people requiring services for noncritical conditions, the PE owners can, and do, staff them mostly (and in some places entirely) with physician extenders and perhaps a nurse. That, too, enhances the bottom line. In the urgent care center that my husband and I have visited several times, there has never been a doctor present, nor have we been attended by a registered nurse.

Urgent care centers can be lucrative for PE houses. For instance, in 2012 Brockway Moran & Partners invested in MD Now, a South Florida urgent care network. It netted four times its investment through the sale of the organization to Brentwood Associates and Blue Sea Capital six years later.[166]

One of the fastest growing urgent care chains, CityMD, was purchased by Warburg Pincus in April 2017 for $600 million.[167] A year later CityMD, through Warburg, acquired Stat Health, a leading UCC in Long Island, for $100 million.[168] In 2019, CityMD merged with Summit Medical Group of New Jersey, one of the largest physician-owned and -controlled multispecialty groups in the United States. With its 120 locations now dominating urgent care in the New York–New Jersey metropolitan area and an extensive network of in-house referrals for primary care and specialty practices, CityMD seems to have a growing lock on all types of medical services in the region. According to Sarah Pringle of PE Hub, it is the first PE-owned urgent care chain to unify UCCs and independent physician practices.[169] Comparable combinations are sure to follow. Can such monopolies be beneficial for controlling national health care costs and improving quality of care?

GoHealth Urgent Care is an example of a joint venture between a PE firm and a hospital system. Founded in 2013 by two physicians, GoHealth was acquired by TPG the following year. Since its purchase, the urgent care company has allied with Dignity Health (San Francisco, California), Legacy Health (Portland, Oregon), and Northwell Health (Great Neck, New York). In 2015, Welsh, Carson, Anderson & Stowe, together with Select Medical Holdings (Mechanicsburg, Pennsylvania), acquired Concentra from Humana.[170] In 2018, MedExpress Urgent Care and Atlantic Health System joined forces.[171] In these cases, the hospitals get to overwhelm their competition and curtail ER visits but receive a steady stream of patients to fill their beds, and they also obtain capital for growth. PE shops, predictably, make lots of money.

PE companies, with their insatiable appetites, have been devouring urgent care clinics. Although the facilities tend to be low margin, by stepping up the number of clients, accelerating the pace of treatment, and lowering the training level of the practitioners, these chains can be, for their owners, like hitting the lottery. Such efficiency tactics come straight out of the PE playbook. But the freestanding clinics are costly for patients, with fees for nonemergency care generally "22 times more expensive than at a physician's office."[172] Just as important, do their moneymaking approaches harm vulnerable individuals who rely on urgent care clinics for their everyday ailments and often crisis situations? Even more, does this type of environment lend itself to accurately discerning routine maladies from more severe, potentially lethal conditions, especially if the midlevel health providers are on their own, without supervision? How many clients are sent home with a bandage when they should have been diverted to more intensive care?

Surprise! Outsourced Staffing and Hospital Bills

Medical staffing companies, long eschewed by PE firms because of the unpredictability of revenues and susceptibility to recessions,[173] have recently come on the PE radar for several reasons. First, to control expenditures, hospitals are increasingly outsourcing their emergency room doctors, hospitalists, anesthesiologists, radiologists, pathologists, neonatologists, and other specialists. The facilities have found that they can better manage fluctuations in patient requirements for specific services by hiring personnel as needed. Second, demand for physicians and nurses is steadily growing while the number of such professionals has declined. Third, a large percentage of practicing doctors are at or near retirement age; the Association of American Colleges and Universities estimates that one-third are older than fifty-five. As vacancies swell, hospitals will require more temporary staff to fill them.[174] Fourth and most important, these subcontracted physicians charge exorbitant fees because they are usually out-of-network and can set their own rates.

As mentioned in chapter 3, one of the oldest PE-owned staffing enterprises is Envision Healthcare, which is also the largest in the sector.[175] It services 6 percent of the $41 billion hospital-based physician outsourcing market. The chain's financial whirl began in 2005, when Onex purchased both EmCare, the leading medical staffing subcontractor in the United States,[176] and American Medical Response, a major ambulance firm, from Laidlaw International for $820 million. After Onex merged the two businesses, renamed it Emergency Medical Services (EMS), and completed an IPO for $113.4 million, the company was taken private again in 2011 by Clayton, Dubilier & Rice (CD&R) for $3.2 billion. Two years later, the PE house merged EMS with Amsurg, a staffing and ambulatory surgery center, and rebranded it Envision Healthcare; CD&R then put the combined assets on the public exchange once more, raising $1.1 billion in the IPO and retaining substantial stock.[177] CD&R steadily sold off its shares until 2018, ultimately earning five times its investment, according to Kevin Conway, vice chair of the PE firm.[178] The yo-yoing continued: in a massive $9.9 billion deal in 2018, KKR took Envision private again, after carving out American Medical Response (see chapter 9).

Envision exemplifies how money-spinning consolidation, where a succession of PE firms each takes a large bite of the apple, inevitably winds up with others paying a huge price. One of the most critical issues has been the exorbitant charges by the chain: somebody must pay for these ongoing financial bites! In particular, the corporation has been embroiled in lawsuits and government attacks over its balance billing (known as "surprise billing") practices.[179] Envision and its PE owners strategically refuse to enter into insurance contracts for its physicians, including those staffing emergency rooms, even if a hospital has a negotiated agreement for its other medical personnel. Consequently, as an out-of-network company, Envision can charge far higher fees than it would otherwise, thereby generating significant out-of-pocket expenses for patients even if they are insured.[180]

An investigation by Yale University researchers confirmed the chain's egregious practices. Their analysis showed that when a facility contracted with Envision's EmCare for its emergency room staffing, out-of-network charges spiraled by more than 80 percent above former rates. In addition, the PE-owned entity engaged in other unsavory schemes. For instance, in 2017, Envision paid roughly $30 million in fines to resolve claims by the US Department of Justice that its EmCare ER doctors received bonuses for unnecessarily admitting patients to hospitals.[181]

TeamHealth, the second largest player in hospital staffing, has had a similar circuitous trajectory and deplorable track record. The company was formed as a platform in 1999 by Madison Dearborn Partners, Cornerstone Equity Investors, and Beecken Petty O'Keefe & Company for $335 million.[182] It was acquired in a secondary management LBO by Blackstone Group in 2005 and then listed on the New York Stock Exchange in 2009 through a $159.6 million IPO. Subsequently, Blackstone Group took the company private again in a tertiary LBO in 2017 for $6.1 billion.[183] TeamHealth, too, has engaged in unscrupulous and hefty surprise-billing practices. The Yale study mentioned above revealed that the company threatened insurers that its physicians would move from in- to out-of-network status if they did not get the fees they were demanding, and as a result, they ended up receiving rates that were 68 percent higher than usual.[184]

Envision and TeamHealth control 30 percent of the physician staffing sector and have enlisted more than 80,000 physicians and mid-level health workers.[185] Additional PE houses are flocking to the niche as well.[186] They eye businesses that already hold market power or can become a platform for local or regional consolidation. With that reach, they can force health insurance companies into paying them higher than usual fees if they want them in their networks. The PE firms also have a hold over patients who, in emergency situations, cannot choose their ER physician or, for surgeries, don't have a choice about the hospital's outsourced anesthesiologist. There also has been a rise in the use of surgical assistants, many of whom bill patients separately. American Surgical Professionals, for example, is the largest US provider of such operating room support. The once-public company, which was taken private by Great Point Partners in 2011, has engaged in appalling out-of-network billing practices.[187]

Overall, as Eileen Appelbaum concludes, "Private equity has shaped how these companies do business. In the health-care settings where they operate, market forces do not constrain the raw pursuit of profit. People desperate for care are in no position to reject over-priced medical services or shop for in-network doctors."[188] The scamming, which is widespread, touches a sizable number of families. According to some sources, about one-fifth of ER patients and 9 percent of elective inpatient care at in-network facilities result in balance billing for patients. An inquiry by Stanford University researchers, based on 12.6 million ER visits, found even higher numbers: in 2016, 42.8 percent of the individuals in their study had received a surprise medical bill.[189] Although about twenty-five states have enacted various levels of protection for consumers, two experts point out that they don't have jurisdiction over self-insured employer plans, which enroll nearly 61 percent of covered private-sector workers.[190]

At the beginning of the summer of 2019, congressional leaders finally took notice of the oversized earnings flooding into PE shops, along with the fleecing of vulnerable patients. Two US House and Senate committees attempted to protect consumers from these surprise out-of-network bills and cap the rates insurers pay for the outsourced services. The Senate Health, Education, Labor and Pensions Committee, through its Republican chair, Lamar Alexander, and ranking Democrat, Patty Murray, proposed Senate Bill 1895, the Lower Health Care Costs Act. Simultaneously, HR 3630, the No Surprises Act, was offered by the House Energy and Commerce Committee chair, Democrat Frank Pallone, and ranking Republican, Greg Walden. Pallone and Walden also later wrote a six-page letter aimed at Blackstone (TeamHealth) and KKR (Envision's EmCare), demanding information about how many businesses they own in the staffing sector; the terms, revenues, and annual returns on these investments; and their role in the management of the companies and negotiations with insurers. Given the PE industry's determined concealment of financial undertakings, the information was not forthcoming. The PE investors put a full-court press against the proposals, including targeting vulnerable legislators supporting them. A "dark money" group, Doctor Patient Unity, spent more than $30 million for newspaper and local TV ads, op-eds, and district meetings to oppose any limits on fees for outsourced practitioners; the legislative acts were disingenuously dubbed as "rate-setting" and "government control" over US health care. Reporters for the *New York Times* soon discovered Doctor Patient Unity's financial backers: TeamHealth and Envision.[191] At that point, KKR and

Blackstone Group had additional considerations sparking their attack. Because of congressional attempts to control surprise medical billing, Envision's solvency was possibly at stake; the $5.4 billion loan to buy the company was steadily losing value.[192] TeamHealth's debt financing was at risk as well.

The legislative offensive was reinforced by Physicians for Fair Coverage (mostly PE-backed by firms such as ValorBridge Partners, Carlyle Group, Onex, WCAS, and Ares), which launched a $1.2 million national ad campaign. The opponents of these bills seemingly were willing to accept an arbitration approach but at higher payment levels than the congressional proposals.[193] The insurance companies unleashed their own group, Coalition against Surprise Medical Billing, the only major corporate American player in favor of controlling balance billing; they were seeking lower rates for hospital staffing services.

The onslaught took its toll on the national policymakers. In July 2019, an arbitration amendment was inserted into the House proposal, which watered down the adverse effects on PE owners; some of their allies in Congress also were pushing other concessions to weaken or scuttle the measures. Additionally, unease had developed among a number of vulnerable lawmakers regarding their 2020 election prospects.[194] Leaders of the House Ways and Means Committee Richard Neal (Democratic chair) and Kevin Brady (ranking Republican) were actively pushing to eliminate benchmarking entirely. Neal's second largest contributor to his 2020 campaign was Blackstone Group, and Brady's topmost financial backer was Welsh, Carson, Anderson and Stowe, two large owners of staffing companies.[195]

After a hiatus of several months, bicameral negotiations among the four key leaders began anew and culminated in a deal that would ban balance billing: insurers would pay the median in-network rate negotiated by doctors in a given geographic area. However, it included an arbitration clause that the staffing companies and their PE owners had sought. As a result, the ranking Senate Democrat on the team, Murray, withdrew her support.[196]

Talks in the House commenced again in early December amid attempts to attach newly revised surprise-billing regulations to the end-of-the year appropriations bill. But that stalled too because of steadfast lobbyists and their provider-friendly legislators, including Neal. Finally, in a last-minute push, Congress concluded a deal that was eventually signed into law by President Trump. Beginning in 2022, patients will be protected against surprise bills from both out-of-network staffing companies and emergency air transit. They are responsible only for their in-network cost-sharing fees and usual deductibles; it is up to insurers and providers to negotiate for the remaining portion of the bill. To the relative satisfaction of providers, including PE-owned health care businesses, there are no rate-setting, cost threshold, or benchmark amounts. If the two parties can't reach an agreement, they submit the charge to an arbitrator, who, among other considerations, takes into account the median in-network fee. Public payers are excluded from the deal, another victory for the PE firms. Nonetheless, it is expected that battles over the details of the arbitration process will heat up. Moreover, ground ambulances were excluded from the ban; sick and defenseless people will still face unexpected, exorbitant bills for their out-of-network ride to the emergency room.

Concluding Remarks

There have been varying points in time in which PE firms moved into particular physician specialties, different motivations for doing so, and a range of investments in each, but nowadays acquisitions and mergers are skyrocketing in all niches. There appears to be no type of doctor's office or medical facility that GPs would eschew. There is seemingly no end in sight as they steadily buy, consolidate, and control the lifeblood of our health care system: physicians, their office practitioners, and ambulatory centers.

The PE shops, which volley the entities from one to another in quick succession, have been paying high valuations but cashing out at lucrative rates of return. Participating physician-owners, too, have found the transactions financially rewarding, though generally at the price of their independence and control over their practice. The ill effects have been experienced mainly by young doctors, midlevel practitioners, paraprofessionals, other office staff, the medical specialties themselves, and especially patients and the larger society.

As I have outlined in this chapter, there are devastating drawbacks both overall and in specific niches. Short-term ownership, for instance, constrains investment in staff training and up-to-date equipment and technologies. It also encourages other strategies that pump up the sale price to a subsequent buyer at the expense of high-quality services. Streamlining, a forte of the PE industry, fosters the increased use of lesser-trained, sometimes unsupervised physician extenders and an assembly line approach to patient care.

Elevated leverage, the mother's milk of PE, is distinctly unsuited to physician practices and their ancillary facilities and products. To boost cash flow, the shops may increase patient volume, encourage unnecessary procedures, and stint on medical supplies. And there's always a chance of bankruptcy resulting from a shift in regulations, payment rates, or economic conditions. Losing Gymboree, Claire's, or Toys "R" Us, as disturbing as it was for the workers and public, is not as shattering as individuals forgoing their dialysis treatments or dermatology patients their cancer therapies. At the current rate of consolidation in certain physician specialties, a PE-controlled chain may be—or may soon develop into—the only game in town.

The moneyed interests are also contributing to rising health costs and inequality of care. Welfare medicine, including the acceptance of Medicaid patients, is antithetical to the PE business model—that is, unless it can unscrupulously speed up treatments and provide shoddy services. The shops also tend to turn their back on sponsoring community events, even if the prior doctor-owners generously funded them.

PE firms are on a roll, pushing full steam ahead in the physician practice, urgent care, and medical staffing domains. What will be the next niche? It seems that the indispensable but long-neglected primary care doctors are on their radar, as are other relatively unclaimed health care spaces.[197] If the trend continues—and I'm sure that it will—medical decisions will be less and less between you and your doctor.

5

Drilling for Gold

Corralling Dentists

DENTAL CARE was one of the initial health care services to stir up PE interest, and leveraged buyouts emerged in the late 1990s. In an early example, APG Partners acquired Aspen Dental Management in 1998, and the company has been pitched from one PE to another ever since. Acquisitions and consolidations in the sector picked up at the turn of the twenty-first century: by 2012, PE firms owned 12,000 dental practices (8 percent of the total).[1] Since then—and at an accelerating pace— more and more offices—have come into the clutches of the financiers.

PE ownership of dental practices is characteristically through a dental service organization (DSO), a "façade shell company" that shields against liabilities and provides tax benefits.[2] DSOs are structured so as to circumvent any regulations over the clinics: a number of states prohibit or restrict nondentists from owning a dental practice and place other constraints on the businesses. As usual, PE shops defend these arrangements by claiming that they are protecting the practitioners from everyday business matters, allowing them to focus on their dentistry. Yet given the purposeful complexity of DSO configurations, it is challenging to uncover who is actually in charge of the enterprises.[3] Jim Moriarty, a dental medical malpractice lawyer, puts it more bluntly: "In reality . . . a DSO is just a dental clinic bought and sold by private equity investors. PEs purchase the practice and then make the dentists employees."[4]

By 2012, DSOs fell under government scrutiny. There had been intensifying concern that they were encroaching on the actual practice of medicine and not just engaging in back office services. In addition, allegations of egregious behavior in at least six states sparked a US Senate investigation that year, which dug deeply into charges that PE-owned practices were performing needless procedures and providing substandard services. The strategies of five companies, in particular, were in question: Church Street Health Management (CSHM), National Children's Dental Research, ReachOut Healthcare America, Heartland Dental, and Aspen Dental Management.[5]

A major PE target was (and still is) Medicaid, the government medical program for low-income people. Sydney P. Freedberg, an investigative reporter for *Bloomberg News*, observes: "After years of complaints that the poor were being deprived of [dental] care under Medicaid, public pressure and class-action lawsuits opened the floodgates."[6] Millions of kids had been denied much-needed dental work and had suffered discomfort, sometimes agony, infections, and related medical conditions.[7] Finally, after years of resistance, states—to varying degrees—began to add dentistry to their Medicaid plans. Naturally, several PE firms used this new flow of money as their personal ATMs.

Medicaid-supported dental clinics, particularly those controlled by PE shops, proliferated. Outlays under welfare medicine rose dramatically, as did PE abuse of the program and the children who were being cared for. Some clinics quickened the pace of treatments by overly sedating kids and using straitjacket-type restraints on them. A 2013 joint report by committees led by US senators Max Baucus and Chuck Grassley documented that these corporate-run practices "overemphasize bottom-line financial considerations at the expense of providing appropriate high-quality, low-cost care."[8] Children were subjected to unnecessary interventions and serious trauma. The DSOs also engaged in "wham, bam, thank you ma'am" dentistry: they sent crews of dental assistants to schools where they treated up to thirty students daily.[9]

The first large bankruptcies were also an issue in 2012: CSHM (owned by Arcapita, Inc., Carlyle Group, and other PE firms associated with the Small Smiles network) filed for Chapter 11, followed by All Smiles Dental Centers (owned by Valor Equity Partners).The PE titans refused to place blame on their exploitive financial gambits or poor-quality care. Instead, they blamed the insolvencies on "senseless litigation" and government investigations.[10]

Dr. Paul Casamassimo, chief policy officer for the American Academy of Pediatric Dentistry, explained that in bankruptcies everyone suffers: patient records are misplaced; young dentists and dental assistants lose their jobs; and patients no longer can be cared for by their usual provider, even if they are in the middle of a procedure.[11] Nevertheless, consolidation is still going strong and shows no signs of stopping.

The sheer size of the market for dentistry is an inducement for private equity, which is like a child gazing into the window of a candy store. Could PE outfits possibly ignore $73 billion, the sweet taste already in their mouths? Just as rewarding, cash flow is predictable and steady, patients tend to be regulars, and dentists contend with fewer regulations than physicians do. And unlike doctors, who have been gobbled up by hospital systems and PE firms alike, roughly 80 percent of dentists are outside the clutches of corporate medicine; it is still a cottage industry.[12]

There are myriad means for extracting windfall profits: augmenting patient volume by mostly using lower-paid paraprofessionals; accelerating patient flow; installing IT systems; adding procedures (i.e., endodontics, orthodontics, oral surgery, periodontics, prosthodontics) and consumer products; selling and leasing back real estate; implementing forceful collection policies; building de novo clinics; acquiring and merging practices; and developing hard-hitting marketing and billing tactics.[13]

As with physician specialties, the use of midlevel staff for certain dental treatments is highly controversial. For example, Dr. Jill Tanzi, president of the Massachusetts Dentists Alliance for Quality Care, said that her group is fighting against proposed legislation in Massachusetts that would allow "dental therapists" to provide procedures such as filling cavities. While these practitioners could help fill the gap in underserved communities, it is also likely that PE-owned practices will hire the lesser-trained and lower-paid assistants to substitute for dentists. Tanzi argued that such replacements would adversely affect patient care.[14]

Dr. Michael Davis, a dentist and observer of private equity investments in the sector, was adamant that the financiers are "only about money" and should not be allowed to take over dentistry (or any physician practices, for that matter). He told me that PE has diverse scams, but they all rely on cheating individuals and taxpayers, overtreating patients, upcoding services, and providing poor-quality care. As an example of upcoding, Davis said that he has heard of dentists placing sealants on patients and then billing for "tooth restoration" or fillings at a far higher reimbursement rate. He also mentioned cases where PE-owned companies have obliged customers to prepay for their care but subsequently provided them with treatments of limited efficacy.[15]

Davis added that PE firms often perpetrate their fraud on the working class. One con is discount dental plans, which a chain may sell as "insurance" but which can only be used at one of its own facilities. These policies are neither registered with nor scrutinized by the government. Its clinics then perform unnecessary treatments but at discounted rates. Companies, he said, get fines for some of their ploys, but the amounts are peanuts for them. If the United States wants to stop the bad behavior, the country needs to move the lawsuits from civil to criminal cases.[16]

Dentists tend to sell their practices to private equity because there are no alternative markets, especially for individuals who are ready to retire. Davis pointed out that students graduating from dental school have incurred such high debt that they are not sufficiently creditworthy to buy an ongoing practice, as had occurred in earlier years. Tanzi echoed that observation: she noted that it is difficult to set up your own office or buy one from someone else when you are $300,000 or more in debt after attaining your professional credentials.[17]

Casamassimo offered additional reasons that dentists off-load their practices. They do not want to be responsible for administration of the business anymore—they are tired of the day-to-day hassles that have nothing to do with actual patient care. They also look forward to having a support system that maintains the equipment and deals with personnel issues.[18]

According to Davis, many dentists who have sold their practice to PE shops not only are sorry but feel embarrassed that they were conned. The dentist-owner was told that the PE company would do the distasteful bureaucratic, insurance, and other managerial tasks, and the dentist would have total control over treatment decisions. It does not work out quite that way, however. Many dentists become "wracked with guilt," especially because of how badly their patients are being served.[19]

Davis spoke to numerous dentists as part of his research on corporate dentistry for articles in *Dentistry Today* and his own blog. He writes, "The overwhelming majority of doctors selling to corporate dentistry [whom I] contacted were either somewhat unhappy or decidedly very displeased in their dealings with DSO practice buyers. Almost none wanted to be interviewed on-the-record, because of nondisclosure agreements signed with corporate dentistry or ongoing litigation. Their feelings ranged from anger, shame, severe frustration, to total burnout."[20] And the dentist, who is now an employee, may have to use cheap, low-quality labs (or the chain's labs) and sometimes low-end dental materials and shabby supplies that are chosen for them. He has even heard of dentists who are forced to utilize expired materials. I asked how often these problems occur. "It happens a lot," he said. "Every dollar must be squeezed out for profits."[21]

Casamassimo confirmed that many of his colleagues who have sold their practices to PE firms have found the new owners exerting more control than they had envisioned beforehand. The PE managers may even get involved in decision-making at the patient level, sometimes "telling [the dentists] what they can put in patients' mouths." According to him, several dentists feel as though they have "sold their soul." Those who had previously performed some dental services gratis or at reduced fees—and Casamassimo maintained that most do a small amount of charity work—can no longer continue the practice under PE ownership.[22]

Another problem, Casamassimo said, is that the corporate chain may promise that a dentist's team will be retained but not how they will be treated. In order to streamline the business, new PE owners may rearrange duties and routines and interfere in so many frustrating ways that the staff becomes disenchanted and leaves. This is a particular problem in small towns where workers may have earlier enjoyed a satisfying interaction with their boss and others in the office, need the income, and have few other employment options. "It is a ripple effect," Casamassimo added. "It affects the dentist, the personnel, and patients." Even if dentists aspire to start again elsewhere, they are stymied by the noncompete clauses they typically are forced to sign.

A larger question is "whether the model funded by Wall Street is having a destructive influence on dentistry itself."[23] Concerned over what is happening to the profession, at least three state dental advocacy groups have emerged. The Massachusetts Dentists Alliance for Quality Care is especially disturbed by PE's assertive recruitment of students and newly minted dentists. The group seeks to connect them to private practitioners so as to provide an alternative to commercialized enterprises, which they believe have "no knowledge or interest in patient care."[24] Concerned Dentists of Washington State also highlights the importance of solo and small group practices, which they "consider to be the backbone of quality dental care."[25] However, Concerned Dentists of Washington also is targeting the insurance industry because it places too many constraints on the provision of care. As suggested above, this indubitably is one of the main reasons some dentists give up their practice to private equity.

A main goal of a third advocacy organization, Concerned Dentists of Texas, is to force the implementation of state laws that prohibit nondentists from owning dental practices. A director of Concerned Dentists of Texas asserts, "It is our belief that if hedge/equity funds and insurance companies own dental practices and employ dentists, many with $450k in debt and working under pressures of company demands for performance, how can we ever preserve the right of our children and grandchildren the freedom to choose their dentist and their right to great dental care?"[26]

The Robber Barons
Church Street Health Management / Small Smiles Dental Centers

FORBA Holdings (the name refers to "For Better Access") was founded in 1928 by Dr. Bruna DeRose and operated the Small Smiles clinics. In 2006, the DeRose family sold FORBA for $435 million to Carlyle Group, Arcapita, and American Capital; the exorbitant price represented ten times EBITDA. By 2011, with centers in twenty-one states, the newly renamed Church Street Health Management, based in Nashville, Tennessee, was the leading dentistry chain treating low-income children. It annually served more than a million kids and collected $161 million in revenue, 90 percent of it from Medicaid and CHIP.[27]

In 2012, inquiries by news outlets and the Grassley and Baucus Senate committee investigating corporate dentistry revealed massive, horrific mistreatment of young patients: children were restrained and inadequately anesthetized.[28] Just as appalling, they received unnecessary procedures, including tooth removals, capping, and pulpotomies (root canals on baby teeth). Many of the kids were "psychologically traumatized as well as physically and cosmetically damaged."[29] CSHM and its PE investors had been preoccupied with the bottom line at the expense of vulnerable children.

In 2010, the chain had reimbursed Medicaid $24 million to resolve financial fraud charges; the company's insurers paid another $39 million in compensation to the affected children. Company executives also had signed a corporate integrity agreement, which they breached repeatedly, leading to more fines. CSHM filed for bankruptcy in February 2012, and three months later the distressed business was bought by Garrison Investment Group and Ares Capital Corporation through a cut-rate $25 million LBO.

The unsavory treatment of children persisted, however, despite the change in ownership and corporate leadership. In 2014, CSHM was excluded from participating in Medicaid and other federal programs for five years. At the time, the US Health and Human Services's inspector general said: "CSHM has committed repeated and flagrant violations of its obligations under the CIA [corporate integrity agreement]— violations that put quality of care and young patients' health and safety at risk."[30] That was the death knell. In February 2015, CSHM filed for bankruptcy again and was soon liquidated. The various PE investors are seemingly none the worse for their ownership of CSHM or its misdeeds.

ReachOut Healthcare America / Big Smiles Dental

Similar to CSHM, ReachOut Healthcare America concentrated its services on young Medicaid patients in their schools through the brand Big Smiles Dental.[31] Prior to its acquisition by Sentinel Capital Partners through a management buyout for $22 million in 2007,[32] ReachOut had been serving only five school districts in Missouri. The PE firm quickly financed the acquisition of two rival companies, including Mobile Dentistry, thereby increasing the chain's patient roster—mainly schoolchildren—by 500 percent.[33] Only three years later, having created sufficient value to sell ReachOut at a healthy rate of return, Sentinel disposed of the assets; Morgan Stanley Investment Management in an SBO became the new owner.

The PE-owned mobile clinics, which had clinched deals with a number of school districts in twenty-two states, roamed from place to place performing as many procedures as they could on an estimated 1.5 million low-income children.[34] By 2012, ReachOut too became a center of attention for its deficient quality and excessive dental treatments. As one source notes, the chain's dentists were "alleged to strap children down forcibly and perform root canals on baby teeth and unnecessarily crown baby teeth with stainless steel caps, when no dental treatment was warranted in the first place."[35] In one case, a mother sued ReachOut for performing unwarranted and improper dental work on her four-year-old son without her permission: the youngster had been given baby root canals and two steel crowns while being held down by three adults. Several school districts subsequently severed their relationship with the enterprise.[36] In 2017, ReachOut went out of business, leaving others to suffer the consequences. Morgan Stanley wiped the company off its website's prior ownership list, as if it had never been associated with the place.

Meanwhile, Morgan Stanley kept Smile America Partners (initially a merger of two companies in Arizona and Georgia), which it had bought simultaneously with ReachOut. As of 2018, Smile America transported mobile clinics to 8,000 elementary schools in nineteen states, serving 500,000 children and employing 350 dentists and 500 hygienists. Roughly 85 percent of its substantial revenue flow came from Medicaid.[37] Not bad for a PE owner that mistreated children through its ReachOut mobile clinics.

Aspen Dental Management

Another serially owned PE dental company with a troubled history, ADM was founded by Robert Fontana; as the ongoing CEO, he has been involved with every transaction to date.[38] In 1997, Fontana sold a majority share to APG Partners. APG scaled the company enormously, from ten locations to a hundred, before it was off-loaded to Ares Capital Corporation in an SBO in 2006.[39] After taking its bite out of the still-growing company, Ares flipped it in 2010 to Leonard Green & Partners in a tertiary LBO for $547.5 million.[40] But PE houses weren't through with the company: it experienced a quaternary LBO in 2015 by American Securities and Candescent Partners, at which time it re-capitalized its financial structure again.[41]

ADM, through its various PE owners, aggressively spread its reach throughout the United States by borrowing millions of dollars, and it has paid its GPs more than $212 million in dividend recaps since 2012.[42] ADM is the second largest dental management organization in the United States. By 2020, it had 850 offices in forty-two states; at the end of the year it signed an agreement with Sun Capital Partners to acquire ClearChoice Management Services, a nationwide network of sixty dental implant centers, for more than $1.1 billion.[43]

It seems that ADM's forceful expansion has not been impeded by its flagrant violation of state laws and ruthless treatment of patients and dentists alike. For example, New York attorney general Eric Schneiderman fined the company $450,000 in 2015 for illegally practicing dentistry. He fully recognized that the clinics, though technically owned by dentists, were subject to extensive control by ADM and its PE investors. They routinely executed business decisions that impacted patient care. The owners "exercised undue control over the clinics['] finances" and "created a financial incentive for Aspen Dental Management to pressure staff in the dental offices to generate revenue."[44] There also were hundreds of consumer complaints related to such matters as misleading advertisements (bait and switch), avoidable treatments, and unclear or incomplete terms for the financing of dental care. Since then, the company has had to make similar settlements with attorneys general in Indiana, Massachusetts, and Pennsylvania.[45]

The chain has encountered class action lawsuits as well. In October 2012, a New York district attorney charged Aspen Dental Management and Leonard Green & Partners of, among other harmful actions, favoring patients who needed the most expensive procedures, bonus programs for dentists and office managers that encouraged financial gain over patient services, and " 'high pressure' sales tactics to develop a treatment plan that a dentist ha[d] to follow even if he did not perform the original plan or the patient ask[ed] for less costly alternatives."[46]

The Center for Public Integrity and PBS *Frontline* also investigated the company's practices. In "Patients, Pressure and Profits at Aspen Dental," they reported that ASD preys on individuals who cannot afford a dentist; it overcharges them, provides excessive treatments, and then locks them into exorbitant debt. Former employees told the researchers: "Aspen Dental trained them in high-pressure sales." They "describe[d] the initial exam as a sales tactic to maximize revenue on each new patient." Managers and dentists alike had goals that were set for them, and "corporate management scrutinize[d] the productivity of dentists and staff daily."[47]

When dentists sell their practice to ADM, as with other PE-owned places, they must sign confidentiality agreements. One dentist anonymously told investigators that he left Aspen Dental because "I couldn't do it anymore. . . . They spend most of their time trying to talk people out of their teeth."[48] ADM mostly expands through de novo office building rather than acquisitions, and it heavily advertises to fill the new facilities with patients.[49]

Consumer complaints have continued unabated, resulting in the formation of another class action lawsuit against the company at the end of 2018. Moreover, on the website *Consumer Affairs*, where people can assess and grade services, the most prevalent rating in 2018 for patient satisfaction, out of 188 responses, was one (scored from one to five). Several people wrote that if allowed they would have given ADM a zero. Their grievances included dentures that didn't fit; uncalled-for procedures; overpriced, poor-quality treatments (after receiving a second opinion elsewhere); pulled teeth without cause; fraudulent billing; high-pressure sales tactics; and injuries caused by the procedures.[50] Lawsuits abound everywhere, and some consumers who were adversely affected by the company organized Boycott Aspen Dental in October 2018.[51] Yet PE firms and banks continue to invest in the company. Why is Aspen Dental Management still around?

Heartland Dental

Prior to enticing private equity investors, Heartland Dental had grown from its founding in 1997 to thirty-four dental offices in five states by 2012. That year, the company was taken over by the Ontario Teachers' Pension Plan at an extraordinary $1 billion, presumably making its founder, Richard Workman, a very rich man.[52] By 2018, having increased annual revenues by 126 percent to $1.3 billion since its acquisition, the pension plan was ready to divest much, but not all, of its investment: KKR became the majority owner for $2.8 billion. Workman was now even wealthier since he retained a 10 percent stake in the company.[53]

It was a convoluted sale, mainly because at that point Moody's Investors Service rated Heartland as junk, owing to its "very high" leverage.[54] KKR worsened the situation: its $1 billion loan to purchase the chain had been obtained through financial maneuvers and with covenant-lite terms, rendering the debt even riskier.[55] KKR's strategy was uncommon in other ways; it purchased Heartland from its "core investments" fund, a new vehicle that is supposed to hold on to establishments far longer than usual—fifteen years or more. But will Heartland survive, given its huge liabilities, as KKR milks it over the coming years?

Heartland is one of the largest dental platforms in the United States, operating 840 practices in thirty-five states.[56] But patients won't recognize that they are being treated by a private equity–owned business since each dental practice has its own individual name. Is this yet another example of what Dr. Michael W. Davis dubs "stealth branding"?[57]

All Smiles Dental Centers

Another company with a problematic past, Dallas-based All Smiles Dental Centers, was ushered into bankruptcy by its minority investor Valor Equity Partners eight years after its founding in 2002.[58] Audited by Texas Medicaid for controversial treatments and financial fraud, All Smiles was forced to sign a corporate integrity agreement in 2012 to upgrade its billing practices and to reimburse Medicaid $1.2 million.[59] In 2011 alone, All Smiles had amassed $1.6 million from Medicaid just for steel crowns. Because of unwarranted and poor orthodontic care, Texas Medicaid discontinued payments to certain clinics as well. Steeped in other controversies, such as strapping small children to boards and treating them with insufficient anesthetics, All Smiles quickly filed for Chapter 11.[60]

Thirteen months later, South Texas Dental bought the chain out of bankruptcy and rebranded it with its own name. The business seemed to be in the hands of dentists, who were fully in charge of patient care. But not for long. In January 2019 South Texas Dental was bought by Western Dental (see below).

Premier Dental Holdings / Western Dental

Western Dental, owned by Robert Beauchamp Jr. and his family, had been tangled in legal problems stemming from widespread overbilling and shoddy care in the chain of a hundred dental offices in California.[61] Indeed, in 1997 state regulators called the company "a 'low-quality dental mill' in which dentists were encouraged to over-treat patients to maximize profits."[62] It was so dangerous for patients that California regulators sought to place the company in receivership. Regardless, in a $380 million management buyout, Court Square Capital Partners and other investors acquired the business in 2006; six years later, New Mountain Capital paid $575 million for it in an SBO. As usual, the PE firm borrowed millions, borne by Western Dental, to purchase pediatric and family dental practices throughout California and elsewhere. In 2017 alone, it bought at least thirty-seven centers.[63] During the next two years the acquisitions continued apace, including the leveraged buyouts of Coast Dental Services and Smilecare Dental Associates in 2018 and the purchase of Guardian Life Insurance Company's dental services organization in 2019.[64] Western Dental is now the foremost Medicaid provider in California and Texas.[65]

The chain's sordid practices seem to have persisted over the years. In 2018, for example, *Consumer Affairs* published 47 verified ratings on its website, and—Western Dental received a one (scored from one to five) for overall customer satisfaction. Some typical comments: "don't care about you just like the money"; "their focus on money rather than dental care is the reason I will no longer set foot in a Western Dental facility"; "substandard workmanship"; "I went in for my regular checkup/cleaning and came out confused and feeling scammed"; "They are pushy people, the REPS that come around and take care of the accounting. They rip people off. They try to sell services and try to charge you for them that you said no to. Not a trustworthy company"; "I'm not one to vent publicly but I have to. My mom is on Social Security and is an elderly lady and she had a tooth that was in pain which needed to be pulled . . . so she goes to Western Dental . . . and without her consent they took out almost 400 dollars from her bank account." There were additional complaints about scheduling issues, aggressive collection of bills, exorbitant fees, and pushing braces for youngsters not ready for them. There were also 345 comments from 2001 through 2017 on the site. Ninety-three percent of the reviewers rated Western Dental a one on customer satisfaction, and—another 6 percent rated it two.[66] Another website, with 790 assessments over a longer period of time, shows similar complaints.[67] This not a reassuring sign for dentistry since Western Dental is still on the go, amalgamating ever more practices, including Benevis.

Benevis (formerly National Children's Dental Research) / Kool Smiles

Another dental platform focused on Medicaid beneficiaries, National Children's Dental Research experienced its first PE investment in 2004 from FFL Partners and Tailwind Capital. In 2010, the business acquired DPMS / Kool Smiles,[68] its main company henceforth, and subsequently was renamed Benevis. In 2018 it was turned over and recapitalized through an SBO to Littlejohn & Company; Tailwind grabbed an additional stake as well.[69] Kool Smiles owns more than 150 practices in seventeen states, mostly in low-income neighborhoods. Indeed, Medicaid and CHIP comprise fully 70 percent of its business.[70]

As with many early PE-owned dental practices, Kool Smiles was a target of the 2012 US Senate investigation of corporate dentistry. The familiar litany of horrific abuses, mainly perpetrated on indigent people, included the overuse of poor-quality, ill-fitting crowns; patient restraints; insufficient anesthesia for painful procedures; avoidable tooth extractions; and other treatments that were performed solely to boost Medicaid payments. Patient complaints emanated from each state in which the company was located.[71] Not surprisingly, Kool Smiles also was accused of Medicaid fraud.

A few years later, five whistleblower lawsuits triggered an investigation by the US Department of Justice. Accused under the False Claims Act, Benevis and Kool Smiles in January 2018 paid $23.9 million to settle charges that "they knowingly submitted false claims for payment to state Medicaid programs for medically unnecessary dental services performed on children insured by Medicaid." The action further contended that "Kool Smiles clinics routinely pressured and incentivized dentists to meet production goals through a system that disciplined 'unproductive' dentists and awarded 'productive' dentists with substantial cash bonuses based on the revenue generated by the procedures they performed."[72] Kool Smiles apparently also falsely advertised one of its principal dentists as a pediatric dentistry specialist.[73] The financial settlement involved not only the federal government but seventeen states.[74]

Benevis/Kool Smiles never admitted wrongdoing but deviously rebranded its clinics with a variety of names.[75] Littlejohn and Tailwind continued to aggressively push the corporation's ongoing growth and to pocket the usual fees. However, drowning in debt totaling $200.5 million, Benevis was unprepared to deal with the short-term declining revenues resulting from the COVID-19 pandemic. In August 2020, the enterprise filed for Chapter 11. Private equity firm New Mountain Capital, along with its affiliate—and Benevis's lender—New Mountain Finance Corporation (a debt buying and direct loan firm), arranged to purchase the business out of bankruptcy two months later.[76]

So, is it now business as usual? As shown above, New Mountain Capital has its own history of substandard care and reprehensible business practices. Moreover, in several years it will dump the assets on the next PE house and garner more financial rewards. What about the children and adults who were damaged by Littlejohn and Tailwind's criminal dental services—and who will continue to be put in harm's way?

Great Expressions Dental Centers

Yet another large dental DSO, Great Expressions Dental Centers has been tossed from PE firm to PE firm since 2008.[77] Given its umbrella over ninety-eight dental practices and revenues of $60 million at the time, the chain was an appealing target: Audax Group and Eagle Private Capital became its first PE owners. Moving like a high-speed train, GEDC acquired fifty-four more offices—a few of them direct competitors—placing exorbitant debt on the company.[78] It also bought certain specialty offices that enabled GEDC to secure its own referrals.

Only three years later, Audax hopped off, taking its lucrative share, and in an SBO OMERS Private Equity jumped aboard. At that point, GEDC was considered one of "America's fastest-growing private companies" on the Inc. 5000 list. The chain's CEO since 1998, Richard Beckman, told USA Today in 2013 that the goal "is to keep growing annual revenue to about $500 million, mostly by acquisitions."[79]

In 2016, GEDC was flipped to Roark Capital in a $675 million tertiary LBO, more than 60 percent financed through debt.[80] The company had at that point increased its geographic footprint into nine states. The latest owner intended to continue the company's steady expansion. As of 2019, GEDC had more than 300 dental locations in nine states.

In May 2019, the Better Business Bureau investigated Great Expressions, "prompted by a pattern of complaints surrounding billing and customer service issues." From 2017 through June 2019 alone, it received 238 allegations against the company for fraudulent billing, overpricing, aggressive collection tactics, charging for treatments that were not performed, and shoddy, overly painful dental work. The Better Business Bureau's website states that it attempted to solve some of these issues, "but the business failed to respond to questions to potentially eliminate underlying issues with consumers. This business has also indicated that it will not work to resolve customer disputes through BBB." The organization gave GEDC an overall rating of F and a similar rating for all its practices.[81] Beckman, who ended his reign as GEDC's CEO in January 2018, surely had played a part in the chain's misdeeds. Nevertheless, in April 2019 he became CEO of Benevis. Is anyone concerned?

The DSO Bandwagon

There are many other large DSOs owned by the PE industry, each consolidating dental care in different regions or, in some cases, competing areas.

North American Dental Group, in which Abry Partners held a minority stake since 2012 and was joined by Riverside Company three years later, acquired 200 dental centers in eleven states. In late 2019, Abry and North American Dental's two cofounders sold their shares to Colosseum Dental via Jacobs Holding for $660 million; it will be the first transatlantic dental group. The chain finally may be in good hands.[82]

Founded in 1991, Dental Care Alliance (DCA) over the years has grown organically and via acquisitions, financed by its several PE owners. Through Quad-C Management in 2012, its first LBO, DCA doubled in size. Barely three years later, Quad-C cashed in. Taking on even more debt in an SBO, DCA was bought by Harvest Partners, Crescent Capital Group (minority stake), and DCA's management team. Harvest firmly ensconced itself on the board of directors, indicating that it was monitoring the business diligently. The PE shop guided the chain through even larger acquisitions, totaling 330 dental practices in eighteen states as of 2020.[83] The buying spree (and the accompanying debts) are ongoing. As with a few other PE-owned DSOs, the business operates through multiple brands, not the corporate name, thereby camouflaging the actual ownership of its practices.

In 2016, Harvest Partners acquired Konikoff Dental Associates, which it kept for less than a year, at which time the PE firm flipped it to New Mainstream Capital. Konikoff's seven offices became the platform for a new DSO, CORDENTAL Group, which New Mainstream formed with two administrators, Dana Soper and Steven Jones, neither of whom are dentists. Soon, CORDENTAL went on a frenzied shopping binge: Chattanooga Dental Care (January 2018); Drs. Melman, Ravett & Associates (June 2018); Lisbeth Bradley DDS (July 2018); Michael Turk, DDS (August 2018); Sirkin, Kruger and Associates (September 2018); John Monaco (May 2019); Elizabeth Johnson Burns (May 2019); and AppleWhite Dental Partners (June 2019), the latter a DSO with thirty-five dental offices. In only a few years, CORDENTAL's geographic footprint spread to five more states. Most of these purchases were from individuals who were retiring, leaving the once dentist-owned and -controlled practices in the hands of financiers.

Chicagoland Smile Group, which formed the foundation of a platform management group for Shore Capital Partners, was purchased in

2015. Renamed Great Lakes Dental Partners, it is steadily spreading throughout Illinois, with the intention of consolidating practices in nearby states as well.[84] One of its acquisitions, Advanced Family Dental and Orthodontist in 2018, doubled its size.

Smile Doctors Braces is the largest orthodontist practice in the United States. Established in 2015, its first PE (minority) owner—Sheridan Capital Partners—grew the company from twelve clinics to more than ninety across eleven states in just two years.[85] In a management buyout in 2017, Linden Capital Partners acquired the chain, and the already heavily indebted company rapidly gobbled up ten more clinics in a number of states.—It is still on a tear.

Smile Brands (formerly known as Bright Now! Dental) has been subjected to a lengthy PE journey, beginning with its first LBO by Gryphon Investors in 1998.[86] Seven years later, the company experienced an SBO for $340 million by the California State Teachers' Retirement System, A. S. F. Co-Investment Partners, and Freeman Spogli & Co. In 2012, Smile Brands found itself in the hands of Welsh, Carson, Anderson & Stowe in yet a third LBO; the deal included a payoff of the company's existing debt but was financed with $340 million in new loans. The chain, however, continued to expand, amassing millions more in liabilities. Again in 2016 its debt was paid off as part of a fourth LBO via Gryphon Investors (which had previously owned the business), financed with fresh loans. The PE shop subsequently snatched $300 million for itself in a 2018 dividend recapitalization, paid for with even more borrowed money. In 2019, Smile Brands had more than 400 dental offices across seventeen states, under the cover of several brands: Bright Now! Dental, Monarch Dental, Castle Dental, A+ Dental, OneSmile Dental, Johnson Family Dental, P3 Dental Group, and DecisionOne Dental Partners. In 2020, Smile Brands was on the market once more.

Jefferson Dental Clinics, founded in 1967, treats mostly Medicaid patients, especially children. It endured its first LBO in 2009 for $100 million through Black Canyon Capital and underwent leveraged recapitalizations in 2012 and 2014. In 2017, via an SBO, Brentwood Associates acquired the business for $230 million.[87] Apparently, Black

Canyon received a 230 percent return on its investment; not bad, given that it was primarily paid for through debt and taxpayers.

American Dental Partners, launched in 1996, was initially funded with venture capital from Summit Partners. Two years later the company was placed on the NASDAQ in an IPO that raised $33.8 million for the PE firm. Summit Partners sold shares in a 2004 secondary public offering, profiting by millions more. American Dental was taken private by JLL Partners in a $420 million LBO in 2012. Since then, it has acquired more large chains, accompanied by continuous debt and refinancing. In 2019, it had 270 dental centers across twenty states. I suspect that JLL will be selling American Dental Partners soon.

PE interest in dentistry has not abated as firms continue to amalgamate the specialty into regional and national chains.[88] The shops are now extending their reach into complementary arenas, particularly cosmetic dental laboratories. Though still in the initial stages, investments in places that manufacture dental veneers, implants, other dental prosthetics, and bleaching products are picking up speed. Sarah Pringle of PE Hub observes that this explosion of PE attention to such businesses is likely because of the "selfie generation," who demand white, straight teeth.[89] Flush with dry powder, to what extent will PE capitalize on other aspects of US dental needs?

Concluding Remarks

Dental practices were one of the earliest health retail niches to attract private equity investments. Similar to the ownership of physician practices, they are set up to circumvent rules against corporate control over the practice of dentistry; in reality, the shops hold sway over clinical decisions, even if indirectly. They have proved willing to enhance their bottom line at the expense of patients, particularly children on Medicaid. Several of the debt-laden chains have gone bankrupt.

The concern over PE ownership of dentistry practices is ongoing, including the adverse effects on patient care, dentists, their assistants, and the profession as a whole. In addition, the Medicaid program is still subject to fraud that not only bilks taxpayers but puts a substantial number of kids in harm's way. Tanzi told me that she has personally witnessed the overtreatment of children who participate in Medicaid.[90]

PE firms continue to acquire and consolidate dental practices; indeed, it is a hot market. In 2017, they purchased more than twenty-six practices and another eighteen by mid-2018, accounting for 16 percent of the US total.[91] Children continue to be a target of PE moneymaking tactics, and it is likely that the shops will appropriate ever more pediatric centers.[92] Midsize DSOs are in high demand from both PE players and larger DSOs, heating up the competition and raising price tags on deals.[93] The persistently high leverage on PE-owned dental chains may foreshadow more failures if conditions in the US economy deteriorate. Will the PE shops remain largely unscathed, as they did in the previous round of bankruptcies, while others face the consequences?

6 |

Frail Elderly and Children

Homecare and Hospice

HOME HEALTH care has experienced widespread growth since the early 2000s as a result of government policies (including the Affordable Care Act), private insurance initiatives, and a vastly increasing demand for services. Not only are we facing population aging, but seniors are living longer than in previous generations. The "old-old" (eighty-five years and over) are the fastest growing demographic in the United States, and the need for long-term care and post-acute care is rising commensurately. Home health spending totaled nearly $103 billion in 2018 and, according to government estimates, is forecast to reach $173 billion by 2026. The annual growth rate—currently almost 6 percent—most likely will rise as well, greater than any other medical-related expenditure.[1]

The exorbitant cost of nursing homes and mounting charges for post-acute care in hospitals have driven payers to press for what they view as less expensive alternatives. Certainly, there is an ongoing shift of services from institutional settings into the home. Medicare has been one of the main drivers of home health care—and nonmedical supports as well. In 2018, the program shelled out $17.5 billion (3 percent) of its total $582 billion budget for such services. As Medicare enrollment rises (30 million elders are expected to join by 2035), home health costs will intensify further.[2] In addition, Medicaid expenditures on home- and community-based services (HCBS) amounted to $82.7 billion in 2018.[3] Significantly, home health agencies (HHAs) rely on Medicare, along with Medicaid, for the preponderance of their revenues: The two public programs comprise roughly 76 percent of total US homecare spending.[4]

Following the Money

Unsurprisingly, PE firms have flocked to the booming homecare industry, envisioning glittering dollar signs in the escalating call for at-home services and open-ended government payment sources. And it has proved to be quite a fruitful area for investment: of all Medicare-reimbursed post-acute care providers, including inpatient rehabilitation facilities, skilled nursing homes, and long-term acute care hospitals, home health businesses have attained the highest earnings, averaging 15.6 percent.[5] According to Emily Evans, a managing director for Hedgeye Risk Management, they can bring in as much as 40 percent profit margins. In-home assistance is among the uppermost industries overall in terms of return on equity, placing sixth in 2017. The average return on equity of for-profit enterprises in Hedgeye's database averaged 38 percent, while HHAs produced 65.9 percent.[6]

Another appeal for PE firms, as usual, lies in the largely fragmented nature of the industry. There are more than 12,400 Medicare-certified HHAs; the leading ten companies only comprise one-fifth of the total.[7] General partners argue that their consolidation of the space serves valuable objectives: by centralizing overhead functions, HHAs can achieve efficiencies; provide leverage in negotiating better rates from insurers; assist with regulatory and other burdensome requirements; enhance referral opportunities; improve staff productivity with technology; and reduce fixed costs.[8] They also claim that it will facilitate partnerships with companies offering Medicare Advantage (MA) plans, the fastest growing insurers of medical care for the aged. One expert in the field maintains, "Expanded MA opportunities have been a driving force throughout the overarching wave of consolidation the home care industry has seen of late." Without scale, he continues, "providers won't get to the table with the MAs or be able to negotiate favorable rates with them."[9]

But the potential for mergers and amalgamation that is so attractive to the PE industry is disadvantageous for people in need of homecare, as well as for society at large. For one, consolidated HHAs can foster higher charges, higher taxpayer expenditures, and excessive amounts of debt, which often generate massive cost-cutting and a lower quality of care. Any savings from efficiencies and enhanced fees do not translate into a reduction in prices for customers but rather line the pockets of the financiers. The PE houses also capture hefty fees and at times dividend recaps from their purchases, robbing agencies of capital that otherwise could be used for quality upgrades, such as more intensive staff training and higher salaries. In addition, the huge debt obligations raise the potential of default, leaving communities with fewer choices or, in the case of rural areas, sometimes no services at all.

From Headwinds to Tailwinds

Federal and state policies have always affected investors' interest in home health and support services, especially since 1980, when Congress opened the elder care market for commercial ownership. Medicare reimbursement rates were then tightened through the Balanced Budget Act of 1997 and its 1999 amendments, which authorized an interim payment system and then a risk-based prospective payment system (PPS). Under this system, HHAs received a fixed basic amount—adjusted for geography, patient health, and the like—for every sixty-day episode. PPS turned out to be lucrative for some enterprises, which were suspected of manipulating the system. Not so much for others: one study notes that as a result of PPS, 10 percent of HHAs closed.[10] In any case, since PE firms are not in the business of subjecting themselves to risky conditions or what appeared to them as capricious government measures, they did not jump into the arena immediately; compared to retail and other investment opportunities at the time, home health care was not their cup of tea.

However, conditions substantially changed, and by 2012 PE players found the financial environment of home services more hospitable, especially because of the push against institutional care by the Affordable Care Act, MA plans, and insurers more generally. The appeal of HHAs was also furthered because the homecare industry lacks robust regulations and enforcement: PE "efficiency" measures probably would not be closely watched. To be sure, it is tricky to monitor the quality of care in individual people's homes. The federal Government Accountability Office (GAO), for example, found that the government heavily reimburses HHAs without being able to substantiate the qualifications of the individuals providing services, how well they perform, or even if they actually show up at the house.[11]

Loaded with $976 billion of dry powder in the US, PE investment in the sector moved into the fast lane, reaching "historically high levels in 2016 and 2017."[12] Joyce Famakinwa, a reporter for *Home Health Care News*, observes that in 2018 and 2019 there were more than a hundred homecare transactions, and private equity accounted for nearly half.[13] In the next several years, acquisitions, add-ons, and mergers are expected to proliferate. Deals are not only quickening but becoming larger, steadily changing the home health and personal care landscape. The earlier trend from nonprofit to commercial providers—reaching 79 percent today—has given way to vulture capitalism. Taxpayer money for sick and frail elders and children has become the PE industry's personal cookie jar.

Beginning in 2020, newly initiated federal rules under the Bipartisan Budget Act of 2018 revamped the reimbursement model again. The intention was to discourage "unnecessary" medical services, especially therapy, by shifting home health to value-based care or the patient-driven groupings model. The regulations also aimed to steadily eliminate prepayments, where agencies could apply for up to 60 percent of their anticipated bill as soon as services commenced. What is more, the new reimbursement system imposed greater hurdles, including doubling billing efforts. These burdens compounded changes enacted in 2017, which added communication and documentation requirements to the CMS Conditions of Participation.[14]

The end result will be more need for technical assistance with the "complicated new documentation and coding processes," less compensation for therapy, a disruption of cash flow (especially for places that do not have sufficient surplus capital), and lower fees.[15] April Anthony, CEO of Encompass Health, expects a 2–3 percent contraction in Medicare rates; another source writes that the revised system could reduce overall payments to HHAs by 8 percent, squeezing profit margins.[16] The industry is not happy, including the not-for-profits, and heavy lobbying is under way.

Large companies have the resources to study utilization patterns, purchase expensive information technology systems, and hire consultants.[17] Encompass, for example, has added roughly twelve new coding positions and is undertaking costly care planning and data analytics.[18] On the other hand, the latest policies may prove more than small to midsize agencies can handle. They will not only suffer disproportionately but may be forced to sell to PE firms and others seeking to consolidate the industry. For example, Stephanie Goldberg argues that a number of businesses will leave the space, and those that stay will aim "to get bigger, triggering consolidation and putting more pressure on smaller players."[19]

Concomitantly, driven mainly by a fever pitch of enthusiasm by PE firms, home health (and hospice) valuations have become exceedingly high, frequently at double-digit levels, as has the amount of leverage required to buy them. Knowledgeable observers are raising questions about whether there can be a workable balance between profit making and the provision of high-quality services.[20] A study in *Health Affairs* suggests that both costs and profits are significantly greater in proprietary HHAs than in nonprofits while the nature of the care tends to be less satisfactory.[21] The authors, however, did not home in on private equity per se. Had they done so, they might have discovered both greater earnings and diminished quality of care. Given the extraordinary prices today, in order for PE shops to obtain outsized returns—the foremost PE objective—the portfolio owners would have to perform magic to pay down huge debts and, at the same time, provide affordable, first-rate services.

There is also an incentive to cherry-pick the clients who are the most profitable. Nina Bernstein, a reporter for the *New York Times*, writes that commercial homecare agencies do not want high-maintenance Medicaid-funded customers because they are not sufficiently profitable.[22] Clearly, the PE financial model is particularly susceptible to eschewing costly patients when feasible.

The labor force is also of concern under PE ownership. The number and preparation of workers are the largest component of HHA outlays and the most essential factors in providing topnotch services. But homecare employees overall tend to be inadequately trained, over-worked, and underpaid.[23] Further, low salaries are linked to high turnover, which is well known to negatively affect quality of care.[24] Yet poor wages, cutbacks in staff, and lesser training are the hallmarks of PE "efficiency" measures after acquiring a home health agency.

PACE: More Homecare Financialization

Nothing is sacred to the PE industry, including programs of all-inclusive care for the elderly. The purpose of PACE, initiated as a demonstration project in 1971, is to provide comprehensive medical care, as well as personal and household tasks, so that nursing-home-eligible elders can remain at home.[25] As envisioned when it was officially authorized in 1990, the Medicare- and Medicaid-funded program pays a fixed monthly fee per client to nonprofit agencies, which in turn provide for all of their participants' needs, both at home and at day centers.[26] These include physician services, medications, hospitalization, rehabilitation, dental treatment, assistance in daily living (meals, bathing, housekeeping), and transportation.

In 2015, CMS tentatively opened the program to for-profit companies, "ending one of the last remaining holdouts to commercialism in health care," as a reporter for the *New York Times* laments.[27] With potential profit margins as sizable as 15 percent and a guaranteed flow of taxpayer cash, a few PE firms, most noticeably Welsh, Carson, Anderson & Stowe (WCAS), immediately took the plunge. In a 2016 leveraged buyout totaling $204 million, the PE firm transformed the nonprofit

InnovAge into one of its profit-making portfolio companies. Apparently, the participants and their families were not even told about the change.[28] Since then, InnovAge has borrowed millions via the PE shop to acquire PACE locations in Colorado, Pennsylvania, Virginia, California, and New Mexico. With three of the eight members serving on the board of directors, which is chaired by one of its partners, WCAS has no intention of losing control of its objectives for InnovAge, at least until it is sold in a few years.[29]

What is a PE house to do with fixed reimbursements to cover all of frail elderly people's needs? How about telemedicine instead of direct physician care? That would save money, but is it the best means for frail people—sometimes with dementia—to receive medical intervention? Would it be less expensive to monitor patients in the home virtually? Perhaps, but that could limit much-needed socialization at the day centers. What about cherry-picking customers to root out those with costly needs? Stinting on services would bolster profits, given the fixed reimbursement rate. Do such fragile beneficiaries really require unlimited therapy sessions? Why not eliminate pricey physical therapy, even though it helps them to maintain mobility?

In 2019, CMS removed all requirements that PACE be administered by nonprofit organizations, along with the mandate that each center hire a full-time primary care physician. Couldn't a lower-cost nurse practitioner or physician assistant substitute for a doctor? Perhaps the centers should hire an MD only part time? Previous requirements for on-site monitoring by government inspectors also have been relaxed. Has PACE become another unregulated playground for the PE industry? Certainly, InnovAge has been lucrative for WCAS, which by the summer of 2020 was estimated to be worth $950 million; at that time, the PE shop sold a 49 percent stake in the business to Apax Partners.

On a Rampage: Hospice

PE-owned HHAs seek to enlarge their cash flow lines and protect themselves against cutbacks in fees or other adverse measures by adding private-pay personal care, newly Medicare-funded nonmedical supports, and telehealth to their mix of offerings. Since 2019, the federal government has allowed at least some at-home support services through Medicare Advantage, and PE firms are aiming for contracts with commercial insurers as well.

However, a foremost target is hospice for the terminally ill, whether at home or in institutional settings (hospitals, nursing homes, free-standing facilities). Hospice is meant to allow those at the end of life to die more peacefully by relieving pain and easing discomfort and stress, whether physical or emotional. Individuals are supposed to receive assistance through a team of professionals (including nurses, physicians, psychologists, social workers, aides, spiritual counselors, and homemakers), who also provide prescription drugs, other medicine, and supplies; medical equipment; therapy when appropriate; and bereavement services for the recipient's family. In return, the patient forgoes curative treatments.

Initially administered by volunteers, local charities, and religious-affiliated nonprofit groups during the 1970s, end-of-life care was authorized for payment under Medicare through the 1983 Tax Equity and Fiscal Responsibility Act. Spurred by the taxpayer-funded bonanza, for-profit entities soon entered the sector. Over the next twenty-five years, hospice transformed into a $17 billion industry; of the several thousand Medicare-certified hospices, for-profit agencies today represent two-thirds. As Reed Abelson, who in 2018 investigated hospice providers for the New York Times, puts it: "hospice, the business of caring for those who are nearing death, has become a booming multibillion-dollar industry that is attracting more and more for-profit companies."[30]

As with HHAs, hospice is well funded by Medicare, and the number of people taking advantage of the benefit has risen noticeably.[31] Roughly 50 percent of deceased beneficiaries had been in hospice care by 2016, up from 23 percent at the turn of the twenty-first century; Medicare expenditures rose in that same period from $2.9 billion to $16.8 billion. The number of hospice providers swelled also.[32] Profits, too, have been exceedingly high.

GPs paid heed, and the incurably ill became yet additional prey for the financial scavengers. Widespread buyouts and mergers ensued, often as add-ons to home health agencies. Some of the acquired places have been huge chains, as I discuss below. The mostly fragmented space, similar to HHAs, continues to face intense consolidation.

The hospice industry is fraught with financial abuse and patient neglect. In a comprehensive investigation in 2014, Ben Hallman, a reporter for the *Huffington Post*, found that quality has suffered enormously. He writes that during one three-year period, more than half of all hospices were cited for violations, mostly related to poor care; 20 percent of the total had more than seventy such breaches.[33] In another report, the US Department of Health and Human Services Office of Inspector General (OIG) makes clear that some hospices skimp on indispensable services and, at times, deliver inferior care.[34] The human cost is inestimable.

Deceptive charges to Medicare are common among hospice providers as well. Hallman writes, "The U.S. government has accused nearly every major for-profit hospice company of billing fraud."[35] The commercial places charge Medicare one-third more per person than nonprofits do, generally through upcoding. Taxpayers pay the price. According to the OIG, overcharging of Medicare by hospice providers has mounted to "hundreds of millions of dollars."[36]

A substantial number of for-profit hospices engage in aggressive marketing, often to grief-stricken families, and recruiting of patients. In earlier days, the focus was on people suffering from terminal cancer. Since 2000, commercial players have sought every type of Medicare-eligible (and frequently ineligible) patient, such as those with Parkinson's disease and dementia.[37] After all, with so much scaling and organic growth, the entrepreneurs have a substantial number of beds to fill. Under Medicare, the only requirement is a physician's signature declaring that a patient has six months or less to live; given the evidence, that clearly is not overly challenging to obtain. Abelson contends, "Much of the hospice care [businesses] now seek higher profits even if that involves enrolling patients who don't need such care, or cutting staff and services to bare levels."[38] The OIG confirms that one of the fraudulent schemes in which agencies may engage is to knowingly sign up Medicare beneficiaries who are not qualified, including hiring recruiters to find them and doctors willing to falsely certify their need for services.[39] Such illegal behavior is seriously injurious to patients since, once they are enrolled in hospice, they give up their right to Medicare-funded curative medical care.

The hospice industry is embarrassingly unregulated, even more so than HHAs and nursing homes, and penalties are far less. Hallman reports that there are no fines or suspensions of payment for wrongdoing; in nearly every case, regardless of the gravity of the situation, all the hospice must do is agree to a corrective action plan. It is possible to revoke an agency's license, but that remedy rarely occurs. Incredibly, the *Huffington* reporter notes, "Federal authorities have failed to take punitive action after discovering that hospice workers repeatedly overdosed patients with morphine, disbursed the wrong drugs and showed up to see patients hours or days late." His investigation unearthed numerous cases where hospice agencies "endangered patients' safety or failed to perform core hospice missions." It also revealed that the typical hospice had not undergone a full certification inspection for nearly four years and almost 20 percent of them for more than six years.[40]

Unfortunately, these studies on hospice do not differentiate between for-profit entities overall and PE-owned portfolio companies. As in many inquiries of corporate misdeeds, private equity involvement is neglected, overlooked, or not even recognized in the first place. Yet the payment and regulatory environment seem ready-made for the PE industry: as the OIG points out, "the financial incentives in the current system also could cause hospices to minimize the amount of services they provide."[41] Hospice reimbursements are based on a fixed daily rate, regardless of a patient's needs or what services are actually delivered.[42] This is fodder for PE firms, which can seek out the most profitable patients, curtail services, and turn a blind eye to quality, all without financial or other penalties. Hospice is heaven-sent for the PE model.

The Winding Road to Mega-Mergers
Kindred Healthcare (formerly Vencor)

Kindred Healthcare is the largest home health and one of the top hospice providers in the United States, owning 5.85 percent and 3.54 percent, respectively, of the businesses.[43] Vencor was founded in 1985 as a long-term care (LTC) hospital for people on ventilators. It grew rapidly, expanding into other LTC ventures. After a $1.9 billion merger in 1995 with Hillhaven Corp. (a nursing home operator), it became one of the largest LTC chains.[44]

Overwhelmed with debt, Vencor filed for bankruptcy in 1999; at the time, it operated 300 skilled nursing homes and 60 hospitals, and had liabilities totaling $1.4 billion. It also had several government suits against it: Vencor had agreed to pay $270,000 to settle a finding by Florida investigators that the company attempted to evict Medicaid residents from its facilities in order to make room for higher-paying clients. The US Justice Department also accused the business of fraudulent charges to Medicare and Medicaid by its hospitals; improper billing practices for ancillary services, such as rehabilitation; "and various quality of care issues in its hospitals and nursing centers."[45] However, the chain had been split in two and its assets transferred to a new REIT, Ventas Inc., headed by William Bruce Lunsford, a cofounder of Vencor.[46] The resources were now safely shielded by Ventas. The US government aimed to recoup $1 billion, but Vencor was hard-pressed to pay because of its Chapter 11 status and lack of assets.

Vencor emerged from bankruptcy in 2001 as a publicly traded company on the New York Stock Exchange and changed its name to Kindred. The financially troubled provider of deficient care to frail and sick older people had a new start. It commenced buying more than thirty-six enterprises, including long-term acute care hospitals, rehabilitation facilities, pharmacy services, home health and personal care agencies, skilled nursing homes, hospice services, and assisted living establishments. Kindred borrowed heavily again for these purchases, and it acquired and merged with large, multimillion-dollar businesses, such as Senior Home Care and Vista Healthcare.[47] The chain also decided to get rid of its low-margin LTC nursing homes and focus on home health, hospice, rehabilitation, and LTC acute facilities. For example, in a hostile 2015 takeover, Kindred acquired Gentiva (renamed Kindred at Home and Kindred Hospice) for $1.8 billion (see discussion of Gentiva below).[48]

Kindred and its subsidiaries once more became the subject of government investigations. In 2016, it paid $125 million to settle charges that RehabCare, which Kindred had purchased in 2011, "engaged in a systematic and broad-ranging scheme to increase profits by delivering, or purporting to deliver, therapy in a manner that was focused on increasing Medicare reimbursement rather than on the clinical needs of patients."[49] In addition to charging the program for therapy at the highest reimbursement levels, regardless of client needs, the company billed for services to residents who were asleep at the time. In another instance, Kindred paid $25 million to resolve a False Claims Act accusation that its affiliate Gentiva charged Medicare for hospice services that patients were not eligible for. Even though the problems had occurred before Kindred's purchase, it failed to correct the violations under a five-year corporate integrity agreement.[50] The chain also had to pay $12 million to settle a 2016 class action lawsuit alleging that by understating the work hours of licensed practical nurses and physical therapy assistants, Gentiva failed to pay them either the minimum wage or for overtime.

Notwithstanding these problems, Humana, TPG Capital, and WCAS acquired Kindred in 2018. The public-to-private LBO amounted to a massive $4.1 billion. As a consequence of the deal, Kindred was split into two divisions: TPG and WCAS took over the LTC hospitals and inpatient rehabilitation facilities; the hospice and homecare businesses were shared among the three partners.[51] Six months later, Kindred acquired the hospice operator Curo for $1.4 billion: the combined enterprise emerged as the largest homecare and hospice chain in the United States.[52]

In 2021, Humana purchased Kindred's entire home health business while divesting its share of the post-acute facilities. LifePoint then agreed to acquire the post-acute division.

It is too early to determine the effects of this enormous consolidation on quality of care. Nonetheless, given the history of the company and the PE firms' need for huge returns on this extremely leveraged investment, I suspect the future does not bode well for frontline workers or their patients.

Curo Health Services

Curo was created as a platform in 2010 by GTCR, and after half a billion dollars in acquisitions, the company was purchased by Thomas H. Lee Partners and HealthView Capital Partners in 2014 via a $730 million SBO.[53] Curo briskly continued its consolidation of hospice centers, piling on millions in debt. Only four years after their purchase, the two PE firms handed over the enterprise to the consortium of owners discussed above, earning $270 million in the process.[54]

Gentiva Health Services (formerly Olsten Health Services)

Before its hostile takeover by Kindred, Gentiva had a long history of chewing up home health and hospice agencies and spitting them out. The company was established in 1946 by William Olsten but did not begin its health service division, Olsten Health Services, until 1971. Throughout the 1990s, it acquired agency after agency, and by the end of the decade it was the largest provider of home health care in the United States. In 1999 Olsten Corporation split off the health care division into an independently traded company, Gentiva Health Services.[55] It continued the aggressive buy-and-sell strategy and in 2015 was acquired by Kindred, which took on its $1.1 billion in debt.

One of Gentiva's largest purchases was Harden Healthcare, which included an array of post-acute care providers. That platform, created at the end of 2001 by Capstar Partners and Lew Little Jr., proceeded to engage in several rounds of debt financing and refinancing. Among other companies, it acquired Girling Health Care (2007), Auxi Health (2007), and Asian American Home Care (2011).[56] In 2013, Gentiva bought

Harden's home health, hospice, and community care businesses for a whopping $408.8 million, surely a home run for Capstar.

In another formidable buyout, Gentiva picked up Odyssey Healthcare in the largest hospice purchase in history. Formed in 1996, the company had accumulated millions from numerous investors for expansion and acquisitions before its 2002 IPO (NASDAQ), which reaped $54 million. Capital from Candescent Partners and others—in a 2010 PIPE (private investment in public equity)—added more purchasing power for the publicly traded company. Numerous financiers had a piece of Odyssey's money-spinning ride over the decade that culminated in the $1 billion take-private buyout by Gentiva.

Aveanna Healthcare

One of the largest home health organizations in the United States, Aveanna Healthcare is the product of a far-reaching scaling of home assistance for children and the financial bleeding of companies serving them in the process. It was formed by Bain Capital in 2017 through the merger of Epic Health Services and PSA Healthcare, two sizable entities in their own right. Epic was a foremost provider of pediatric home health services, specializing in children with complex and costly conditions, such as cerebral palsy, cystic fibrosis, congenital heart defects, and cancer. PSA brought to the table pediatric home services in 110 offices across twenty-eight states.

Epic Health Services

Established in 2001, Epic Medstaff Home Healthcare caught the eye of Webster Capital Management in 2010, and Webster acquired the company in a $50 million LBO, using $21.6 million in debt financing. Webster soon rebranded the enterprise Epic Health Services. In a dash to scale its purchase, Webster proceeded to pile up Epic's liabilities, including a $30 million dividend recapitalization for itself in 2013, which "enabled Webster to more than recoup its initial investment."[57]

During the Webster years, Epic expanded to a national, billion-dollar conglomerate, snatching home health businesses from corporations, other PE firms, and small to midsize agencies;[58] it also varied its service lines as it pressed on. The company added places that offer adult home services; pediatric therapy; personal care; behavioral education; autism services; enteral nutrition therapy; medical staffing; pharmaceutical services; medical equipment and products; speech, occupational, and physical therapy; and respiratory care.[59]

As a result, revenues grew 25 percent annually, from $60 million in 2010 to $750 million in 2016.[60] From an initial $50 million purchase, Webster obviously did well in its 2017 sale to Bain. The money was siphoned from places serving the nation's at-risk children and adults, mostly funded through Medicaid and Medicare. Epic, via Bain, was after the homecare division of Maxim Healthcare Services: the proposed $1.25 billion transaction, according to bond rater Moody's, would have increased the company's already heavy debt burden to $2 billion.[61] After an intensive investigation, the FTC nixed the deal in January 2020 because of its potential anti-competitive effects.

PSA Healthcare

In 1989, Joseph D. Sansone purchased Ambulatory Services from Charter Medical, renaming it Pediatric Services of America. Five years later, through a public offering, he placed the enterprise on the NASDAQ. Sansone was determined to grow the publicly traded company through local and regional acquisitions of pediatric services. In four years, PSA became the largest provider of home-based pediatric services in the nation.[62] Similar to Epic, the company steadily added new medical service lines to its repertoire, along with paramedical testing services—which it divested in 1999.

In 2007, the company was acquired by Portfolio Logic (an investment management company) for $10 million in a public-to-private transaction. PSA next was purchased by J. H. Whitney & Company in a 2015 LBO of nearly $200 million. Portfolio Logic obviously made a ton of money on the deal. Also in 2015 PSA and Portfolio Logic were forced to pay a $6.9 million fine and sign a corporate integrity agreement with the US Department of Health and Human Services' inspector general for falsely submitting claims for homecare services to Medicaid.

Among other problems, PSA had failed to document monthly visits by its registered nurses, overstated the number of times staff provided care, and did not repay money it owed to the public program.[63]

J. H. Whitney purchased the company regardless of the transgressions and continued the ongoing consolidation of pediatric health services during 2016.[64] In the process, it bloated the portfolio company with millions in debt. As mentioned above, the following year, in yet one more LBO, PSA was merged with Aveanna through their respective owners, J. H. Whitney and Bain.[65]

Individuals receiving care through Aveanna, mostly children, have not fared well under PE ownership. An investigation of the chain by *Bloomberg News* shows that seven youngsters died under its care in 2018. In these fatalities, "health officials found that Aveanna nurses failed to check vital signs, follow emergency procedures, appear for their shifts or give the proper doses of medicine." Moreover, in interviews with *Bloomberg* reporters, "more than a dozen former Aveanna employees described how the pressure to meet financial goals jeopardized the quality of care for children." For example, the company often refused to send out nurses who would have to be paid overtime and neglected to match employees with patient needs if it meant lower revenues. The researchers discovered that in Texas Aveanna was responsible for 85 percent of the state's total violations by HHAs from mid-2016 through May 2019. Further, after Bain took over, 90 percent of branch-office bonuses were tied "to earnings growth, the hours of patient care it provides and cash collection."[66]

I spoke to Kevin Zepp, founder and CEO of Liberty Healthcare Services, one of the places purchased during Webster's ownership of Aveanna. He indicated that he had no qualms about selling his business and suggested that the company had been taxing work, both financially and emotionally. He said that he, as did others in the field, experienced constant staff turnover, competition (especially over salaries), and difficulty in obtaining financing. He told me that a bank he had worked with for years had been burned by another agency's homecare loan and no longer would fund him or the homecare industry generally. In selling Liberty Healthcare Services, he had realized his investment and could now move on.[67]

Zepp defended the sale to Webster by explaining that homecare entities require greater volume and consolidation to gain efficiency; negotiate more effectively with insurance companies, which squeeze the margins whenever possible; implement improvements; and install the latest technology. I asked him about the downsides of the sale, and he replied that there weren't any. When I suggested that Aveanna has had serious quality issues, including the deaths of children, he claimed that he did not know about that. Could it be the nondisclosure agreement he had to sign?

The massive chain seems to be unstoppable, like the Energizer bunny, in its pursuit of purchases—and infirm people—to exploit.

BrightSpring Health Services (formerly ResCare)

ResCare is another homecare company with a long, complex history of financial squeezing by a variety of entrepreneurs. Established in 1974 by James R. Fornear, the Louisville, Kentucky–based establishment began its life as a provider of services for at-risk youth (education, training, and treatment programs) and soon added a second division that assisted people with disabilities (residential support, vocational training, and group homes).[68]

At the end of 1992, the flourishing company (which operated in six states) issued an IPO and began trading on the NASDAQ. Through more and more acquisitions funded by private placements, it expanded both divisions, and by 1999 enjoyed revenues of $800 million and had a presence in thirty-two states.[69] At that point the chain was a treasure trove, and Onex Partners wanted in. In 2004, it anted up $114 million in development capital, thereby capturing 24 percent of the stock; six years later Onex purchased the rest of the company in a public-to-private LBO for $292 million. ResCare was now a PE portfolio company.

In 2005, through a flurry of activity, ResCare entered full force into the business of homecare for the elderly, including medical and support services; that year ResCare bought more than seventeen agencies. Over the next eight years it acquired at least thirty-five more places of various sizes and geographic reach. As of January 2018, it had accumulated nearly $1 billion in debt, and three months later it underwent a debt refinancing for $390 million, adding $300 million more in revolving credit from twenty-four lenders.

This highly desirable moneymaking machine (funded partly by Medicaid), however, has a sordid history. Prior to 2000, in a qui tam lawsuit filed under the Texas Medicaid Fraud Prevention Act, ResCare was accused of financial misdoings in its billing practices, including charging for mental health services that were either unnecessary or never delivered; doctoring patient records; and backdating documents. The financial fraud, of course, had detrimental effects on clients. As one observer puts it: "patients were receiving less care than they should have received."[70] The company paid $2.2 million in 2005 to settle the charges, a pittance given its revenues.

In 2007, the company and one of its homecare subsidiaries in Georgia faced a class action lawsuit for purportedly violating the federal Fair Labor Standards Act by neglecting to pay its workers for their travel time between homecare sites.[71] At the end of 2009, a jury in New Mexico found ResCare guilty of violating the state's Resident Abuse and Neglect Act and imposed a fine of $53.9 million in damages.[72] Unrelenting accusations against the company have flown as fast as its growth. In West Virginia, there were thirty-two substantiated complaints from 2012 to 2016 concerning ten of its agencies. The state's Office of Health Facility Licensure and Certification charged ResCare with neglect, severe understaffing, and not adequately training its frontline workers; a thirteen-year old had died, allegedly because of inadequate supervision.[73] In 2018 the South Central Workforce Development Board of Bowling Green, Kentucky, terminated ResCare's $1.8 million contract because, as its president and CEO remarks, "ResCare simply wasn't providing the type of services for adults, dislocated workers and youth that were expected."[74]

And there is more. California investigated allegations under the False Claims Act that ResCare was falsely billing Medicaid for attendants that never showed up.[75] An additional class action lawsuit, this time in Kentucky, alleged that the company did not pay its employees for overtime.[76] In Iowa, ResCare had to pay $5.6 million for failing to have physicians certify that Medicare- and Medicaid-funded home services were medically necessary.

According to a report by Baton Rouge radio station WBRZ, the Louisiana Department of Health determined that a ResCare group home "failed to protect clients from physical and psychological abuse, neglected to seek medical treatment after the incidents, and found they couldn't provide evidence that the abuse was thoroughly investigated." Further, WBRZ investigated job listings for ResCare and discovered that its workers were not required to have "any formal skills or training to take care of these special needs clients."[77]

I had firsthand experience with ResCare because my mother received at-home support services from the company from 2009 through 2012. Its deficient, centralized billing center occupied more than a few hours of my time as I attempted to sort out the incomprehensible and often dubious monthly charges. To make matters worse, I was paying ResCare $16.50 per hour plus mileage, while our homecare aide, I later found out, earned only $9.00. She received no health insurance or other benefits besides employer contributions to Social Security, and she relied on Medicaid for her three children.

Typically, in order to cover up its ignominious reputation, ResCare was rebranded BrightSpring in 2018, at which time it was on the auction block again. A year later KKR snapped it up through its portfolio company PharMerica for $1.32 billion.[78] Regardless of ResCare's serious abuses, Onex received roughly $1 billion—including $218 million in prior dividend recaps—on its initial $204 million investment.[79]

PharMerica is no neophyte in unlawful practices. Formed in 2007 by the merger of AmerisourceBergen Corporation and Kindred Healthcare and shortly placed on the New York Stock Exchange, it offers institutional and specialty pharmacy services. It quickly spread geographically as the company purchased and merged at least twenty-one pharmacies over the years; it became the second largest nursing home pharmacy in the United States.[80] The chain was accused of soliciting kickbacks from Abbott Laboratories in exchange for promoting its prescription drug Depakote for nursing home residents, a violation of the Anti-Kickback Statute. PharMerica paid $9.3 million in 2015 to settle the charges.[81] In an additional instance, the company had to pay $31.5 million for consistently administering narcotics, such as oxycodone and fentanyl, to patients without valid prescriptions and submitting false claims to Medicare for the illegally dispensed medicine; it also had to enter into a corporate integrity agreement for five years.[82]

Prior to KKR's acquisition of PharMerica, the compromised chain had experienced two failed attempts to take it private, in 2012 and 2016. Apparently, KKR has fewer reservations than others do about the integrity of enterprises it purchases: at the end of 2017 it paid $910 million for PharMerica in a take-private LBO.

Encompass Health (formerly Advanced Homecare Management and HealthSouth Corporation)

Encompass Health is one more leading chain of home health and hospice services that has seized small and midsize agencies as it seeks to enrich its several PE owners. Formerly known as Advanced Homecare Management, the enterprise was founded in 1998 by April Anthony, and in 2004 it was acquired by Apax Partners.[83] With at least $7.5 million in debt funding, Advanced Homecare expanded its offerings to include nursing, therapy, intensive care units, hospital ERs, and nursing homes through its acquisition of Healthcare Innovations (2005); Advantage Home Health Services, in an SBO from Capital Partners (2006); and WellCare Home Health (2007).

In less than three years, Advanced Homecare, renamed Encompass Health, experienced an SBO by Cressey & Company, KarpReilly, and Northwestern Mutual Capital. Characteristically, the new PE owners went full steam ahead with scaling the business: they debt financed more than fifty mergers, acquisitions, and add-ons over the next eight years. Encompass bought large and small as it propelled its way through the states; it was not shy about buying sizable, spread-out places at highly leveraged prices or branching out across the post-acute care continuum.

By 2015, Encompass had become more than ripe for the PE shops to realize their profit; it was merged with HealthSouth through a $750 million private-to-public transaction. Encompass was now a publicly traded company, joined with a chain consisting of 235 agencies in thirty-six states, the fourth largest provider of Medicare home health and hospice services. Unfortunately, it was now linked with a company that had a scandalous history.[84] In 2018, the entire business was rebranded Encompass Health. It is still expanding its footprint as a publicly traded company, including with the purchase of Alacare Home Health & Hospice in 2019 for $217.5 million.[85]

Elara Caring

The ninth largest homecare provider in the United States, Elara Caring ensued from a mega-merger of three companies, Great Lakes Caring, Jordan Health Services, and National Home Healthcare. The transaction among their respective PE owners in 2018 encompassed a debt package of more than $1 billion. Although part of the Elara network, each of the three enterprises has kept its own brand name. The intention, of course, is to scale and consolidate even further beyond the sixteen states Elara currently serves.[86]

Great Lakes Caring (formerly Great Lakes Health and Hospice)

Cofounded by Cheri Deary in 1994 to provide home health and supportive services, the Michigan-based Great Lakes Caring began its PE journey down the tracks when it was acquired through an LBO and recapitalization by Pauschine Cook Capital Management in 2007. A major purchase in 2010, In-House Hospice and Palliative Care, added end-of-life services in Michigan and Ohio to its offerings; Beringea was a second investor.

The next stop of the PE train was Wellspring Capital Management, which captured the company through an SBO in 2014. During this brief layover, Great Lakes and its new PE owner added to their roster Angels at Home Healthcare, a home health company with locations in Massachusetts and Illinois. Moving on, the subsequent stay was with Blue Wolf Capital and Constitution Capital Partners, which purchased Great Lakes in November 2016 in a tertiary LBO. The following month the company added Grace Hospice, thereby expanding the business to the Midwest. But Jordan Health Services stood out as the most significant purchase prior to the mega-merger.

Jordan Health Services (formerly known as Northeast Texas Health Services)

Jordan Health Services has been on a parallel odyssey with Great Lakes, though starting a bit earlier. Established in 1975 by Joe and Jean Jordan, the Texas-based company provided home health and personal services to Medicaid recipients. Jordan Health's first encounter with private equity was growth and recapitalization financing through Trinity Hunt Partners in 2007, whereby it added at least four enterprises. Jordan was picked up by Palladium Equity Partners and W Capital Partners in 2010 via an SBO. The investors apparently were forced to retain the business until 2018, since attempts to sell Jordan in 2014 and 2016 failed, allegedly due to lower bids than the PE firms were willing to accept. During Palladium and W Capital's holding period, Jordan borrowed more than half a billion dollars to refinance its debt and purchase additional places. It acquired more than thirty-four companies in eight years, spreading its home health offerings across Texas, Oklahoma, Louisiana, Missouri, and Arkansas.[87] The chain was then well positioned for a sale.

National Home Healthcare

The third piece of the triumvirate, NHHC, provides home health and staffing services along with other types of at-home help in the New York metropolitan area, northern New Jersey, Connecticut, and Massachusetts.[88] Founded eight years after Jordan Health Services, NHHC was placed on the NASDAQ (unknown date) and in 2007 was acquired by Eureka Capital Partners and Angelo Gordon & Company in a $104.9 million public-to-private transaction. At the end of 2016, Blue Wolf

Capital stepped in through a $65 million SBO. Finally, after more debt financing and purchases, NHHC merged with Great Lakes Caring and Jordan Health Services.

Additional Musical Chairs
Abode Healthcare

Taking advantage of the initial Medicare and Medicaid thrust away from institutional care to at-home services, Colorado-based Abode Healthcare was established in 2012. The company began its expansion with $16.5 million in development capital from its PE owners, Frazier Healthcare Partners and Heritage Group.[89] It quickly added three hospice agencies in additional states—Hearts for Hospice, Hospice of North Alabama, and Premier Hospice and Palliative Care—and in 2016 refinanced its debt, taking on $29.5 million in new liabilities.

Since then, two other PE firms took a bite of the apple: Tailwind Capital and ICG Enterprise Trust acquired Abode in an SBO and recapitalization in 2018.[90] Fourteen months later, more debt was placed on the enterprise: $15.5 million for additional acquisitions. Slightly more than a year later, the chain was off-loaded to Summit Partners in a tertiary LBO. What a windfall it must have been for Tailwind and ICG to have the luxury of selling the company so quickly—and at the expense of taxpayer-funded programs.[91]

Compassus (formerly CLP Healthcare Services)

Established by James Deal and Robert Holder in 1979, the Tennessee-based CLP Healthcare, which offered hospice and palliative services, has been shuffled around in a game of musical chairs.[92] Since its first PE management buyout in 2006 by Cressey & Company, its value has swelled as the enterprise has purchased ever more hospice agencies.

After Cressey extracted sufficient gains, the music stopped in 2014, and the PE house passed the business to its next temporary owners, Formation Capital, Audax Group, and Safanad. Because of the more than $300 million purchase, the new PE firms had to push hard to reap financial rewards. Apparently, they achieved their goal with the acquisition of such places as Life Choice Hospice in Pennsylvania, Optum Palliative and Hospice Care in Minnesota, Hospice Advantage in Michigan, and the health and hospice operations of Genesis HealthCare.[93] The music stopped again in 2019: TowerBrook Capital Partners and nonprofit Ascension Health captured the company for a remarkable $1 billion. Whoever thought people at the end of their lives would prove to be worth a small fortune?

During its journey among PE shops, Compassus has had its share of fraud allegations, particularly from 2007 to 2013 when it was still under Cressey's ownership. Its Optum add-on—then called Evercare Hospice—engaged in deceptive practices aimed at boosting the number of hospice patients it could bill Medicare for. Tactics included dissuading doctors from discharging elders from hospice if they were no longer qualified and neglecting to fully document patients' conditions.[94] The New York Times reports that Evercare hired agents to secure potential patients from hospitals and nursing homes, even if they weren't entitled to hospice services.[95] After purchasing Evercare, Formation and Audax rebranded the company Optum Palliative and Hospice Care, ostensibly to wipe clean its sordid history.[96] I wonder if the GPs were concerned when they bought such a troubled company. Or was the temptation of huge earnings too blinding?

Simplura Health Group (formerly All Metro Health Care)

Established in 1955 to provide HCBS in Long Island, All Metro spread throughout New York like a wildfire, focusing on care for participants in two Medicaid specialty waiver programs. Brown Brothers Harriman Capital Partners invested in All Metro at the end of 2005, and over the next nine years the company steadily expanded its locations. Nautic Partners eventually came sniffing at its door and bought the chain in 2014, partnering with management. A year later, the PE firm pocketed $132 million in a leveraged dividend recap that included fifteen lenders. Obviously satisfied with its rate of return, Nautic off-loaded All Metro to One Equity Partners in 2016. Shortly thereafter, the company was renamed Simplura Health Group.

One Equity proceeded to build the value of its acquisition through further buyouts, spreading the geographic footprint from New York, New Jersey, and Florida to three more states and increasing its lines of services to include daycare facilities, hospice, and home health care. In rapid succession, it purchased Multicultural Home Care (Massachusetts), Independence Healthcare (Massachusetts), SaraCare of Jenkintown (Pennsylvania), Keystone In-Home Care (Pennsylvania), Helping Hand Home Health & Hospice (Pennsylvania), and Personal In-Home Services (West Virginia). One Equity Partners also purchased the real estate of VillageCare, a not-for-profit agency offering at-home and community-based services along with managed LTC options.

Throughout its history, All Metro / Simplura has been primarily dependent on Medicaid for its revenues. The succession of owners for this leading supplier of homecare—and there are sure to be more—have feathered their nests at the expense of elderly and disabled poor people, along with US taxpayers.

AccentCare

An umbrella firm, AccentCare offers home health, personal assistance, rehabilitation therapies, and hospice services. It has a relatively long history of debt, refinancing, and recapitalization since its inception in 1999 as a start-up supported by venture capital. With each round, AccentCare accumulated both millions in liabilities and more investors, such as Mission Ventures, Cardinal Health, Piper Jaffrey, Salix Ventures, and in 2001 Highland Capital and Three Arch Partners. Along its venture capital voyage, AccentCare purchased such agencies as Continue Care (2000), Alliance for Health (2002), and SunPlus Home Health Services (2006).

The entity was then sufficiently ripe for PE notice: it was attained by Oak Hill Capital Partners in 2010, with the LBO generating $180 million in new debt. Over the next nine years the corporation raced through acquisitions as though it were on a speedway, starting in 2010 with the purchase of Guardian Home Care Holdings, itself no stranger to PE ownership; this was its third leveraged buyout.[97] With millions more in debt financing ($205 million in 2011) and then refinancing ($162.7 million in 2015, $227.1 million in 2017, and $300 million in 2018), AccentCare piled on business after business. In 2018 it bought seven places. By mid-2019, the Dallas-based enterprise had become the fifth largest home health and third largest personal care company in the United States.[98]

Those numbers whetted the appetite of Advent International Corporation, which procured AccentCare in June 2019; the LBO required fourteen lenders. Oak Hill Capital Partners had hit the jackpot. But the chase for buyouts is not over. The chain is aiming for a $3 billion valuation through its new PE owner and is adding new service lines.[99]

Interim HealthCare (formerly Medical Personnel Pool)

One of the earlier homecare agencies, Medical Personnel Pool—rebranded Interim HealthCare in 1992—is now the US division of Caring Brands International.[100] A franchiser of in-home medical and personal services, along with health care staffing, Interim has had its pockets picked regularly by PE firms since the late 1990s. The LBO ball started rolling in 1997 when the establishment was first acquired by Bank of America, Cornerstone Equity Investors, and Ridgemont Equity Partners for $134 million. Nine years later, in a management buyout by Sentinel Capital Partners, it faced its second turnover. A tertiary LBO transpired in 2012, when Halifax Group took control; two years later in a leveraged recap, Halifax awarded itself a juicy dividend. After a few years of adding more franchises, in yet another swap, Interim was relinquished in 2015 to Levine Leichtman Capital Partners, which proceeded to dip into the corporation through a dividend recap three years later. There will be more predators in coming years, draining off capital on the backs of the frail elderly and disabled populations.

Senior Helpers

Launched in 2002, Senior Helpers has become one of the leading homecare franchises in the United States; today the enterprise operates in more than forty states, with more than 320 locations. Senior Helpers had modest beginnings: Peter Ross and Tony Bonacuse decided to build a business together and sought a sector with recurring revenues. They met one afternoon, each armed with ten preferred industries, and senior care was at the top of both lists.[101] They started with one agency in Baltimore and presently opened another in California. Ross expressed to me that they viewed Senior Helpers as mission-driven: not only do seniors desire to age in place but that is the best situation for them.

By 2012 they decided that if they could attain a certain multiple, they would sell the business, especially since Bonacuse was ready to retire. Senior Helpers was apparently a red-hot item because, according to Ross, they received thirty-one initial bids when it was put up for auction, and he gave twenty-seven management presentations. "It's an audition for them and you," Ross said. They ended up choosing Levine Leichtman Capital Partners (LLCP) because the PE firm offered them the most money.

LLCP hung on to Senior Helpers for only four years. After granting franchises throughout the nation, the company was turned over to Altaris Capital Partners for $125 million, with LLCP earning four and a half times its investment. The multiple was so high that the GPs received a small "deal of the year" award. LLCP, like many other financiers, had brought in the money from homecare; now it was Altaris's turn, and it continued the trend.

Ross insisted that he never felt encumbered by LLCP executives. As long as he met their financial goals, they left him alone, he said. But near the end of their timetable, they were more reluctant to invest in new types of opportunities. Altaris, on the other hand, was ready to go and "took the handcuffs off growth. . . . Altaris is a joy to work with," he enthused. The PE firm brought expertise to the table, especially on how to improve the business. "They follow a model and can get on your case if you deviate from that model." I guess there was PE control over the business after all, but Ross did not seem to mind. I could not sniff out from him the effect of the PE firm's model on front-line workers and quality of care.

Through Altaris, Ross and Senior Helpers have engaged in four new directions. One of them, Town Square, offers day facilities for elders. It is a group option that he would rather call "adult enrichment centers" since "daycare" for adults, in his view, is not an appropriate designation. As of 2021, Senior Helpers had 317 franchises and was ready for more.

The Gold Rush

As mentioned above, private equity attraction to the homecare space has reached historically high levels since 2016, including first-time buyouts: a number of long-standing businesses were brought into the fold through LBOs. Linsalata Capital Partners in 2016 acquired H. H. Franchising Systems, Inc. (Home Helpers), an entity that had been established nineteen years earlier.[102] Care Advantage did not encounter PE for twenty-nine years.[103] The enterprise, which provides at-home health and supportive services in Virginia, was acquired by BelHealth Investment Partners in 2017—and immediately went on a tear. In less than three years it bought eight homecare agencies throughout Virginia and one in Maryland.[104] Always Best Care Senior Services, launched in the mid-1990s, was not captured by private equity until 2016, when it was purchased by Gemini Investors: the franchising firm provides homecare aides.[105]

An additional relative newcomer to PE is Synergy HomeCare, although it has had venture capital investments since 2015. Founded in 2001 by Peter Tourian, Synergy was bought in 2018 by NexPhase Capital in an $80 million LBO. Andy Kieffer, a NexPhase partner, envisions boundless growth with minimum capital expenditures because of the franchiser's exclusive focus on nonmedical services. He also notes the limited reimbursement risk the company faces since most customers pay out-of-pocket, and "these are needed services, not desired services."

Kieffer adds, "On the franchise side, [Synergy] has over 700 territories in which to sell. If we could open up another 200 that would be great. There's so much white space. There is more business to be had than any of us [franchisers] could possibly serve."[106] The chain already has 300 locations nationwide. NexPhase continued capitalizing on new opportunities with Medicare Advantage as it began offering the supportive services approved in 2018 by the federal government. Synergy already has joined efforts with three MA plans in eight states.[107]

+ + +

After twelve years of private ownership, Charter Healthcare Group, founded in 2006 by Fred Frank and Sabina Del Rosario, became a portfolio company of Pharos Capital Group through an LBO and recapitalization in 2018. Offering hospice, home health, and transitional services in California, the establishment had received $1.6 million in 2016 from Medicare for serving just 324 beneficiaries.[108] Charter now serves as a platform for Pharos to scale and consolidate in additional states, raking in more taxpayer money, until Pharos has enhanced the corporation's value sufficiently to sell.

+ + +

Tiana Zang, an experienced hospice provider, and two silent partners formed Sage Hospice and Palliative Care in 2013. Within a few short years, it expanded to become the third largest hospice in the Phoenix, Arizona, metropolitan area. Zang said that much of its growth is attributable to "word of mouth" about the exceptional, compassionate care Sage provides. The success of the enterprise received national attention and, inevitably, PE interest. At that point, despite a workforce of 140 people, Zang still engaged in hands-on work, relationships with clients, and everything else regarding the place. But in her words, "it had become a grind" even though she very much cared about Sage and its employees. And she needed financial help.[109]

By 2018, hospice care had become a hot commodity, and Zang received a significant number of phone calls. She had envisioned selling Sage to a strategic buyer, but then the PE shops came knocking at her door. She did not know very much about them or their business model. "I was naïve," she told me (like so many others who have sold to PE).

She found H. I. G. the most appealing because its executives told her that Sage would become the platform and future acquisitions would assume the Sage name: other PE shops would have absorbed her company under their brand. H. I. G. intends to spread Sage not only regionally but nationally. Zang sold her firm in 2018, retaining a small stake. "There would be more resources for everyone," she said.

I asked Zang about her experience with H. I. G. in the years she had been with the firm thus far. "They are a good group," she avowed. "But they are all about the numbers." She explained that the hospice profession is "all heart," unlike financiers where patients come second. According to her, H. I. G. does not get involved in Sage's operational functions; the company stays off her back as long as what she wants to do doesn't cost the PE shop any money and the chain is meeting its financial goals.

There have been noteworthy cultural shifts within Sage. In an attempt to standardize everything, for example, the new PE-chosen CEO rewrote the policies and procedures previously put together by her team. They had been working well, Zang said, and everyone was insulted by what they viewed as unnecessary interference. H. I. G. even attempted to revise the long-standing mission statement. There also has been a loss of control over the treatment of both clients and staff. In one instance, she wanted to give the employees a bonus, but she had to ask permission to do so. Moreover, the new regime moved to vendors who were less expensive rather than stick with the reliable ones she had been working with for years. The cheaper wholesalers took longer to deliver items, and their quality tended to be inferior. For the first time, Sage received complaints from its customers about products. But that CEO suddenly died, and she began working with a new one whom Zang regarded as on the same page as her.

Overall, she said that it had been a bittersweet experience, though she did not regret her decision to sell. Since the deal with H. I. G., Zang has talked to other founders in the homecare and hospice sectors who sold their businesses to private equity. "I don't know anyone who said it went well," she reported. The former owners lost control over their enterprises, including quality of care, and then they left. On the other hand, she added, there were proprietors who never cared about hospice in the first place, so they just took the money and ran.

In 2020, H. I. G. doubled down in the sector with its purchase of St. Croix Hospice from the Vistria Group for $580 million. Founded in 2008, St. Croix had been acquired in 2013 by Clearview Capital, which held the business for only three years. At the time of the H. I. G. leveraged buyout, it had twenty-one locations in five midwestern states.

+ + +

ComForCare, a nonmedical and private duty nurse franchise company since 2009, was taken over by Riverside Company in 2017. ComForCare then bought At Your Side in 2017, CarePatrol in 2018,[110] and Blue Moon Estate Sales (a leading moving liquidation service) in 2019. The acquisitions were bundled under one trademark, Best Life Brands. Together, there were 700 locations throughout the United States and Canada in 2020.

Riverside has sought substantial expansion and invested heavily in sales and marketing.[111] During the COVID-19 pandemic, it added to its traditional techniques through the use of texting, social media, and virtual interviewing; in 2020 ComForCare established forty-two new franchises. It also offered health screening for local businesses, thereby generating extra revenues.[112] Its intention is to become even larger through strategic partnerships (like the one it has already worked out with Kindred at Home), organic growth, and acquisitions. Yet does such ongoing enlargement and consolidation benefit older people in need of affordable, high-quality supportive services? Of course, Riverside Company will thrive.

+ + +

In one more first-time LBO, Varsity Healthcare executed a growth investment in Angels of Care in April 2019. Established in 2000 by Bonnie West, the business offers home health services to youngsters with complex illnesses. Angels of Care currently owns eighteen agencies in Texas and Colorado and is gearing up to scale and consolidate even further.[113] How does consolidation benefit children in need of affordable, quality services? Varsity, too, will thrive.

Private Equity Influence through Stock Ownership of Publicly Traded Companies

Listed homecare businesses have not escaped PE influence mainly because the entrepreneurs may retain some or a significant percentage of stock after they initiate an IPO. Three such enterprises were among the top home health providers in 2017: Amedisys (which holds 4.54 percent of the home health industry), LHC Group (2.1 percent), and Almost Family (1.7 percent), the latter of which was purchased by LHC in 2018. Amedisys also owns 1.7 percent of hospice businesses in the nation.[114] Another publicly listed chain, Addus HomeCare, a leading source of personal services, has substantial PE stock ownership in the aftermath of its IPO.

Amedisys

The second largest player in the home health sector, Amedisys was established in 1982, and twelve years later was placed on the NASDAQ. The fast-growing company, based in Baton Rouge, Louisiana, has rolled up more than fifty-four establishments over the years. It also began a geographic expansion and diversification into personal care and hospice services. For example, in 2019 it acquired Compassionate Care Hospice for $340 million, which rendered Amedisys the third largest hospice provider in the United States.[115]

Beginning in 2013, KKR accumulated shares in the highly profitable company, amounting to slightly more than 14 percent of the total by 2017. That year, KKR sold half of them for $178 million. The PE firm has been represented on the Amedisys board of directors since 2013 by Nathaniel Zilkha, a KKR partner.

LHC Group

Launched in 1994 by Keith Myers and Donna Lejeune as a solo home health agency, LHC Group today is the third largest home health provider in the United States, just behind Amedisys; it operates agencies across thirty-seven states.[116] The chain has four divisions that serve the post-acute care needs of Medicare beneficiaries: facility-based services; home- and community-based care; home health; and hospice.

In 2001, LHC was acquired by the Catalyst Group, which placed the company on the NASDAQ five years later. The IPO raised $67.2 million for the PE firm, and a second public offering the following year generated $77 million. LHC at the time was a healthy entity, valued at $232 million, and Catalyst retained substantial shares. By 2012 the GPs were ready to sell; TPG showed interest, but for reasons that are not publicly available the public-to-private deal was canceled. Instead, over the next several years Catalyst steadily sold its shares. Nonetheless, the PE shop has been a strong presence on LHC's board of directors through Ronald Nixon, one of its founders.

Addus HomeCare

Addus HomeCare, founded in 1979, experienced a short history of PE ownership prior to its IPO on the NASDAQ. The chain, which provides personal care, hospice, and home health services across its three divisions, was acquired by EOS Partners through a $100 million LBO and recapitalization in 2006. A 2009 IPO by the shop, which raised $54 million, was followed by two more: one in 2018, which earned $123.9 million, and another in 2019 for $159 million.[117] Though Addus is publicly traded, EOS retains a large share of stock, 11.5 percent, which can exert enormous power over the business. In addition, Mark L. First, an EOS partner, sits on Addus's board of directors.

Social Impact Investing

A few PE firms have raised social impact funds in the twenty-first century. The goal is to invest in companies that address social and environmental issues alongside their profit-making activities. Bain closed on its Double Impact fund in 2017, raising $390 million. KKR's Global Impact fund accumulated $1.3 billion while TPG, through its Rise Fund, procured $2.1 billion in 2017 and later $1.7 billion for a second vehicle.

Arosa+LivHome is one of the Bain Double Impact fund's portfolio companies, purchased in 2018.[118] The PE formed the platform through a merger of North Carolina–based NurseCare, launched by Ari Medoff in 2012, and California-based LivHome, founded by Michael Nicholson and five investors. The business offers nonmedical and skilled nursing services at home and in institutional settings.

Medoff told me about his journey to becoming CEO of Arosa+ LivHome. After a stint in private equity and then business school, he set out to buy a company. He decided on homecare because he viewed it as sufficiently fragmented that he could potentially outcompete or acquire competitors. Ultimately, he bought NurseCare, which he grew while keeping the well-being of its labor force in mind. Several years later, Bain came to him with a buyout offer, which included a significant stake in the enterprise for Medoff. He and Bain hit the ground running in 2019: two months after the leveraged buyout and merger with LivHome, in quick succession they acquired Partners in Senior Care, Forever Young Home Care, Cameron Group, Senior Care Management Associates, Companion & Home Care, and Lifelinks. They moved into 2020 with the purchase of Lifecare Innovations. The chain seems unstoppable.[119]

Medoff told me that caregiving is one of the hardest jobs; management must give the caregivers more respect as well as communicate better. Workers also require health insurance and a stable schedule. Better care follows, he added. Treating employees well also helps with the high industry turnover. He noted that thus far Arosa+LivHome is doing far better than the average, although he did not offer an exact percentage. Medoff views himself as having a calling to help society, and one of his goals is to create decent jobs. "We can do better for workers with our business model," he said. He believes that there are limits as to what government can accomplish; on the other hand, the private sector needs to rejuvenate itself and find a mission. He acknowledged that private equity ownership is too short term for his liking.

He said that Arosa+LivHome offers medical, dental, and vision insurance to its caregivers, but unfortunately it is not the best of plans because "healthcare insurance is insanely expensive" for such a low-margin sector as homecare. At the same time, offering a "401(k) is tough because most of our caregivers do not have the luxury of putting aside 3 percent of their income to qualify for the 1.5 percent company match we make." He indicated that the chain is seeking to do more for its frontline staff. It will be interesting to see if over time, the caregivers are indeed cared for. Ari Medoff seems interested in doing so, but he must work within the confines of Bain's Double Impact investing playbook.

Nonprofit Homecare Agencies
Heartland Hospice / HCR ManorCare

My mother was at Heartland Hospice, an arm of HCR ManorCare, where she was receiving end-of-life care; it is the third largest hospice in the nation, comprising 2.3 percent of the total. The aides, nurses, and other personnel who took care of my mom were caring, thorough, and available to her and me for the many months that we had been signed up with Heartland. A guitarist arrived weekly to serenade my mom with her favorite songs as did the massage therapist who relaxed her entire body. "Perhaps I am wrong about private equity," I thought. They were doing everything possible to make my mother comfortable during her last days of life. Then I learned that Heartland had become nonprofit. Aha!

HCR ManorCare has experienced a sinuous financial whirl since it was established in 1959 by Stewart W. Bainum Sr., who opened one nursing home in Wheaton, Maryland, under the trademark ManorCare. After its IPO in 1969, the company targeted nursing homes with private pay or Medicare customers, eschewing Medicaid. In 1980, ManorCare merged with Quality International Hotels, later renamed Choice Hotels, which it then spun off in 1996. With the acquisition of Cenco, Inc., in 1982 for $209 million, ManorCare became the fourth largest nursing home chain in the United States.[120]

In mid-1985, the company threw itself into a dynamic nursing home building phase. By 1993, it climbed to the third largest nursing home chain: its annual profits totaled $59.4 million on revenues of $1 billion.[121] In addition, the entity's $1.98 billion in assets as of 1997 included a number of subsidiaries: ManorCare Health Services, ManorCare Realty, Vitalink Pharmacy Services, and In Home Health (Heartland Division). It also operated assisted living facilities under the names Arden Court and Springhouse.

In 1998, ManorCare merged with Health Care and Retirement Corporation (HCR), and the combined enterprise was renamed HCR ManorCare in a deal valued at $2.9 billion, including $478 million of ManorCare's debt. As part of the consolidation, ManorCare joined HCR as a public company on the New York Stock Exchange. As of March 2000, it had vast real estate holdings, more than sufficient cash flow, and a stock market value of $3.7 billion. Just as important, according to Wall Street Journal reporter Robin Blumenthal, it "was unscathed by the reimbursement-fraud scandals that had affected other nursing homes in the late 1990s and pushed some of its competitors into bankruptcy."[122]

That all ended, however. In December 2007, HCR ManorCare joined the ranks of PE-owned portfolio companies when it was taken private in a whopping $7 billion LBO by Carlyle Group. Since HCR ManorCare owned rather than leased its facilities, Carlyle borrowed against the properties to finance the purchase, leaving the chain with more than $5 billion in debt.[123] Carlyle Group then split the real estate from the nursing home operations and reorganized the chain so that each facility would be responsible for its own liabilities.[124]

The story becomes even more convoluted: in 2010 Carlyle Group sold the real estate of HCR ManorCare to a REIT, HCP of Long Beach, California, for $6.1 billion, giving itself an ample dividend recap in the process. HCR ManorCare subsequently had to lease its 338 post-acute care, skilled nursing home, and assisted living properties from HCP and continue to operate them.[125] The once-lucrative business began to suffer financially, weighed down by overleveraged liabilities from the initial Carlyle buyout and the crushing rent payments.[126] In 2012, HCP sold the assets to Quality Care Properties, a publicly traded REIT. At that point HCR ManorCare tried to renegotiate the leases but failed, and the situation worsened. By mid-2017, the enterprise was on the brink of bankruptcy.

In a 2018 investigation of HCR ManorCare's chain of 230 nursing homes, the *Washington Post* uncovered untenable financial practices and egregious conditions. In their review of financial statements from 2009 through 2016, the researchers found that violations rose just after Carlyle pocketed the dividend recap, selling nearly all of the chain's real estate to do so, which meant HCR ManorCare was paying huge, unsustainable rents to the new owners. From the dividend alone, Carlyle had recovered the $1.3 billion of equity it initially paid for the deal, and it gained $107 million more in diverse fees, including annual advisory payments. To deal with the growing debt, siphoning of cash, and massive rents, Carlyle began its cost-cutting initiatives, including slashing the number of nurses and other frontline employees, switching to cheaper supplies, and refusing to repair crucial equipment, such as Hoyer lifts.[127]

According to the *Washington Post* reporters, during the five years before bankruptcy the number of health-code violations rose 26 percent, including "not preventing or treating bed sores; medication errors; not providing proper care for people who need special services such as injections and colostomies; and not assisting patients with eating and personal hygiene." In one Pottsville, Pennsylvania, facility, state inspectors alleged that as soon as they entered the place the "signs of neglect were conspicuous." The daughter of one resident said, "It was dirty—like a run-down motel. Roaches and ants all over the place."[128] The short-staffing was considerable; at times there was one aide for sixty patients, according to a frontline worker.

The chain was attacked from all sides. Despite the bankruptcy threat, its CEO was demanding $100 million in deferred compensation that Carlyle had promised to pay him as part of the initial deal. At the same time, the establishment was under investigation by the US Department of Justice, which alleged that the company "routinely submitted false claims to Medicare for rehabilitation therapy services that were not 'medically reasonable and necessary.' " HCR ManorCare soon defaulted on its loans and filed for Chapter 11; in March 2018 it was taken over by Quality Care Properties, which put together a prepackaged plan for the corporation's future.[129]

Four months later, HCR ManorCare emerged as a nonprofit entity: in July, the not-for-profit health system ProMedica and the REIT Welltower entered into an 80-20 joint venture to acquire Quality Care Properties. Welltower paid $2.2 billion for the real estate, while ProMedica acquired HCR ManorCare's operating entities, including the home health and hospice division, for $1.3 billion.[130] As part of the deal, HCR ManorCare's for-profit facilities were converted into not-for-profit assets. With total revenues of $7 billion, the combined venture became the fifteenth largest not-for-profit health system in the country. HCR ManorCare also is the second largest provider of nursing homes in the nation. And its Heartland businesses in 2017 were the third largest hospice (2.3 percent of the total) and thirty-first largest home health company, with more than a hundred locations in twenty-three states.[131]

At the beginning of 2020, HCR ManorCare divested itself of two divisions, its physical rehab segment (Heartland Rehabilitation) and a medical staffing platform (Milestone), and sold them to a new PE firm, Grant Avenue. The two entities operate under the brand H2 Health. Heartland Rehabilitation has more than sixty outpatient centers in seven states. Interestingly, the PE firm has established a nonprofit foundation focused on health care–oriented charitable organizations, which will receive a percentage of the shop's net income and carried interest.[132]

Bayada Home Health Care

The seventh largest home health enterprise in the United States, with 1 percent of the sector nationwide, Bayada generates more than $1.2 billion in revenue annually. Based in Moorestown, New Jersey, the company offers home health, personal assistance, and hospice care, with 35 percent of its business devoted to pediatric services.[133] After forty-four years of ownership, J. Mark Baida, its founder, in 2019 gifted a majority of the corporation to a nonprofit foundation. He told me that he chose the nonprofit route in order to ensure that Bayada and its high-quality caregiving model would endure long term. He had always wanted a business that could make a difference, and he views Bayada in that light. One of its distinctions, he said, is that the staff is treated respectfully. In fact, prior to donating the enterprise, he distributed $20 million among his employees as a thank you for their hard work. There is so much competition in the industry for workers, and he hoped that the bonus would serve as an incentive for them to stay on. I asked Baida about the reaction of other people in the industry to his generosity. He described it as "incredulous" and "surprised." On the other hand, his children, who work in the business, are supportive of the decision.[134]

Concluding Remarks

Home health and hospice care, which are two of the fastest expanding industries in the nation, have proved to be a gold mine for private equity. Over the decades there has been a transition from nonprofit to commercial agencies and then to PE ownership. Since 2016, GPs have been acquiring platforms and engaging in a rapid progression of add-ons and mergers, steadily scaling the once-fragmented sector. Ironically, the main government motive for moving away from institutional settings has been to combat rising costs. But PE firms are now in a position to raise fees and siphon off large slices of the gains for themselves. Significantly, the bulk of their revenues accrues from taxpayers through Medicare and Medicaid.

The care of fragile elderly people and children is increasingly in the hands of providers whose main goal is outsized profits, with their clients' well-being of secondary importance at best. Unquestionably, public policies have been a critical impetus in the transformation of the homecare and hospice landscape. Even a sacrosanct program, such as PACE, has been opened to private equity, handing the notoriously rapacious firms free rein as to the type and level of services.

As the for-profit side of the industry surged, increasing numbers of homecare and hospice chains engaged in financial fraud and exploitation of patients, and this has only worsened since the flood of PE investors entered the scene. Several companies have even re-branded their identities in order to camouflage their unsavory histories. Characteristically, the most vulnerable populations are trapped in a quickly revolving door of PE owners, and each time it turns one or two of them snatch valuable resources meant for disabled or dying elders and kids.

7 |

Public Crisis, Private Gain

Substance Abuse and Eating Disorders

SUBSTANCE ABUSE, whether it is heroin, cocaine, opioids, or alcohol, continues to be a crisis in the United States. Roughly 2 million people are addicted to prescription painkillers and another million to heroin and other illegal drugs; more than 72,000 die annually of overdoses, mostly due to opioids.[1] Just as tragic, the 2015 National Survey on Drug Use and Health reported that 6.2 percent of adults eighteen and over (15 million individuals) suffer from alcohol use disorder, and 88,000 die annually from it.[2]

Over the years, only a fraction of people desperately requiring help have received it, and the number of addicts is spiraling.[3] States, localities, and nonprofit agencies have not been building sufficient rehab centers to meet the need, creating a void that profit-making companies are satisfying. Only a decade or so ago, more than 60 percent of recovery clinics were either nonprofit or government-run; nowadays, most of them are commercial enterprises. PE firms especially are pouring billions of dollars into the market and are not shying away from purchasing nonprofit agencies and converting them. PE-backed Acadia (discussed below), for example, had no qualms about bringing into its fold nonprofit establishments, including Abilene Psychiatric Center (purchased in 2007) and Discovery House Group, an outpatient substance abuse treatment facility (purchased in 2015).

Behavioral health is one of four sectors preferred by private equity today, and addiction services in particular have proven to be hugely profitable. Reporters for the New York Times call the sector "one of the most lucrative health care industries to emerge in a generation," valued by the US Substance Abuse and Mental Health Services Administration at roughly $35 billion.[4] It has become big business. According to one source, earnings can reach as high as 25 percent for some clinics, and valuations are rising commensurately.[5] And it is the financial success of treating the substance abuse tragedy that has sparked the appetite of private equity firms, which never shy away from feeding on other people's desperation. At an investor conference, Joey Jacobs, CEO of Acadia, put it starkly: the rising use of heroin is a "favorable industry tailwind."[6]

PE shops have been taking advantage of this public health calamity since the early 2000s. From 2006 to 2013, they entered into sixty-two deals related to rehab, totaling more than $2.2 billion. Even at that time, treatment centers were considered valuable investments, with profit margins reaching 20 percent or more.[7] As usual, the fragmentation of the industry appealed to the GPs, who aimed to scale their purchases into regional or national powerhouses. In 2014, even the largest commercial owners controlled relatively few places, leaving ample room for them to step up their acquisitions and mergers. According to the Braff Group, forty-eight PE firms have purchased rehab businesses since 2014; in 2016 alone, they invested $2.9 billion in the industry, and the total has been mounting since then.[8]

Politicians Step In

Since the early 2000s, there has been greater political attention paid to mental health issues, including dependence on alcohol and drugs, especially prescription painkillers. Beginning in 2008 and strengthened in 2013, the Mental Health Parity and Addiction Equity Act has mandated that insurers cover behavioral and mental health benefits equivalently to physical conditions. Although parity has not yet been achieved, the bill opened the money valve sufficiently to draw the attention of the financiers.[9]

In 2008, Congress also enacted the Medicare Improvements for Patients and Providers Act, which advanced access to mental health services in public programs such as Medicare and Medicaid. The Affordable Care Act of 2010 turned the tap further by expanding the percentage of adults and youngsters with insurance and requiring health plans to provide benefits for substance abuse and mental health disorders, including for individuals already suffering from the conditions.

But as Dr. Timothy Brennan pointed out, "It is the opioid crisis that has shown the bright light on addiction."[10] By 2016, drug dependency had become a national legislative priority, resulting in the rapid enactment of three bipartisan bills. The Comprehensive Addiction and Recovery Act and the 21st Century Cures Act address overdose prevention and provide slightly greater access to treatment and medication, especially naloxone, which reverses overdose effects. The Comprehensive Addiction and Recovery Act also extends the right of office-based nurse practitioners and physician assistants to prescribe buprenorphine, an effective and safe drug for weaning users from their addiction, and increases the number of patients these providers can serve at any one time.[11] What is more, the bill opened up greater entrée for Medicaid patients by increasing fees to mental health and substance abuse agencies. The 21st Century Cures Act, which centers on a number of diseases and advances evidence-based therapies, specifically expands medication-assisted treatment for drug abuse. (The use of buprenorphine and at times methadone—in conjunction with behavioral therapy—is the evidence-based standard for treatment of addiction and reduction of relapse.) The third bill also passed with overwhelming bipartisan support: Congress enacted the Opioid Crisis Response Act in 2018.[12] Among its measures, the statute augments access to treatment for Medicare recipients by rescinding several restrictions that had rendered it challenging for elders to receive help. It also requires state Medicaid programs to cover medication-assisted treatment and associated therapy costs.

Who Pays?

The United States has always provided only a limited number of drug and alcohol rehab facilities financed primarily by state and local governments, along with nonprofit agencies relying on charity.[13] During the 1980s, commercial insurers began picking up part of the tab, and more recently Medicaid has become one of the principal payers. Nonetheless, PE-owned providers generally do not accept welfare patients in their residential establishments; lower-income people tend to be shunted into day clinics with limited, if any, therapy. Since the 2016 and 2018 legislative initiatives, Medicare has joined in and funds services for older addicts.

But none of the latest bills pays for an extensive expansion of public-sector treatment centers. Cost remains a considerable obstacle for the vast majority of the addicted population, even those with insurance coverage. Desperate families still spend more than $35 billion out-of-pocket on substance abuse treatment, and this is expected to grow considerably in the coming years.[14] The price tag for services can be devastating, depleting bank accounts, imposing massive debt on families, or wiping out house equity through second mortgages. Anne Fletcher, author of *Inside Rehab*, writes that many people are forced to use their retirement savings. Much of this money, however, is paying for "posh residential treatment at astronomical prices with little evidence justifying the cost."[15]

The Wild, Wild West

Because the US health care system has neglected to provide sufficient public clinics to meet the rising need of addicts seeking help, individuals and families have no alternative but to fall back on costly commercial providers. Nonetheless, the PE-owned companies have proven to be sorely inadequate. Researchers at the National Center on Addiction and Substance Abuse at Columbia University contend that few patients secure treatment that is based on scientific findings about its effectiveness. In a five-year investigation, they found that "the vast majority of people in need of addiction treatment do not receive anything that approximates evidence-based care."[16] Brennan confirmed that an overwhelming percentage of commercial clinics do not practice evidence-based medicine. They certainly are not following a medical model. He told me that unlike any other disease, there is substantial heterogeneity in treatment for identical conditions.[17]

Another expert in the field, Dr. Thomas D'Aunno, said that while vastly improved medications have been developed over the years, his research shows that there is not much improvement in the quality of care. He said that although methadone and buprenorphine are critical to successful recovery, patients require more than achieving sobriety. To sustain recovery, they need counseling, job assistance, nutritional guidance, help in rebuilding their social structures, and other psychosocial supports prior to their discharge—and similar help afterward. According to him, prior to the rush of PE investment in substance abuse treatment, profit and not-for profit clinics had similar goals and means of serving their clientele. However, research indicates that PE-owned opioid centers often provide medication-assisted treatment but nothing else.[18] PE shops are attentive only to the financially rewarding aspects of substance abuse, and supplementary but vital services are often either neglected or trimmed to the bare bones.[19]

The disparity between what researchers demonstrate is optimum for recovery and how rehab establishments provide treatment is remarkably jarring. Lacking adequate government regulations, PE portfolio companies have few, if any, standards to which they must adhere; they generally take the most profit-making approaches.[20] For example, even though individual therapy has proven to be most efficacious, many places substitute less expensive group therapy. Because of the widespread failure to use proven methods, the fraction of the addicted population that actually gains entry into rehab is faced with conditions that often do not help them remain drug-free in the long term. Without serious national or state guidelines and with limited inspections, there is no guarantee that recovery centers are even safe.[21] In California, for instance, there are sixteen inspectors for approximately 2,000 facilities.[22] Nor do the businesses have independent, impartial data on the long-term effectiveness of their programs.

Because of extremely high valuations for clinics, GPs are paying top prices, and to meet their expected rate of return they frequently prune operating expenditures accordingly. Staffing, of course, is a foremost PE target for the sharp knife, and addiction centers are no exception. Since most states do not mandate either advanced-level educational requirements for addiction counselors or any medical schooling, the PE-owned clinics can be staffed almost entirely with low-paid workers; all they need in a majority of states is certification as an alcoholism and substance abuse specialist, and there are no particular licensing requirements in the rest of the country.

Anne Fletcher notes that about half of rehab residents have a "dual diagnosis," a mental disorder independent from their substance abuse.[23] Despite the fact that comorbidities are usually associated with addiction, and substance abuse itself is considered a disease, the treatment workers seldom receive medical supervision. Further, in many places staffing is so insufficient that patients are left unattended, at times leading to dire consequences.[24] Lean and mean is feasible since, as Fletcher notes, the PE-owned enterprises tend to get the identical reimbursement from public and commercial payers regardless of staff levels, education and training of employees, the nature of their therapy program, or the extent of offered services.[25]

Certain substance abuse providers turn to outright fraud by gouging anguished families that have few other places to which they can turn. Rohit Chopra, chair of the Federal Trade Commission, points out, "When an investor is highly motivated to drive up operating margins in a short time period for an eventual sale, it can lead to predatory practices that put families and honest competitors at risk."[26] An investigation of addiction centers by the Southern California News Group found a prevalence of excessive billing practices, kickbacks, and other financial abuses.[27] Owners can also profiteer on medication. According to the National Institute on Drug Abuse, the rehabilitation businesses themselves decide what to charge patients. In the case of methadone, providers pay approximately $4,700 annually per person but have been known to bill residents up to $9,600.[28]

Another exploitive tactic, especially when a PE shop is expanding existing clinics and acquiring new ones, is "body brokering": the company pays intermediaries to lure patients in, not always using savory methods. In these cases, the specific needs and expectations of the addicts may be at odds with those of the broker, who places them only in clinics that compensate him.[29] In a nine-month investigation, Julia Lurie, a reporter for *Mother Jones*, found that "recovering users are wooed aggressively by rehabs and freelance 'patient brokers' in an effort to fill beds and collect insurance money. The brokers, often current or former drug users, troll for customers on social media, at Narcotics Anonymous meetings, and on the streets of treatment hubs such as the Florida coast and Southern California's 'Rehab Riviera.' " Lurie notes that although some states have enacted anti-brokering laws, their enforcement is lax.[30]

Moreover, the marketing techniques of substance abuse entities tend to be quite sophisticated, including fancy brochures and exotic websites. Brennan told me that he receives at least one or two emails weekly from PE or venture firms. He suspects that they are interested in gaining intelligence from him to enhance their advertising strategies. He also said that they often pay call centers, staffed by for-profit marketers, to sign up referrals: these are camouflaged to appear as a neutral source. "They can use very shady practices," Brennan emphasized.[31] As John Oliver and his researchers discovered, it is challenging to find unbiased information on the internet, since sites are mostly paid for by the rehab companies themselves.[32]

The substance abuse industry is unrestrained and chaotic, and is only worsened by the moneymaking pursuits of PE firms. Their rehab businesses are often revolving doors, with relapsing patients going in and out of care. Lanzone Morgan claims, "One of the most perverse issues revolving around addiction rehabilitation centers is that there is a financial incentive for failure."[33] The owners are not liable for ineffective treatments or inadequate support services, and when their patients relapse, they can charge them for yet another cycle of expensive therapy.

Milking Addicts

PE firms first entered the substance abuse arena in the first decade of the twenty-first century. Nearly all of these portfolio companies, such as Camp Recovery Center, Acadia Healthcare, New Season, and Foundations Recovery Network, have engaged in unsavory practices to various degrees in order to pump up their PE earnings. For the most part, they have been subjected to short ownership time frames, multiple sales, fast-paced expansion through de novo locations and acquisitions, extreme levels of debt, and elevated rates of return. None of the PE owners paid the piper for the company's wrongdoings despite the suffering experienced by patients, families, and employees.

Taking advantage of the government-declared opioid crisis, enlarged sources of public and commercial revenues, the easy availability of low-interest credit, and prior evidence of the industry as a gravy train, the latest round of PE ownership, largely since 2014, persists in its breakneck speed of acquisitions and profitability. The evidence is not yet in on the quality of care provided to patients, but the earlier history of PE takeover of the space does not augur well for the future. Indeed, PE-owned City Line Behavioral Healthcare and its Liberation Way centers faced accusations of substandard care shortly after the chain was established in 2018; a year later it declared bankruptcy.

Camp Recovery Center Health Group

Camp Recovery Center (CRC) is one of the oldest, largest, and arguably most problematic rehabilitation chains. Founded in the mid-1990s by Barry Karlin as a small California center, the business met its first PE (minority) owners, Apollo Global Management and Caltius Structured Capital, in 2001. The following year, North Castle Partners and aPriori Capital Partners acquired the company. By 2006, after piling up a series of acquisitions, CRC served more addicted people than any other provider in the United States. It was time to sell, and at a price of $723 million the PE firms earned more than three times their equity investment in only three years.

The new owner, Bain Capital, purchased CRC by placing $446 million of new debt on the corporation (62 percent of the total cost).[34] The PE house also received $6.3 million of Acadia Healthcare stock through the deal. Over the next several years, the portfolio company went on a buying spree, purchasing twenty rehab facilities, including Habit OPCO.[35] By 2014, CRC was the largest provider of substance abuse and behavioral services in the nation.[36]

CRC proved to be a jackpot for Bain, especially its methadone clinics, which according to one observer served as its "cash cow." In the first five years, Bain grabbed $20 million in management-related fees alone.[37] The United States got an intimate peek at its profiteering, despite the PE firm's notorious secrecy, because Mitt Romney (a Bain partner) divulged his taxes when he ran for president in 2012. That year, he reported securing between $100,000 and $1 million in dividends, interest, and capital gains from one of the Bain funds holding a portion of CRC, as well as income from two other vehicles with investments in the organization.[38]

With three Bain managing directors on CRC's board, the PE house maintained tight control over the company's moneymaking progress. To fuel CRC's enormous ongoing growth, it engaged in nonstop borrowing; in 2014 it owed $775 million, with interest at $49 million annually.[39] The chain, of course, required substantial cash to pay down the debt. Therefore, CRC hiked the rates of both drugs and services, "expand[ed] the client base through slick, aggressive marketing," and skimped on staffing and other operating costs.[40] Total revenues swelled accordingly—$450 million in 2012.

The well-being, safety, and quality of services for the vulnerable addicts under its care evidently were not on Bain's radar screen. In 2012, *Salon* investigated CRC residential facilities across the nation, using government reports, complaints by families and staff, and interviews with prior residents and employees; it discovered claims of abuse and neglect in at least ten of them. *Salon* also reported that subsequent to the suicide of a patient at a $40,000-a-month center in Arizona, regulators found forty-two severe violations that put residents at risk. Many other places were seriously overcrowded.[41]

In the case of the original Camp Recovery Center of the mid-1990s, immediately after Bain acquired it, according to *Salon*, "safety and quality eroded, while state agencies periodically reported increasingly more troublesome findings after 2006 regarding conditions at the camp." The article notes that fees were increasingly raised from $6,000 to sometimes triple that amount. To fill the place, nurses were compelled to admit even the sickest patients, though Camp Recovery was not licensed for medical services. The provider reduced staffing levels, limited the purchase of drug-testing kits, and lowered other costs while simultaneously boosting caseloads. The investigator adds that one previous director dubbed CRC "the slumlords of treatment."[42]

In a 2013 *Bloomberg* article, Physicians for a National Health Program recount that take-home doses of methadone from CRC clinics were sold on the black market; at times, the consequences proved deadly. The piece also excoriates CRC for sorely insufficient staffing and counseling.[43] Similarly, a series of articles in the *Tennessean* described how in 2011 a whistleblower exposed practices at New Life Lodge, also a CRC establishment, after three residents died. New Life was fined $9.25 million and prohibited from admitting new patients for six months because of defrauding Medicaid and providing substandard care. The Bain-owned facility had billed TennCare for services never provided, jammed in more patients than allowable, was understaffed, and employed unskilled and inadequately trained frontline personnel.[44]

As usual, it was time for rebranding: CRC was renamed Mirror Lake Recovery Center, and its sordid history was wiped clean with a swipe of the hand. In February 2015, the chain was off-loaded to Acadia Healthcare for $1.3 billion, including $905 million in debt.

Acadia Healthcare

The Acadia Healthcare platform was formed at the end of 2005 by Trey Carter and Waud Capital Partners to build a network of behavioral health care facilities, including substance abuse centers. During six years of Waud ownership, Acadia participated in more than fifty leveraged buyouts. To take advantage of the opioid crisis, beginning in 2010 Acadia aggressively acquired clinics; growing from 6 that year, by 2016 it owned 587 in the United States and the United Kingdom.[45]

In 2011, the PE firm cashed in through an IPO; via a reverse merger, it combined with Pioneer Behavioral Health. At the time, Waud sold 8.3 million shares valued at roughly $59 million. The PE steadily traded in its stake, reaping millions of dollars as the value of the chain rose. KKR, which had held stock in Acadia since 2005, also steadily unloaded its vastly appreciated shares, as did Bain Capital, a stock owner since 2015.

The chain continued to expand, with revenues and net income from ongoing operations reaching $3.4 billion and $224.9 million, respectively, in 2018.[46] Apparently, people with behavioral problems and substance abuse are exceptionally lucrative. Taxpayers have been generous to Acadia: Medicaid funded fully 25 percent of its revenue in 2018, with another $4 million derived through the 21st Century Cures Act.[47]

It seems that Acadia, too, was unconcerned with patient care as it hastily bought and consolidated behavioral health and substance abuse treatment centers across the nation. For example, Highline Medical Center, purchased in 2013, had eighty-six reviews on Yelp; since 2009 it had received one star (on a scale from one to five) from 72 percent of respondents. Likewise, Delta Medical Center, also bought by Acadia that year, was rated negatively by 68 percent of the forty-seven reviewers on rehab.com, who included comments such as "misdiagnosis," "poor accommodations," and "dreadful treatment by staff."

Allegations against Acadia rolled in: a fourteen-month study of the company by Seeking Alpha found serious malfeasance, including sexual assaults, patient neglect and abuse, and even wrongful deaths.[48] USA Today in 2017 described egregious treatment of patients at Park Royal Hospital, another Acadia facility. Its chief medical officer had resigned in protest over the low quality of care. The place also had been sued for not preventing attacks on patients, failure to check on people, and insufficient staffing.[49] Moreover, the Seeking Alpha report noted a steady sell-off of stock by Acadia's officers and directors, dropping their ownership from 30 percent to under 1 percent.[50]

The publicly traded chain (NASDAQ) is currently sidestepping the charges; it is also burdened with $3.2 billion in debt. Yet KKR, TPG Capital, and other PE firms were eyeing it for a public-to-private buyout in 2018. A deal never materialized; perhaps the shops were looking to buy on the cheap, something Acadia stockholders were unwilling to do.[51]

New Season (formerly Colonial Management Group)

Colonial Management Group, a network of outpatient methadone clinics, is another for-profit chain capitalizing on the opioid crisis. Founded in 1986 by John Steinbrun, its first PE (minority) investor, Warwick Capital Group (unknown date of investment), provided growth capital for acquisitions. By 2013, Colonial had purchased fifty-seven opioid and other drug treatment centers in eighteen states.[52]

As with many other chains, Colonial skimps on services after it acquires a business, but the company seemingly is particularly egregious in its wrongdoings. In some places its clinics have been dubbed "dose and go" operations.[53] Shapiro Law Group reports that state agencies have accused a number of its facilities of malfeasance, including "failing to properly monitor the dosage patients receive, resulting in patients receiving too much medication and selling the extra on the street. Nearby areas reported increases in fatal overdoses at the same time." It is also charged with "taking on too many patients, beyond the amounts approved by the state"; "failing to administer drug tests, leading to adverse drug interactions with patients on other substances"; "failing to provide counseling"; and "failing to keep accurate and up-to-date records."[54] Ella Nilsen, a reporter for *Sentinel Source*, concurs, adding that less than 2 percent of Colonial's clients had been "weaned off the drug or successfully discharged from the program between 2011 and 2012."[55]

The litany of grievances across the nation is endless. Excessive caseloads, insufficient staff training, and lack of accountability for methadone are common concerns. In Daytona, Ohio, for example, inspectors noted that caseloads were double or triple what is permitted under state regulations. The situation in many Colonial centers has been so lax that take-home doses of methadone could be sold on the street, leading to misuse of the drug. The US Department of Justice imposed a $95,000 fine on a clinic in Alabama "because the clinic couldn't account for 3,423 doses of methadone."[56] In 2010, a class action lawsuit against Colonial accused the company of charging patients cash fees for methadone without providing any detox, counseling, or other services to assist them with ending their addiction. The lawyers for the complainants declared: "It is nothing more than legalized drug dealing."[57] The case was settled out of court.

In 2015, Colonial was taken over by Behavioral Health Group, an outpatient opioid addiction treatment network that has been handed from one PE to another over the years. Created as a platform in 2002 via the Cambria Group and others, in 2011 it experienced an LBO and recapitalization through Frontenac Company, which proceeded to acquire a large number of centers. Colonial Management was included in the sale and renamed New Season. Hocus-pocus yet again: Colonial got a new start, leaving the suffering of addicts and their families in its wake.

But Colonial's journey was not over. In yet another LBO, Behavioral Health Group (including New Season) was acquired by Vistria Group and HCSC Ventures for $250 million at the end of 2018. Behavioral Health Group has forty-six opioid addiction centers across eleven states, while numerous PE firms have collected outsized profits at the expense of their addicted clients.

Foundations Recovery Network

Foundations Recovery Network, which prides itself on treating people with dually diagnosed substance abuse and mental health disorders, is an archetypal example of just how financially gainful the addicted population can be for the PE industry.[58] Acquired by Sterling Partners in 2007 via a $22 million LBO and sold to Nick Pritzker Capital Management five years later in an SBO, Foundations's price escalated to

$350 million in 2015, when it was purchased by Universal Health Services (UHS). In only eight short years the company's value had increased by a factor of sixteen.

Since then, Foundations has served as a growth platform for substance abuse treatment facilities by the publicly traded UHS.[59] Unfortunately for individuals with addictions, UHS (the largest provider of behavioral health care in the United States) has been mired in abusive practices. A 2015 report by the Service Employees International Union, "Universal Health Services: Behind Closed Doors," delineates appalling conditions at the facilities, including unsanitary and unsafe environments, sexual assaults, and acute staff shortages at every level: mental health workers, registered nurses, licensed practical nurses, and frontline employees. The report also describes the shocking number of deaths and suicides, and how workers were fired for informing superiors of dangerous conditions or other health concerns.[60] A federal investigation of twenty-five facilities beginning in 2013 found rampant criminal and financial fraud as well. For example, UHS settled several lawsuits alleging that it billed for services that were not up to par, such as lower levels of therapeutic care than charged for.[61]

Nevertheless, at the time of these investigations UHS was receiving $2.2 billion in fees for its behavioral health division from Medicare and Medicaid and $395 million from the military; government payouts accounted for more than half of the company's revenues. Nearly 25 percent of its total proceeds was pocketed as profit.[62]

Following the addition of Foundations Recovery Network, UHS's substandard conditions in its psychiatric hospitals continued unabated, as outlined in several inquiries.[63] One can only assume, given UHS's ongoing short-staffing, inadequate training, attempts to keep its places at full capacity, and huge profit margins, that Foundations's substance abuse treatment facilities are not in the best of hands.

Pinnacle Treatment Centers

Founded in 2006 by venture capital firms Celerity Partners and Gemini Investors, along with Dr. Ken Kessler, the Pinnacle platform set out to become a regional opiate treatment chain.[64] During this ownership phase, the company expanded more than ten times its size through both acquisitions and de novo locations, accumulating substantial debt along the way. It also built a central corporate infrastructure. In 2013, the PE firms and Kessler were prepared to collect their loot, but the sale failed to materialize.

In 2016, with inpatient and outpatient centers in five states and a growing opioid crisis, Pinnacle was well situated to try again, and Linden Capital Partners acquired the company that year.[65] Since joining Linden's portfolio, Pinnacle has purchased Family Counseling Center for Recovery in Virginia; Addiction Medicine Care, an office-based opioid treatment provider in Ohio (400 per day patient flow); and in early 2020 Aegis Treatment Centers.[66] It also stretched its turf by purchasing Practice Management Associates, a medical billing and coding business.

I spoke with Matt Rice, the founder and CEO of Recovery Works Drug and Alcohol Rehabilitation Center, a treatment center that had been purchased by Pinnacle in 2012, and asked about the company's history. Apparently, in 2006 he and a wealthy psychiatrist borrowed money, which they personally had to sign for; it was not leveraged on the business. "I signed my life away," he said. But they were successful.[67]

The first center, in Georgetown, Kentucky, was set up like a psychiatric hospital, which was unlike the usual addiction treatment settings. He wanted something different because he saw that what others had in place was not working well, including for his father and brother, both of whom were drug addicts. Individuals should stay in a facility for at least thirty days, he noted, and his place provided what they require.

I asked Rice why, after six years of ownership, he decided to sell his business to Pinnacle. "They were the first one to approach me," he said. He had decided that it was time to move on, and his partner, who was sixty years old, was ready to retire. It seems that Rice never regretted the move: he had signed on with Pinnacle to stay for two years and, after a brief hiatus, remained in various positions for more than four years. He also sold the small stake in the enterprise that he had received in 2012 as part of the deal.

According to him, the private equity firms have been mainly interested in taking Pinnacle into new territories through acquisitions, mostly in Indiana, Ohio, and Kentucky, and not much else. "Private equity has had little impact on the company except growth," he said. And the expansion has been focused and not fast-moving. Clearly, the previous owner of Recovery Works views the ongoing consolidation by the PE firms as sufficient for earning their outsized fees and profits.

Lakeview Health

An additional drug and alcohol rehabilitation company that has quickly changed hands, Lakeview Health was first bought at the end of 2012 through a $73 million LBO (including a debt of $37 million) by Greenridge Investment Partners, C3 Capital, and Trinity Hunt Partners.[68] After two more cycles of debt financing in 2014 and 2016, which was used to renovate its luxury Florida campus and build a fifty-four-bed women's center, the PE firms sold Lakeview to the Riverside Company and Triangle Capital in an SBO at the close of 2016; the substance abuse treatment business found itself with $18.6 million in new liabilities. Further debt financing followed as its latest PE shop opened a de novo facility in Woodlands, Texas, that offered partial hospitalization and outpatient services. Lakeview, like so many lavish PE-owned facilities, thrives on commercial insurance and private pay; its doors are not open to the addicted Medicaid or Medicare population.

Delphi Behavioral Health Group

Founded in 2016 by Blue Ox Healthcare Partners and Ryan Collison as a platform for alcohol and drug addiction treatment, Delphi Behavioral Health Group was ripe to take advantage of money flowing through both government and insurance sources. It rapidly purchased seven relatively small facilities over the next twelve months. At the end of 2017, Blue Ox was obviously sufficiently pleased with its rate of return that it placed Delphi on the market: Halifax Group, through a $130.2 million management LBO, recapitalized the company.

As the acquisitions continued, the chain became so lucrative that it attracted more PE shops—FFL Partners and Lee Equity Partners—which bought minority shares.

Summit Behavioral Healthcare was one of its most substantial buyouts.[69] Summit had received growth capital via Flexpoint Ford beginning in 2015 and more debt financing from Golub Capital for additional buyouts.[70] And acquire it did: from 2014 through 2017 the company bought Valley Recovery Center (California), Victory Recovery Center (Louisiana), the Ranch at Dovetree (Texas), Mountain Laurel Recovery (New Jersey), St. Joseph Institute (Pennsylvania), Turning Point Treatment (Pennsylvania), English Mountain Recovery (Tennessee), and Canyon Vista Recovery Center (Arizona). Now a substantial chain in its own right, Summit was merged with Delphi, taking on its name.[71] The LBOs march on.[72]

SUN Behavioral Health

Established with $19 million in venture capital by Petra Capital Partners in 2014, SUN Behavioral Health expanded through the steady infusion of debt financing and refinancing via a number of PE shops from 2015 to mid-2019.[73] With more than $100 million in total investments, the PE-owned SUN has built four psychiatric hospitals.

According to Steve Page, its founder and CEO, the hospitals are transitory facilities; residents, who are in crisis, stay from three to fifteen days, averaging about seven. The company also provides partial hospitalization in which patients return home in the evenings. Page informed me that more than half of SUN's customers have both substance abuse challenges and behavioral conditions. However, the business is not licensed for long-term treatment of drug and alcohol disorders, though there is a possibility it could move in that direction. Page has a clear game plan, of which he is only in phase one: he ultimately intends to offer the full continuum of care for behavioral health. First, he finds a locality with unmet needs and builds a hospital. The institution then becomes a solid base for recruiting professionals to the area, which allows it to expand the types of services it offers.

I questioned Page about PE involvement in the company. He made no bones about the fact that they are in control of certain aspects of the business. The PE firms could sell SUN anytime they wanted to, he noted. They ultimately decide on acquisitions. And they expect the management team to meet agreed-upon performance goals. But he explained that the PE shops are the ones funding everything. "Where else can you get that kind of money? The banks won't do it." He told me that SUN is going into underserved localities and building free-standing hospitals that "nobody else wants to fund." He was adamant that the PE partners do not exercise operational control. "They wouldn't know what to do even if they wanted to." Nonetheless, if he functions in ways that are not acceptable to them, they will fire him, he said. They could change the top team on a whim, including him.

He voiced some concerns about the PE model itself. He is particularly frustrated by its brief time frame, which is not, in his opinion, appropriate for his type of business. They have short-term financial objectives that compromise some of what he wants to do. Page would like to have ten years with the PE firms, but he can sense that they are already "itching" to move on. He also expressed that "there is some bad behavior out there."

Beach House Center for Recovery

Launched in 2014 by Glenn Cohen, Beach House is a five-acre recovery center in Juno Beach, Florida. In 2018, BelHealth Investment Partners acquired the campus with the intention of expanding its capacity and, of course, increasing its footprint geographically. For individuals paying out-of-pocket, Beach House charges $24,500 to $34,500 for a thirty-five-day stay. I was told by a company representative that for people who are covered, insurance generally pays most of the cost.[74] In order to enhance its visibility and help fill the facilities, BelHealth named Chris Christie (ex-governor of New Jersey) as executive chair of the Beach House board of directors, and Tom Ridge (ex-governor of Pennsylvania, the first secretary of Homeland Security, and an advisor to BelHealth) as a member of the board.

BayMark Health Services

Also on target to take advantage of the opioid crisis, Webster Capital established BayMark Health Services by merging its portfolio company BAART Programs with Capital Resource Partners and CHL Medical Partners's MedMark Treatment Centers in 2015. Thus began BayMark's journey as an outpatient medication-assisted opioid treatment provider. In a series of debt financing and refinancing ($213 million in debt refinancing in 2017 and $11 million the following year), the organization via its PE shop bought multiple medication-assisted treatment and detox centers throughout the nation. These include Applegate Recovery (Louisiana), the Coleman Institute (Virginia), Health Care Resources Center (Massachusetts), Canadian Addiction Treatment Centers (the largest provider in Canada), Tri-City Institute (California), SpecialCare Hospital Management (Missouri), Metamorphosis Opioid Treatment Program (Utah), and Counseling Solution (Georgia and North Carolina).

By the end of 2018, BayMark owned roughly 209 locations and had surpassed Acadia as the largest opioid treatment provider in North America. With an estimated $1 billion valuation in September 2019, Webster was ready to cash in and sought a new buyer, but none was willing to pay the price it demanded.[75] It continues to finance ever more BayMark acquisitions.

Crossroads Treatment Centers

Revelstoke Capital Partners joined the opioid cash-cow bandwagon in 2015, at which time it acquired Crossroads Treatment Centers.[76] As many other PE firms do, Revelstoke held sway over its network of medication-assisted outpatient clinics through its two representatives on the board of directors. Over the next four years, with ample debt financing, Crossroads expanded considerably, and by mid-2019 it was administering methadone and suboxone through ninety-six clinics in ten states.[77] Revelstoke apparently enhanced Crossroads's value satisfactorily since it put the company up for sale in 2019 and sold it to Yukon Partners early in 2020.

Kolmac Outpatient Recovery Centers

Consisting of outpatient clinics for drug and alcohol addiction, Kolmac Outpatient Recovery Centers was established in 1973, and fully forty-five years later it was purchased and recapitalized by WindRose Health Investors. The PE firm and the company's founder, Dr. George Kolodner, seek to build and acquire centers on the US East Coast and eventually across the nation, as well as increase market share for its existing clinics.[78]

Kolodner had established Kolmac after designing an intensive outpatient therapy program that, according to him, was thriving in Maryland. Since he viewed himself as a clinician and not an entrepreneur, he brought in a CEO to scale the enterprise. Kolmac soon expanded to five other states, serving roughly 2,000 patients. Subsequently, he decided to make his treatment model more geographically available and marketed the business to PE firms. Kolodner advised me that patients are spending too much money for residential therapy, and his technique can assist addicts just as effectively at a lower cost. With sufficient intensity of therapy and appropriate medication, people can recover with a 20 percent lower price tag.

He wanted to enlarge the enterprise through de novo offices and acquisitions but required assistance in finding and building centers and in funding the expansion. He found plenty of eager PE investors, but they wanted to absorb his company into their models of care. Sixty PE firms showed initial interest, thirty made offers, and Kolodner met with ten of them. He was concerned about linking his company with a PE firm because he wanted to scale it without ruining the quality of his method. Eventually, he chose WindRose.

Kolodner admitted that he was quite wary of private equity at the time. He said, "I have heard horror stories about owners who were kicked out of their own business." Others, he noted, were made so miserable by the private equity investors that they just wanted to get out. He is satisfied with WindRose because the PE firm collaborates with, rather than controls him. I prodded Kolodner about the inevitable sale and the next PE shop, which may not be so accommodating. "I'm concerned," he said. "But I could always retire."

City Line Behavioral Healthcare

There is a short but disastrous LBO saga about City Line Behavioral Healthcare, which was created as an alcohol and drug treatment platform by Fulcrum Equity Partners in 2018. Simultaneously, Fulcrum melded its existing portfolio company, Liberation Way, into City Line, along with its newly acquired Life of Purpose Treatment business.[79] Fulcrum had bought a majority share in Liberation Way at the end of 2017, two years after it was launched, for $42 million. The founders more than doubled the profitability of the company, and now snatched millions from the sale to Fulcrum.

The miracle surge in earnings, however, was dependent on the maltreatment of clients and financial abuse.[80] The Pennsylvania attorney general, a grand jury, and the *Reading Eagle* all investigated Liberation Way. They found substandard, nonexistent, and unnecessary treatments; redundant testing; overcrowding; unsafe conditions; patient recycling (sometimes six or more regimes of treatment); insurance fraud; and poorly run, unlicensed facilities. One supervisor told the *Reading Eagle*, "It was a great business model, but an awful treatment model."[81] A month after the *Eagle* story, Fulcrum erased any trace of the Liberation Way brand by absorbing its clinics into Life of Purpose; it hoped that the tainted company would just disappear.[82] It also denied any involvement in Liberation Way's misdoings although GPs are well known for their thorough due diligence before purchasing a business.

City Line Behavioral Healthcare filed for bankruptcy in April 2019. Eleven people were charged with insurance fraud, including the cofounders and former executives.[83] Hundreds of addicted individuals had been put in harm's way. Employees suddenly lost their jobs. Fulcrum wiped the drug and alcohol treatment chain off its website.

Eating Disorders

Anorexia, bulimia, binge eating, and other eating disorders (ED) are just as devastating as—and sometimes worse than—substance abuse. The National Eating Disorders Association estimates that 30 million Americans, mostly women, have experienced a "clinically significant" ED.[84] As one reporter emphasizes, "It's a big population to prey upon: One in five American women suffers from some type of ED."[85] Eating disorders are not only among the most difficult mental illnesses to manage but can be the most lethal, especially anorexia; the effects of starvation are grueling on the body. Suicide is not uncommon.

During the 1990s, the growth of managed care organizations fostered shorter hospital stays for ED, and small treatment centers proliferated. Residential centers were scarce; there were only twenty-two of them in 2006. By 2016, however, ED had swelled to a $2.7 billion industry, boasting seventy-five facilities.[86]

Like with substance abuse, the moment proved propitious for PE firms to enter the space. The demand for services, which outpaced availability, certainly left a gap for commercial players to move in. As usual, the fragmentation of the market, composed of small-scale businesses, also was appealing to GPs, who were eager to consolidate the industry. Most important, there were more free-flowing dollars to pay for services. Earlier, there had been substantial resistance from commercial insurers, even after the enactment of the Affordable Care Act; however, the US Court of Appeals for the Ninth Circuit, which deemed the treatment of eating disorders a "medical necessity," mandated that insurers reimburse clients for treatment in California because of its parity law.[87] This ruling opened the door for other states with similar statutes. Successful lawsuits pushed insurers into covering ED. Attorney Lisa Kantor has been one of the foremost advocates driving the litigation process. In 2007, the lawyer obtained a ruling in which the court's California mental health parity decision had to be applied to its residents who seek treatment in other states.[88] Since then, she and her firm have taken endless legal actions against insurance denials of treatment for eating disorders.[89]

Kantor provided me with some background on her work with ED, which she calls the "stepchild of mental illnesses." She handled her first such case in 2006 when a student, insured through Kaiser Permanente Insurance Company, was told there would be a three-month wait for a psychologist. The undergraduate subsequently found a provider, and after a month of treatment she improved markedly, but Kaiser refused to pay. After losing the case at the lower court level, Kantor petitioned the Ninth Circuit Court of Appeals and won, achieving a huge victory for people suffering from ED.[90]

The lawyer has advocated in other ways as well. She reached out to eating disorder clinics in California, such as Monte Nido, and trained owners on how to contend with reluctant insurance companies. She also attempted to assist them in collaborating with each other to obtain higher payments. In addition, Kantor lobbied across the United States to convince facility owners to take a chance on at least one patient periodically and provide them with unreimbursed treatment while she took on the case; she often argues ED cases pro bono.

Around 2014, according to Kantor, came the private equity crowd. Just after the implementation of the Affordable Care Act, PE interest in the sector spiked. "The money thrown around was obscene," she informed me. Everything changed when private equity took over: there was constant employee and company turnover; a money-driven philosophy prevailed; attitudes changed; and quality of treatment declined. She attended conferences everywhere, she said, in an attempt to push back against the deteriorating standard of care, but the leaders in the field could not (or would not) unite. So many already had sold or intended to do so. The extreme valuations of their businesses proved to be too enticing for many owners to hold out.

The financial margins of 20–30 percent for ED clinics have been irresistible to PE shops.[91] One source points out that although there was ongoing consolidation on a small scale prior to 2015, ED treatment is now so financially rewarding that even some of the PE bigwigs, who generally seek multibillion-dollar deals, are aiming to position themselves for growth and consolidation in the area.[92] Naturally, as they expand, the PE-owned companies must elicit more customers, and that involves such endeavors as central call centers and professional salespeople to hawk services. The financiers use sophisticated approaches "that target clinicians and include promotional gifts."[93] Unlike some other industries, there are no laws controlling such practices. To lure residents, the PE owners also tend to prettify the places with resort-like facades.

There is evidence that ED programs should emphasize meal-based refeeding and weight restoration.[94] Nonetheless, the lack of definitive best practices in treating the disorders, inadequate documentation of clinical outcomes, slipshod licensing standards, and limited government oversight allow an open field for PE firms to institute whatever procedures bring them the greatest return.[95] Erica Goode, a reporter for the New York Times, finds, "The quality and form of treatment varies widely across centers, and in some cases includes approaches—equine therapy, for example, or 'faith-based' treatment—with little or no scientific evidence behind them."[96] Despite the probability of comorbidities and digestive maladies, the facilities customarily lack psychiatrists, gastroenterologists, or primary care physicians.

Dr. Evelyn Attia, the director of the Columbia University Center for Eating Disorders, told me that there are evidence-based strategies, but they are not used in most profit-making enterprises. Beginning in the 1990s, a new model of residential care cropped up:—freestanding for-profit facilities. Many patients do not require twenty-four-hour care, she said, and there are far fewer regulations and accountability for these entities. They also tend to have no physicians and a smaller number of registered nurses than academic ED centers do. "We don't even know what training the staff is getting," she added.[97]

Attia emphasized that what private equity does best is marketing, and the firms often showcase their beautiful settings and "unique" techniques, such as equine therapy, that have no proven effect on outcomes. Customers can be fooled by telling them that the treatment center's plans are effective, even when there is no evidence that they are. These freestanding enterprises just need to keep their beds full, and if the treatment does not work, readmission surely doesn't hurt that objective, she said. They are very savvy in their presentations and put pressure on families to sign up.

The for-profit centers mostly target teenagers who, in her view, do not require a residential stay. For those in the first stages of an eating disorder, all they need is a strong family-based approach once a week. Attia maintained that proper outpatient family-based treatment can have a 75 percent chance of recovery or near-recovery after a year as opposed to the more common 50 percent rate in residential facilities. She added that the profit-making places do not accept Medicaid-supported patients and can use the institution for mental disease exclusion to justify it.[98] Therefore, they only take in people paying out-of-pocket or those with commercial insurance, both of which generate higher fees. According to Attia, academic centers tend to get the poorest and sickest individuals, who are challenging to care for, and at the same time they receive low Medicaid reimbursements to do so. As a result, many such places have shut down and others face closure or take in fewer patients.[99]

Another expert on eating disorders whom I interviewed (they asked to remain anonymous) argued that one of the largest issues is the lack of authentic data for long-term outcomes. This person said that cognitive behavioral therapy works best, especially at early ages and in conjunction with the child's family. One of the problems with commercial enterprises, the specialist said, is that they want to keep their paying customers so they may give in to residents' conflicting desire to get better but not by having too many restrictions placed on them. Consequently, the centers will do what patients want and not what they need; overall, PE-owned facilities tend to be less behaviorally oriented. Similar to Attia, this expert told me that they are more attuned to marketing, with beautiful websites that capture the attention of consumers, and they target patients with the least complications. The interviewee also pointed out that eating disorders are expensive to treat. Many patients are in a no-man's-land: private facilities do not want them if they are enrolled in Medicaid or even Medicare because of low payments, and nonprofit and academic institutions who do take them struggle financially to maintain their programs.[100]

The bottom line is that substandard treatment means that individuals with eating disorders suffer measurably and could possibly die. As one observer puts it, "Ultimately, . . . the blame for inadequate treatment circles back again to Wall Street, to money, to eating disorder treatment chains seen as a good investment—patients are seen as a commodity, rather than [as] individuals dealing with a mental health issue."[101] The impressive-looking but often ineffectual residential facilities are quite pricy, generally more than $1,000 per day. The length of stay is variable, but individuals typically remain an average of eighty-three days, thus paying more than $83,000. Without insurance coverage or adequate, well-implemented state parity laws, most families must exhaust their savings and hock everything they own to garner such resources.[102]

Single-Specialty Eating Disorder Companies
Alsana (formerly Castlewood)

Castlewood, acquired by Trinity Hunt Partners in 2008, was one of the first PE buyouts of ED facilities. Castlewood had been launched by psychologist Mark Schwartz and his wife, clinical social worker Lori Galperin, nine years earlier; the $25 million LBO included significant equity in the place for the founders. Despite the beautiful fifteen-acre landscaped surroundings, Castlewood provided deplorable care. Between 2011 and 2014, the company paid millions to settle at least four malpractice and personal injury cases out of court, all of which were resolved with gag orders attached. As grievances piled up, including lack of supervision at the facility, Schwartz's license was suspended and the couple left.

Even after the discredited Castlewood was bought by Riverside Company in an SBO and recapitalization at the end of 2016, the allegations persisted. In mid-2018, a number of former residents and staff contended that Schwartz had told patients they had multiple disorders or dissociative personality, and many of them took part in satanic cult rituals. He was also charged with implanting false memories through a controversial reprogramming technique that is not accepted practice in the field.[103] Despite losing their licenses in Missouri, Schwartz and Galperin continued operating another facility, Harmony Place in Monterey, California, which also treats ED-afflicted residents. According to Castlewood Victims Unite (CVU), the abusive treatments continue in Monterey.[104]

In 2011, the cofounders of CVU, Bobby and Irene Lerz, had placed their sixteen-year-old daughter in Castlewood, but they soon discovered that she was steadily distancing herself from them, which ultimately ended in complete estrangement. "All of a sudden everyone in her life had abused her," Bobby Lerz said. "It was total indoctrination, a cult." Castlewood would not even let him visit her, even though his insurance company was paying the bill.

After forming CVU, the Lerzes became part of a community of people who either had been "brainwashed" or had a relative who had been; most believed that a family member had maltreated them. According to Lerz, "There has never been any corroboration of these claims . . . not even one substantiation." At least seventy or eighty women—a significant percentage of the total population at Castlewood at the time—have not only recanted the accusations of abuse but explained what happened to them in the facility.[105] They were overmedicated and hypnotized, and the debacle left shattered individuals and destroyed households in its wake. Lerz has a mission: to help as many of these families as possible to heal—and hopefully reunite.

In response to the unsavory reputation of Castlewood, the new PE owners changed its name to Alsana, and "all references to Castlewood have been scrubbed from its website."[106] Since the purchase, Riverside has hired several public relations firms to counteract the lawsuits and adverse revelations. Under its Alsana name, and despite the complaints about staff and treatment methods, the company has expanded to new locations in California and Alabama.

Further, as one CVU member points out, in January 2018 Alsana promoted Nicole Siegfried as its chief clinical officer despite the fact that she was "still on probation and under practice supervision" for having an exploitive relationship with an eating disorder patient and other ethical violations.[107]

Though patient mistreatment has been carefully documented by CVU and others, and two people lost their state licenses for malfeasance, Trinity Hunt Partners, which was complicit in the wrongdoings—or at least did not stop them—washed its hands of the company with no repercussions, selling it for three times its investment.[108] Riverside, too, most likely will bear no consequences for any role it plays in future treatment transgressions, and then it will kick the business to the next owner at an even greater value. One PE associate insisted to me that the negative press had been put behind Alsana.[109]

Eating Recovery Center

Just two years after its Castlewood buyout, Trinity Hunt Partners invested in Eating Recovery Center (ERC) as a minority partner, and in 2012 became its majority owner.[110] Dr. Ken Weiner, who established ERC in 2007 with $1.2 million from several backers, retained equity in the company as it made its consolidation voyage via three PE firms in nine years. After amassing considerable debt financing to open new centers, the Trinity-owned ERC acquired the Moore Center for Eating Disorders (soon renamed the ERC of Washington), the largest eating disorder clinic in the state of Washington. By the end of 2012, ERC had facilities in California, Illinois, Texas, and South Carolina and had grown its profits threefold.

Then, only two years after its investment, Trinity was ready for a sale: Lee Equity Partners and Stellus Capital Management bought and recapitalized the chain for $141.5 million in 2014. They expanded de novo clinics and acquired businesses until the next LBO to CCMP Capital three years later, which brought Lee Equity and Stellus a return of four times their investment.[111] The eating disorder enterprise was now worth an estimated $550 million–$600 million but was saddled with $295 million in new liabilities from the deal.[112] CCMP was not finished; in early 2019 the PE added another $30 million in debt to ERC's ledger. That the initial $1.2 million company had reached a whopping value of $550 million or more by 2019 suggests how much PE shops can exploit a sector that caters to vulnerable people, including adolescents.

Monte Nido

Another residential facility centering on eating disorders, Monte Nido caught the attention of Centre Partners at the end of 2012. As a growth investor, the PE firm supplied debt financing that drove the company's expansion from seven facilities in California and Oregon to include centers in Massachusetts, Pennsylvania, Florida, and New York.[113] As with other eating disorder businesses, Monte Nido was so profitable that it was flipped in less than three years: Levine Leichtman Capital Partners purchased the company, including its $44.8 million debt, via an LBO in 2015. Acquisitions, of course, proliferated as Levine continued to consolidate the chain, reaching into additional states. Most likely, the PE shop is readying the golden goose for its next buyer.

One of the cofounders of Monte Nido, Carolyn Costin, agreed to talk to me but warned that she had to be careful in what she divulged because of the confidentiality agreement she had signed with the PE firm. Nonetheless, it became clear that she had not been pleased with subsequent events. Costin herself had recovered from an eating disorder as a child. She and her husband, Bruce Martin, established Monte Nido in 1996 with the expectation of helping other kids. "It was a passion of mine," she told me. She said that early on they had implemented a ten-year outcome study, contacting former clients regularly; the results indicated that Monte Nido had an 80–85 percent recovery rate. She and her husband now needed a financial partner, but they intended to expand their mom-and-pop shop slowly so as to maintain the individualized, high-quality treatments they were offering.[114]

Costin maintained that with their first PE firm, Centre Partners, there weren't too many difficulties, especially since she still had a significant financial stake in the enterprise. Her husband remained as CEO, and she was the chief clinical officer. "We ran everything," she lamented. "It was a rat race." Costin said that she was working way too hard, more than eighty hours per week. She was not sure why she even needed the PE firm except for its ability to attain funding. But now they had a board of directors, something she had not faced before. In fact, the evidence suggests that Centre may have been steering the ship more than Costin could admit to me: the PE firm held two out of the three seats on the board. I suspect that Centre Partners was driving growth at a considerably faster rate than was comfortable for her, and debt was piling up. Costin mentioned that before their involvement with the PE shop, she and her husband never had any debt.

The next PE owner, Levine Leichtman, seems to have been a more troubling experience, and it moved Monte Nido into a different direction than the Costins had anticipated. They had been assured that there would not be any stark changes but were unpleasantly surprised by the transformations imposed. Carolyn Costin wouldn't (or couldn't) say more. She and her husband (who had suffered two heart attacks by then) left the business. In early 2017, she opened the Carolyn Costin Institute, which trains practitioners in eating disorders treatment. In this new endeavor, she said, "I am not beholden to investors."

Veritas Collaborative

Established in 2010, Veritas's three founders amassed their own debt financing prior to its acquisition by Vestar Capital Partners in 2015.[115] Since then the business has gone the whole hog in borrowing millions every year (sometimes more than once), and added a new minority investor, Lunsford Capital, in 2017. In only four short years, the Vestar-owned company aggressively established five ED facilities in North Carolina, Georgia, and Virginia. Although the Veritas executive team may have grand plans for expanding the chain's geographic footprint further, the clock is ticking for Vestar.

Multispecialty Companies

PE-owned chains with well-established mental health, behavioral health, and substance abuse facilities bring in eating disorder businesses as add-ons to their portfolio companies. For example, Acadia, through Waud and later as a public company, began acquiring places that also included ED treatment.[116] Another chain, Odyssey Behavioral Healthcare, formed by Nautic Partners and CEO Scott Kardenetz in

2015, secured Magnolia Creek, based in Rhode Island, the following year. Among other women-centered services, it helps individuals with eating disorders. In 2017, Odyssey acquired the Indiana-based Selah House Eating Disorder Treatment Centers. The whole package was rolled over to Carlyle Group in a $200 million LBO at the end of 2018.

Conversely, Center for Discovery, founded in 1997, commenced as an eating disorder business and wound up as a company encompassing the gamut of behavioral and addictive diseases.[117] The ED business was first acquired by Webster Equity Partners in 2011 through an LBO and recapitalization, which added $13.28 million in debt to the facility. Subsequently, Webster piled up at least five more rounds of debt financing and refinancing, totaling more than $210 million, for aggressive expansion across the United States. One of its purchases, Cliffside Malibu, is a diversified luxury mental health and substance abuse center that has been lampooned by John Oliver on his political comedy show, Last Week Tonight. The company charges $73,000 monthly for what Oliver's researchers found to be unscientific treatments based on unsubstantiated claims of success.[118]

In early 2016, Webster attempted but failed to sell Center for Discovery—renamed Discovery Behavioral Health—for what it sought, at least $200 million. The PE firm subsequently continued to acquire profitable, wide-ranging mental and behavioral health establishments. As of 2021, Webster still held the company, and I suspect that the PE firm is chomping at the bit to auction it off for a hefty valuation.

Another eating disorders enterprise, Remuda Ranch, was established in 1990 on a scenic 150-acre estate, replete with a pool, horses, yoga, acupuncture, meditation, and beautiful views. The facility has had a circuitous history, enriching several PE houses along the way. Remuda had its first LBO via Prairie Capital and Prospect Partners in 2001 and five years later was turned over, in a $50 million SBO, to Haven Behavioral Healthcare, a platform created by Thoma Bravo and FCA Venture Partners that year.[119] By 2013, in yet another LBO, Remuda was absorbed into the Meadows of Wickenburg, a portfolio company of American Capital, and renamed Meadows Ranch. That lucrative investment lasted only about three years, whereupon Kohlberg & Company acquired the Meadows for $97 million.[120] American Capital realized 2.6 times its equity investment in Remuda, a 28 percent compounded annual return.[121] By becoming part of the Meadows of Wickenburg, the eating disorders facility became just one division of a business that also treats clients with alcohol and substance abuse; sexual disorders; depression and anxiety; psychological conditions; posttraumatic stress disorder; work and money issues; affective disorders; and compulsive behaviors. In other words, if you can pay the big bucks, they will treat you. The prosperous company serves celebrities, the rich, and others who can afford to pay $28,000 a month; it does accept some insurance.[122]

Standing Firm: Avalon Hills

Avalon Hills, located in Logan, Utah, was established by Dr. Benita Quakenbush, who long ago recovered from an eating disorder. According to Lisa Kantor, Quakenbush is adamant and passionate about not selling her place to a PE shop, despite potentially huge financial rewards. She remains true to her mission, which is to discover the best possible techniques for her patients. She collaborates with various specialists and uses neurofeedback to inform Avalon's treatment protocol.[123] Quakenbush is obviously willing to forgo the big bucks in favor of using her company to discover the most efficacious treatment for teenagers and others struggling with ED.

Concluding Remarks

A spiraling demand for substance abuse treatment, expanded coverage for services, a movement in criminal law away from locking up addicts, and the opportunity to consolidate a particularly fragmented area of health care has attracted the voracious appetite of PE shops for massive profits. Investing in the full range of care settings, they have been enriching themselves at the expense of substance abusers and their families, taxpayers, and commercial insurance customers, who face rising premiums. In a nation already overwhelmed with escalating health care expenses, PE entrance into the substance abuse arena has only worsened the situation.

Despite the best intentions of the addicts who enter rehab, those not treated with evidence-based interventions and support most likely will relapse, having an immense adverse effect not only on them and their relatives but on society overall. Substance abuse figures prominently in crime, child and spousal abuse, accidents, unemployment, and poverty.

Eating disorders, although not as headline grabbing as opioid abuse, can destroy individuals and their families just as much. ED was first held as a "medical necessity" by the US Ninth Circuit Court of Appeals in 2014, and subsequent state parity statutes and successful lawsuits resulted in a flood of treatment dollars.[124] But the lack of established procedures and limited industry oversight have left a gaping hole for PE firms to step through and use whatever treatments provide them with the highest margins in the shortest period of time. In fact, the moneyed interests have feasted on a banquet of riches, at times even more profitable than substance abuse, while serving their food-challenged clientele.

The evidence suggests that the United States needs a fundamental structural change in the approach to treating substance abuse and eating disorders. In my view, even greater regulation of the enterprises, though surely essential, would not be sufficient given the financial model of private equity firms. We also require far greater funding to combat these diseases, which are shattering households and debilitating millions of individuals. But throwing money at businesses beset by so many PE firms intent on preying on them is counterproductive at best. The nation must provide support to struggling academic centers and founding owners seeking to assist the low-income population suffering from substance abuse and ED, buoy up nonprofit agencies so that they are not forced into commercial buyouts, and enact legislation rendering it financially unrewarding for the PE industry to profiteer from people in crisis.

8 |

Capitalizing on Children with Autism Spectrum Disorders

NEITHER MEDICAL nor educational professionals can define autism spectrum disorders (ASD) precisely, and there is no consensus on what they actually are. There are even different gauges to diagnose the condition used by physicians, psychologists, and education specialists, thereby blurring the overall eligibility for services.[1] Further, each person has distinct behaviors and needs, rendering ASD a challenging syndrome to treat. In children there are several usual commonalities, but these vary in severity, intensity, and how often they are expressed. Symptoms include diminished eye contact, repetitive behaviors, flapping of hands, difficulty expressing emotions, dearth of communication and social skills, and a deficiency in reading nonverbal cues, such as body language.[2] Individuals with ASD generally face one or more comorbid medical or other indications, including intellectual disability, depression, food and sensory sensitivities, chronic sleep problems, anxiety, epilepsy, gastrointestinal diseases, and attention deficit hyperactivity disorder.

Since there is no definitive medical diagnosis, for example a blood test or MRI, it is unknown exactly how many people are experiencing the disorder or whether the incidence is increasing. Regardless, the number of people labeled as autistic is climbing, along with a greater demand for services. As of 2019, according to the Centers for Disease Control and Prevention, 1 in 59 children were identified as having ASD, up from 1 in 2,000 during the 1970s and 1 in 150 in 2000.[3] John J. Pitney, author of *The Politics of Autism*, suggests that the ASD population will only become larger, especially as children on the spectrum mature, thus expanding the number of adults with the condition. Some experts in the field view this forthcoming growth as a "tsunami."[4] There are already 5.4 million people age eighteen and older living with the condition.

There is no known cure for ASD nor is there a drug to ease its symptoms. However, applied behavior analysis (ABA) is the most evidence-based technique for helping youngsters cope with everyday life by modifying their behavior and teaching them various skills. Despite some controversy over the treatment, especially its rigorous attempt to "normalize" children, the method became the gold standard for early intervention by the late 1990s.

There are multiple sites of service for children with ASD: families can receive help at private clinics, at schools, and at home. Nonprofit agencies, the self-employed, and small agencies provide most of the hands-on therapy; even school-based and social service organizations typically enter into vendor agreements with private contractors.[5] In educational settings, students can also receive speech and occupational therapy, case management, and a personal paraprofessional assistant. Indeed, the treatment of kids with autism tends to outweigh all other per pupil costs.[6]

Who Pays?

Autism did not attract much public attention until the late twentieth century, and there were few, if any, services for people affected by the disorder. Families were, for the most part, on their own in both diagnosis and treatment. After ASD began receiving greater notice from politicians, scientists, interest groups, and the media, Congress in 1990 enacted the Individuals with Disabilities Education Act, whose part B authorized, among other mandates, school districts to offer free and appropriate public educational services for all disabled children between the ages of three and twenty-two years old; autism, for the first time, was named as a distinct entitlement.[7] Through part C, the legislation granted access to government-funded early ABA programs for infants and toddlers under age three. Also in 1990, Congress passed the Americans with Disabilities Act; despite its value for disabled individuals, autism was not a main focus.

Shortly after the launching in 2005 of Autism Speaks, still the foremost advocacy group for people with autism spectrum disorders, Congress approved the Combating Autism Act (2006); it was reauthorized in 2011, and in 2014 it was renamed the Autism CARES Act (Autism Collaboration, Accountability, Research, Education, and Support Act). Since then, federal funding for ASD has reached more than $3.1 billion, but most of the money supports basic research rather than services per se.[8] By 2010, because of intense lobbying, ASD captured the notice of local political communities. Subsequently, state by state, legislators began requiring commercial insurers to cover ABA as a benefit in their plans. Currently, 94 percent of insurers have some form of specific mandate for the therapy, thus shifting some early intervention costs from the government to insurance companies.[9]

Nonetheless, Medicaid and CHIP are significant sources of funding, especially for children. Through state plans and waivers, more than 50 percent of children with special needs, including autism, and another 45 percent of nonelderly adults with disabilities (who qualify for SSI) receive at least some services. During 2017, 2.9 million children and 8.8 million adults obtained such aid. In most states, Medicaid pays for the largest portion of at-home and community assistance for children with autism.[10] The 2010 Affordable Care Act expanded financing for programs under the Americans with Disabilities Act as well, mostly by enlarging the Medicaid-eligible population and disallowing denial of insurance coverage based on preconditions, including autism. In addition, more babies are being screened and diagnosed with the condition since the legislation requires the availability of preventive services at no charge.

According to Bryna Siegel, an expert in the field, there are more services, and more costly services, for children with autism than for those with any other developmental disability or disorder. Expenditures for in-home ABA early intervention, generally fifteen to thirty hours of treatment per week, can be high.[11] However, families muddling through the bureaucratic labyrinth of programs and financial assistance soon become aware that the availability of treatment is seriously limited relative to the need; in some places, there are long waiting lists. Dr. Lynn Koegel, a professor at Stanford University, clinician, and author of several books on autism, explained that families who are not satisfied with their children's therapy tend to stay anyway out of fear they will not find a spot elsewhere.[12]

The ability to procure education-based assistance often depends on the willingness of and resources available to states and local school districts. Certain households may have to forgo assistance through Medicaid because their state has not expanded coverage under the Affordable Care Act or is stingy with its coverage of care for children with ASD. In reality, most help provided to youngsters with autism comes from parents, many of whom must sacrifice their jobs and financial well-being.

Whetting the Appetite

The increase in both ASD funding and the number of people diagnosed with the disorder, along with the prolonged treatment for them, certainly has not escaped the attention of the private equity industry: firms are rushing for the gold. Indeed, autism therapy has the potential to be extremely lucrative. As with other human needs in the United States, such services are viewed as just another market good, with more than $10 billion in annual revenues for community-based ABA providers and more than $7 billion for those that are school-based.[13]

PE interest in the sector was noticeably sparked by the states' legislation requiring commercial insurance companies to pay for ASD treatment. That essentially opened the spigot, allowing for free-flowing cash. But the other main sources of funding—school-based treatments, Medicaid, and CHIP—also guarantee an ongoing, stable flow of money, a main criterion for PE interest in a sector. Low labor costs, too, are enticing. Registered behavior technicians (RBTs), who can be assigned most of the hands-on therapy, do not even need a college degree. By and large, the businesses pay them an average of $31,000 a year while procuring far more from the various funding sources for themselves. According to one source, autism therapy firms earn between $15 and $80 billion annually, or up to $60,000 per child.[14] The average gross revenue of ABA centers is slightly under $825,000.[15]

There are more than 4,000 nonprofit and private behavioral health service companies, many of them relatively small and none publicly traded. To date, there are few relatively large multistate establishments that provide ABA programs, but more places are spreading their reach. Nevertheless, autism is still mostly a cottage industry; there is an assortment of regional and local providers, no one enterprise dominates, and only a handful have a national presence. All of this is precisely what makes ASD so attractive for the PE business model: it is ripe for consolidation.

PE firms tentatively entered the ASD sector in the early 2000s with Trimaran Capital Partners's acquisition of Educational Services of America (rebranded as ChanceLight) in 2004. By 2016, and especially during 2018 and later, such deals skyrocketed despite high market prices. PE firms have been gobbling up and merging pieces of the pie, building financial value for themselves. They are on an autism rampage, ready to increase their market share and geographic footprint. Thus far, according to Provident Healthcare Partners, PE buyouts have been immensely profitable.[16] The industry has discovered autism, but its entry into the space is just beginning, and ultimately general partners intend to take over as much of the sector as possible.

I have been told by founder-owners of autism treatment centers that they are barraged with material from PE firms seeking to talk about buying their businesses. John McEachin, cofounder of the nonprofit Autism Partnership, has received at least a dozen unsolicited requests. He suspects there would be a lot more if his company were larger. He will not turn it over in any case, he said, because the purpose and values of the private equity industry—mainly its focus on maximizing profit—clash with his own and his staff's concern for children with autism.[17] Other individuals I have talked with related stories of aggressive sales tactics, especially if their business is well suited for a PE shop's overall growth plan.[18] Many founders, whether they are near retirement or not, are selling their relatively small agencies to PE firms because they can get substantial cash from the deal and hold on to an equity stake; this has proved to be financially worthwhile, especially given the high valuations nowadays. They can also realize even more money, along with the GPs, each time the business undergoes another LBO.

On the other hand, myriad nonprofit and small private agency owners have not yet succumbed to the lure of PE dollars. Dr. Bridget A. Taylor, a founder and CEO of the nonprofit Alpine Learning Group, told me that she just ignores letters of interest from PE firms. She made it clear that it is crucial to pay attention to identifiable outcomes for children, something that PE-owned places tend to ignore; they are mostly interested in growing businesses. Taylor added that ABA professionals are deeply concerned about the increasing takeover of ASD treatment by the PE industry.[19]

Another founder-owner I spoke with, Dr. Julie Crittendon, said that she receives information every day from PE firms interested in buying her out. "It is ongoing, and I try to screen them out." She admitted, however, that she would consider a sale to a PE house when she is ready to retire. She indicated that there are no alternatives beyond just closing up shop, a refrain I have heard from many other owners of small health companies and doctor practices.[20]

Crittendon began her career as a professor at Vanderbilt University, engaging in research on autism. Intensely interested in hands-on involvement, she left academia in 2015 to start her own company, Autism Center for Children. In addition to clinical work, she has designed a model training clinic to prepare others to be competent clinicians. Crittendon views that as her main mission: to do a small part in enhancing autism treatment. Her clinic is debt-free, the usual situation for most autism clinics—until GPs get their hands on them.

She was emphatic on why so many others surrender their companies to PE. "It's the insurance industry," she told me. "It's 100 percent grief in dealing with them. They just drop kids without explanation." Crittendon provided a few examples of what she (and everyone else in the autism treatment business) must deal with. One child she had been working with for a year, providing thirty-five hours a week of therapy, was simply cut off. She had to spend a month writing appeals to reinstate insurance payments for his therapy. "Kids regress if you simply stop," she said. In another case, there were two children in the same family being treated. They were illegally denied benefits after a certain amount of time; Crittendon treated them for months without pay while she and her lawyers disputed the termination. Eventually the insurance company paid, but she explained that others in the same situation, who do not have someone willing to fight for them, would have to forgo treatment to which they are entitled.

Sacrificing the Children

Undoubtedly, autism therapy has become a hot market for PE firms, and whether they are generalists or specialists in health care, they are rapidly moving into the sector. Though ASD enterprises largely attract middle-market investors, some of the largest shops in the world have entered the arena, such as Blackstone Group, KKR, and TPG Capital. As I detail below, a wide range of PE firms have been drawn in, all with one goal: an exceptional return on their investment.[21]

Many of the factors that have caught the eye of PE houses also render them unsuited to providing high-quality care to individuals with the disorder. For example, the lack of clinical standardization for ABA treatment and clashes over strategy among parents, people with ASD, government officials, and lobbyists create a huge opening for offering the least expensive but second-rate services. Dr. William Frea, a clinician, educator, and cofounder of an autism treatment center, Autism Spectrum Therapies, stressed that there is no standard ABA strategy.

There can be varying amounts of hours, types of supervision, collection of outcome data (if any), and level of personnel training.[22] Indeed, according to Koegel, the implementation of ABA therapy is not systematic nor has it been perfected. For instance, should providers start with verbal or nonverbal issues? How much time should be devoted to each? What other concerns should be targeted? What is best for long-term outcomes? Far more research is required, she explained.[23]

In her 2018 book, *Autism Matters*, Dr. Ronit Molko concurs, arguing that there are many versions of ABA-based service delivery, some more watered-down than others. Many providers "also often lack in quality assurance measures." She also observes, "ABA service providers have yet to establish agreed-upon standards of measurement when it comes to determining the outcomes of intervention. ABA is the process, not the outcome: the change in behavior or the acquisition of skills is the measured outcome."[24]

The treatment of ASD is unique among disorders, John McEachin of Autism Partnership told me; it requires considerable expertise. One needs to follow the child's lead without precise directions, and that takes experience and know-how. He is particularly concerned about the negligible qualifications of RBTs, the frontline workers who apply the therapies. Since 2014, they only need to be eighteen years old, have a high school degree, and participate in forty hours of training, which he argued is seriously insufficient.[25] Koegel agrees. She observed that implementation is a large problem since companies are increasingly placing employees in hands-on positions who are not equipped to deal with autistic children or their families; high rates of turnover exacerbate the problem. She stressed that in autism services, the more experience a paraprofessional has the better; some of them, she told me, "feel like they are just babysitting." They do not know what to do until a supervisor arrives, and that could take some time since in many places supervisors are overburdened. Many enterprises are not keeping up with the latest evidence-based ABA procedures, she added.[26]

GPs tout their contribution to aiding children with autism by pointing out the previous dearth of services that they are now supplying.

This is a common refrain throughout the PE industry: its leveraged buyouts, growth capital, and consolidations have led to the rapid availability of ABA treatment for countless more children across the nation. Unfortunately, bigger doesn't necessarily mean better. Alongside the proliferation of centers and the number of therapists have come detrimental economies, such as less intensive training and supervision, cookie-cutter approaches to treatment, and lack of reliable data collection, all of which lead to mediocre care, at best.

Molko, for instance, observes that while "growth has increased access, it has diluted the quality and integrity of the implementation of ABA in the field." And that means that many of the children with ASD will be funded for ABA services, but not receive the type of therapy that would enhance their well-being or help them achieve greater independence and control over their lives. She cautions that "ABA in the wrong hands can be detrimental and even counterproductive."[27]

Koegel is troubled by the role of higher profits in the rapid expansion of autism clinics; she has noticed that many students in the field now aim to establish a private business rather than engage in research to improve ABA techniques.[28] Others, too, decry the disturbing attitude of young professionals who are obtaining a degree just for the purpose of building an autism therapy chain, with the intention of selling it later at an inflated price. According to Frea, a number of these newly minted graduates think that they can outcompete other owners with greater efficiencies. He believes that children with autism need protection against businesses that do not have their best interests in mind.[29]

The US government mandates an entitlement to services for children on the spectrum but does not guarantee that these will be of the best quality. And there are no external checks on the effectiveness of services.[30] In the PE industry, a mainstay of building a company's value is fostering efficiency. Clearly, GPs seek to devise the most cost-effective ABA treatments, regardless of the human consequences. They tend to rely more extensively on less experienced, low-wage frontline employees, assign two or more children to a therapist concurrently, and provide substantially less supervision. After all, since labor represents most of the cost of serving individuals with ASD, there are few other places to cut dollars and increase cash flow to pay off hefty LBO debt or grab a dividend recap or two.

Such cost-saving measures also could be quite attractive to local school districts and state Medicaid programs, all of which have been under financial pressures for years. However, as McEachin pointed out, low-quality ASD programs will ultimately cost Medicaid more in long-term care expenses.[31] Further, as nearly all experts agree, to attain optimal benefits from ABA, the therapist should be skilled, well trained, and have time to develop a meaningful relationship with the child.[32] Sophisticated ABA is expensive: it requires one-on-one assistance, is laborious, and involves regular measurement and adaptation. Such high standards are not well suited to the PE business model, where finances, marketing, and growth trump all other concerns, unlike most founder-owners who value supporting youngsters with ASD and providing high-quality care.

The Financiers: Leading the Way
Autism Learning Partners (rebranded from Pacific Child and Family Associates)

One top company, Autism Learning Partners (ALP), provides ABA treatment along with occupational, physical, and speech therapy in the full range of sites. Founded in 1988 by Dr. Ira Heilveil in Southern California, the company was a sole proprietorship before he entered the PE world in 2009 with investments from Great Point Partners and Jefferson River Capital. According to Heilveil, at the time ALP was a relatively small entity, with $1.12 million in revenues.[33] In 2010, the company received more development capital, $12.65 million, from a third investor, Hercules Capital, followed in 2013 by a fourth investor, Scopia Capital Management.

Much of the money was used for leveraged buyouts, accumulating debt along the way. In 2011, ALP acquired Children's Learning Connection. Founded by two speech and language pathologists in 2000, the small enterprise was added to Great Point's portfolio company along with Autism Services North. In a 2013 buyout, ALP extended its geographic reach farther with the purchase of Autism Intervention Specialists from its founder, Nassim Aoude. Three years later, the chain bought Proof Positive ABA Therapies from its original owner, Heather Grimaldi, and in 2017, Aspire Autism. These, too, were tucked into the portfolio company. Heilveil told me, "ALP was massively in debt, and some people questioned whether the company would survive."[34]

Nonetheless, Great Point and the other investors had added financial value for themselves through the acquisitions and consolidations, and they were ready to collect. At the end of 2017 they sold the company in an SBO to FFL Partners for more than $270 million; the deal was at such a high valuation that it pricked up the ears of the PE industry overall.[35]

Heilveil pointed out that Pacific Child and Family Associates was one of the first autism ABA companies sold to a PE firm. He had received mass-mailing inquiries at the time from ten houses and obtained concrete offers from three of them, mostly because of the company's 15 percent gross margin and track record of growth. After more than twenty years at his establishment, he had been ready to sell, and there were few other options available. He stayed on as CEO for three years, as required by his contract. However, he immediately clashed with Great Point as it attempted to slash costs as much as possible; the PE firm had different values than he had. Heilveil was particularly upset by its efforts to cut employee health benefits. Later, the PE firm exerted massive pressure to "produce numbers" by incentivizing supervisors to increase productivity. At the same time, frontline workers experienced significantly less training and guidance, all of which stressed them considerably. He indicated that because of his respectful treatment of employees, his retention rates had been quite high for the industry; after PE involvement, there was extreme turnover, leading to inferior care. Given the generally low pay in the autism field, the staff tends to be motivated to help children and families, not to grow a company, he said.[36]

The new PE-appointed CEO steadily replaced management with "money people" who cared only about earnings. ALP's quality of care deteriorated: "It was just not the same company." Heilveil pointedly said of Great Point and its administrative team: there was "nothing they wouldn't do [to make a buck]. . . . They have no morality. . . . It is an amoral world. Beyond cruel in some ways." He could not provide more details about his time with the PE shop because he had signed a nondisclosure agreement.

Great Point's website touts ALP's gains under its ownership: locations grew from three to thirty states; hiring increased from 300 to 1,800 therapists; revenues rose by 30 percent annually; and speech, occupational, and physical therapies were added to its offerings. The PE shop proudly announces that the chain became the largest provider of ABA treatment in the country.[37] Nowhere in the section on how Great Point helped ALP is there anything it did to improve services for autistic children and their families.

Since the end of 2017, it has been the turn of the new owner, FFL Partners, to squeeze cash out of ALP's autism services for children. Aaron Money, FFL's representative, told PE Hub that its intention, before exiting, is to increase the company's value by expanding nationwide and augmenting places of service, especially where reimbursements are highest.[38] The buying spree goes on, with no particular advantages—and many disadvantages—for the beneficiaries of its services.

Invo Healthcare Associates

Founded in 1993 by Mary and Patrick McClain in Jamison, Pennsylvania, Invo Healthcare Associates is one of the earlier therapy staffing providers for autism spectrum disorders secured by a private equity firm. Mary McClain informed me that her husband, an occupational therapist, perceived a gap between the demand in schools for services and their availability. In those days, professionals were even hesitant to diagnose autism in children. The McClains established Invo in their basement and grew it to a robust company. Its offerings included occupational, speech/language, and physical therapies in addition to autism treatment; she was adamant that a focus on autism alone is not sufficient for children on the spectrum.[39]

When the McClains sought an exit strategy, they received more than twelve offers for the enterprise. In 2013, Post Capital Partners acquired the place through a management buyout and recapitalization. With no particular expertise in ASD or even health services, Post Capital at the time also invested in EC Waste (waste management); BHS Specialty Chemicals (for the food processing and water treatment industries); DTT Surveillance (assistance for quick service restaurants); and ABRA (auto body and glass services). It is unclear what advantages the PE firm could have offered Invo beyond debt financing for acquisitions, especially given the short time it held the company. Apparently, except for assisting with the company's database of therapists, that is all Post Capital did.

I asked Mary McClain how much control she and her management team retained after the buyout. She claimed that they continued to lead Invo during the short time she stayed on. Post Capital had required her to sign a two-year, renewable contract "because they don't know how to run [an autism treatment] company," she said. "They need you there." But she had to justify expenditures that did not explicitly add to the bottom line. For example, she wanted to sponsor a Special Olympics in Pennsylvania, but the PE firm questioned the outlay. In another case, McClain hired additional therapists, thereby cutting the profit margin that year. The PE firm grilled her on that as well. In fact, whenever she changed any budget item, she had to defend its financial benefit. "[Post] Capital Partners was always concerned about getting a good return on its investment," she remarked. Sometimes the managers said no to her when she introduced changes that were not in the PE's plans. In other words, the focus was always primarily on earnings and selling the company at the maximum value feasible.

I also questioned McClain on her view of the mounting financial liabilities that Invo was taking on through its ongoing LBOs.[40] She was clear that the company had no debt prior to its acquisition by Post Capital and that she was uncomfortable at first. But the company was growing at about 15–20 percent a year and was able to pay the obligations down. Nonetheless, McClain observed that she could have continued operating the company without the PE shop; Invo was profitable, and she really did not need the loans except for growth.[41]

In short order, Invo continued its PE odyssey. In a second management LBO at the end of 2016, Wicks Group, another shop with no expertise in ASD, acquired the enterprise. Researchers at PitchBook estimate that not only did Post Capital "earn" 6.5 times its four-year investment, but it retained a minority share in the place. The Jordan Company, which finances everything from consumer products and aerospace to automotive and chemical products, invested in Invo the following year, placing $70.8 million more debt on the business.

Eager to grab agencies in the new rush for ASD treatment providers, Invo (through Wicks) acquired more businesses, including Autism Home Support Services (AHSS) in 2017. AHSS provides ABA services in Illinois, Michigan, and Colorado. Employees seem to have noticed the change, as indicated by two typical reviews on glassdoor.com:

> Behavioral technician who worked full time for five years at AHSS (March 2019): "If you had asked me 18 months ago I would have had a ton of pros but since they were bought by Invo there are no pros. I guess the one pro is they don't care if you quit even after 5 years. Company does not care about employees[;] we are just a means to an end to get money from insurance. Focus moved from being client focused to fulfilling the most amount of hours even at the cost of your own sanity. BCBAs [board-certified behavior analysts] are given an unethical amount of clients to try to manage and are expected to also train and supervise new employees. RBTs are hired in at ridiculously low amounts and most are unqualified and terrible at their jobs. . . . They force out most full time RBTs in favor of part time new hires and they can't staff half their clients. They are bleeding quality staff and desperate for anyone to work with them and they under pay so you get what you pay for when it comes to staff."

> Current employee, an RBT (October 2018): "All about the bottom line, no longer about the client—this is proven by how many employees have left the company because of administrative issues! Constant struggle for hours. Erratic schedule[.] Growing too much too fast. Hiring cheaper, less

experienced part time staff which is taking away hours from full time staff—full timers are leaving the company left and right. A year ago I would have said the senior management and culture/values were all PHENOMENAL—since we've 'merged' with Invo things are changing for the worse and fast."[42]

By 2018, Invo provided therapy staffing services, including ABA, in twenty-seven states. Wicks continued its shopping spree, and debt mounted, reaching $229.4 million in early 2019. That Fall, Golden Gate Capital acquired the chain in a third LBO. Although the sale price is not publicly available, with such a hot market, the PE investors undoubtedly earned a pretty penny.

Stepping Stones Group (rebranded from MyTherapyCompany)

The Stepping Stones Group (SSG) is another company that has led the charge in demonstrating the enormous value of the autism market. A foremost staffing company that provides occupational, speech, physical, and autism treatment therapists for schools and private learning centers, by 2019 it served more than 400 school districts and employed 1,300 clinicians and special educators in more than thirty states.

In 2014, Shore Capital Partners (along with Resolute Capital Partners and BPEA Private Equity) invested in MyTherapyCompany, founded by Dr. Michael McBurnie, an expert in the field; it was soon renamed the Stepping Stones Group.[43] During Shore's short ownership, roughly three and a half years, SSG acquired AlphaVista Services (2016) and Staffing Options Solutions (2017).[44] McBurnie told me that the PE approached him about selling the business; he hadn't even thought about putting it on the market nor did he have much interest in enlarging it. He would have been content to keep MyTherapyCompany as it was, or perhaps expand it slowly. His concentration was on helping children with autism and other developmental disorders.[45]

When I asked McBurnie about Shore Capital's contribution to the company, he said that the PE brought in experts for building it up, provided a strategy for growth, and supplied capital. In other words,

Shore did little more than scale MyTherapyCompany by acquiring places from founder-owners and seeking debt financing. It certainly did not improve services, although McBurnie emphasized that there is a shortage of staffing for schools, and Shore Capital's investments added to the supply. He also stated that Shore did not pressure him to cut costs, though he's unsure what the next PE owners will do. In the end, Shore Capital "earned" seven times its investment when it sold SSG to Five Arrows Capital Partners at the end of 2017.[46]

The new owners continued the consolidation of ABA therapy companies. Two months after its SBO, SSG acquired Cobb Pediatric Therapy, based in Kennesaw, Georgia. In 2019, the chain spread its reach to New York City with the leveraged buyout of the Perfect Playground, which serves public schools.[47] Five Arrows then purchased StaffRehab (2019), New England ABA (2019), STAR of CA (2020), Ardor School Solutions (2020), and EBS Healthcare (2021).

The Stepping Stones Group has emerged as one of the fastest growing autism treatment providers. Similar to other PE-owned chains in the sector, it has bought businesses that for the most part were founded by clinicians, many of whom were passionate about their work. The ongoing fixation of Five Arrows on acquisitions, consolidation, and readying the Stepping Stones Group for sale does not bode well for the welfare of the youngsters it serves.

LEARN Behavioral (rebranded from Learn It Systems)

Founded by Michael Maloney in 2007, Learn It Systems—renamed LEARN Behavioral in May 2018—treats children with ASD and other special needs through programs in schools, in private clinics, and at home. By 2018, it had services in thirty states and 200 school districts.

Since its first private equity LBO and recapitalization in 2010, the company has bounced to two more PE firms. In the initial one, Milestone Partners (a minority investor) had no expertise in health services; rather, it concentrated on three main sectors: financial services, tech-driven manufacturing, and tech-enabled solutions. Nevertheless, during Milestone's investment in Learn It, there were four PE representatives on its board of directors. As usual, financial gain had become Learn It Systems's top priority. During Milestone's ownership the company initiated a course of acquisitions and mergers that continued throughout its later PE investor years. The initial Milestone-backed LBOs included Trellis Services (2014), Autism Spectrum Therapies (2014), and Beach Cities Learning (2015).[48]

I spoke with Dr. Kathy Niager, founder of Trellis Services (the first of the companies purchased via Milestone), about the transaction and its aftermath. She, like many other founders, had been doing well but decided that Learn It (and presumably its PE owner) could provide both administrative and financial support to assist in Trellis's growth. There was great demand in schools and the community for autism services, she said, and she wanted to accommodate that need. At the time she was being wooed, Learn It seemed to her to be the perfect balance between high-quality care and commercial success. But she was quickly disillusioned: Milestone did not treat her well afterward and was quite disorganized. Niager told me she became frustrated: the PE firm was supposed to be the financial expert, but it did not perform simple tasks like paying bills on time. Moreover, during her ownership of Trellis Services the company had no debt. She later learned that Learn It was in financial distress.[49]

Despite Niager's decades-long experience with children with ADS and with ABA, the PE owner was not interested in hearing about clinical issues; it was only concerned about the bottom line. She had created Trellis Services, working hard for ten years; Niager stated that during that time, she and her staff had continuously advanced the company's ABA treatment model and training. Trellis was "her baby," and now that the investors had taken charge her expertise was ignored. Additionally, prior to the sale, she and her team had felt like family. Niager maintained that there had been a supportive and caring culture, and the staff struggled against the altered tone and the pressure to focus exclusively on finances. The best people subsequently departed. She left six months after the sale.

Learn It Systems's subsequent PE investor, LLR Partners, added $26 million in new debt for its SBO (2016). During its brief involvement,

LLR and Learn It went on a shopping tear, acquiring Behavioral Concepts, Inc. (2017), Advances Learning Center (2018), Play Connections (2018), and Total Spectrum (2018).[50] Less than three years later, after piling up debt and building the financial value of the company, LLR was ready to dump the assets. In 2019, the company was handed over to Gryphon Investors through a lucrative third LBO.

To learn more about Learn It Systems and its PE-financed acquisitions, I interviewed Frea, the cofounder of Autism Spectrum Services, a company bought through Milestone Partners. He said that it began as a mom-and-pop shop in Los Angeles. He had directed an MA training program for autism professionals at California State University and became acutely aware that public schools were in dire need of knowledgeable therapists; that engendered the creation of Autism Spectrum Therapies in 2001.[51]

He stated that by 2006 he and his partner, Ronit Molko, had grown the company large enough to spark the curiosity of PE firms. He was barraged with unsolicited interest in Autism Spectrum Therapies. GPs would show up at various conferences on autism and offer to buy founder-owners dinner or offer similar enticements to talk about acquiring their company. He said the PE shops were focused on the big fish, and the first thing they would ask owners is how much revenue their place brought in. He was more intent on helping children on the spectrum than in being taken over by another company. By 2014, however, Frea was ready to move on, and he and Molko sold Autism Spectrum Therapies to Learn It.

Molko stayed on the management team for two years and then left. Frea said that PE firms generally keep previous executives only for as long as they need them for the transition but then bring in people who are more in line with their financial goals. He pointed out that founder-owners tend to be opposed to certain efficiency measures, such as curtailing staff training, hiring unlicensed professionals to perform therapy, and diluting treatments. It became clear to him in his discussions with other PE-owned autism providers that PE shops are not interested in the ABA clinical process or anything other than streamlining the company and extracting as much money as possible. He maintained that in the autism business there is just so much that can be trimmed without negatively affecting children. And staff often leave when that occurs. People who establish and build an ABA company, on the other hand, tend to spend time regularly assessing clinical outcomes and enjoy the challenge of improving them.

His cofounder, Molko, had a different take on the situation. She told me that though there are some bad actors out there, PE firms can augment the autism industry—especially by providing funds for expanding access to children and families in need of treatment. She added that there are financiers who care about the quality of autism services, and with the right team, they can put together high-level clinical designs that take outcome measurements into account.[52] On the other hand, she wrote in her book, *Autism Matters*: "The large players in the market have generally but not always, done a better job at executing growth, but many forgo clinical quality and meaningful long-term outcomes in favor of that growth. Investors see the value and strong return in this rapidly growing marketplace but may not be putting enough emphasis on the importance of clinical integrity, adhering to best practices, and long-term quality outcomes."[53] She also admitted to me that she is concerned about the high level of debt imposed on some autism treatment chains.[54]

ChanceLight Behavioral Health, Therapy and Education (rebranded from Educational Services of America)

One of the earliest providers of special programs for kids with behavioral disorders that was plucked by private equity, Educational Services of America was established in 1999; nearly five years later it was sold to Trimaran Capital Partners in a $35 million LBO. Through the backing of Trimaran, Educational Services of America—rebranded ChanceLight—engaged in multiple rounds of debt financing to purchase a host of places.[55] In the process, Trimaran extracted at least $3.8 million for itself, most likely through dividend recaps.[56] The PE firm had no special interest in kids with autism; its investments over the years include packaged ice, cabinetry, fast food chicken restaurants, and a community hospital.

At least one of ChanceLight's early acquisitions was subjected to a lawsuit under the federal False Claims Act. The cofounders of Early Autism Project and its director of clinical services were indicted on charges that from 2007 to 2016 they padded the hours that therapists were billing Medicaid and Tricare for autistic treatments and charged them for services that were never rendered. Nine million dollars in taxpayer money had been squandered by the largest provider of care for children with ASD in South Carolina, and the youngsters had been seriously shortchanged. The cofounders and the director also pleaded guilty to kickbacks and bribes to clients. In addition to paying millions to settle the case, ChanceLight had to agree to an independent oversight of Early Autism Project's future claims.[57]

Mark Claypool, the founder of ChanceLight, notes on the company's website that he is "focused on the needs of kids first."[58] The author of two books on autism and related disorders also states in a 2017 *Huffington Post* interview: "Some people ask why I didn't try to operate ChanceLight as a not-for-profit and I tell them that would have required an endless pursuit of fundraising that would have diverted attention from the company's mission. As a social entrepreneur, I formed ChanceLight as a private company, giving me access to capital and other resources that allow ChanceLight to focus on its mission in the most effective and sustainable way possible."[59]

All the same, ChanceLight was in the hands of a zombie PE firm; since its acquisition of the chain, Trimaran Capital could not raise a third fund. In 2012, it had requested an extension for exiting its second one which, according to Dan Primack, a reporter for *Fortune*, "would allow Trimaran to collect millions in management fees over the next several years. And would also erase a clawback that Trimaran owes to its investors for charging carried interest on specific deals, even though the broader fund has not met its minimum hurdles for such payments." Without the extension, Trimaran "threatened to simply distribute illiquid shares in Trimaran's remaining portfolio companies, thus washing its hands of any future responsibility."[60] Finally, the PE shop unloaded ChanceLight to the Halifax Group for $125 million in 2018, with the LBO piling on $58 million in new debt. By that time, Trimaran had also grabbed ample earnings from the business and held millions in shares.[61]

Community Intervention Services

Established by H. I. G. Growth Partners and Kevin Sheehan in 2012, "CIS was formed to acquire, develop and operate a national network of specialized mental health and substance abuse facilities and programs."[62] Its first acquisition, South Bay Community Services, served as its platform for future buyouts. The founder of CIS, Dr. Peter Scanlon, who became chief clinical officer of South Bay, received more than $31 million from H. I. G.'s leveraged buyout of his company.[63] With ABA treatment as part of its initial offerings, in subsequent LBOs CIS acquired several agencies specifically focused on services for kids with ASD.[64] In addition to Massachusetts and Pennsylvania, by 2018 it had expanded to localities in Connecticut, Georgia, North Carolina, and South Carolina.

It is unclear what H. I. G. had to offer CIS in terms of expertise in autism, behavioral health, or substance abuse. The PE firm's portfolio companies, past and present, range from aerospace/defense and manufacturing to media and business services. Eric Tencer, H. I. G.'s chief representative for CIS, also spreads his attention widely: he works on digital, media, and business services as well as health care.

H. I. G. Growth Partners is yet another example of how PE shops can exploit their portfolio companies at the expense of children with mental disabilities and developmental delays. CIS and South Bay, along with Sheehan and Scanlon, were accused of hiring unqualified mental health workers and inexperienced supervisors to serve Medicaid patients in seventeen Massachusetts health centers from 2009 to 2015; the directors of the individual clinics, too, were deemed unqualified and without proper credentials. It was alleged that Sheehan and Scanlon had been fully aware of the fraudulent activities, which affected more than 35,000 children annually. In 2018, CIS was forced to pay $4 million to settle a federal whistleblower fraud case and undergo an internal compliance program.[65] Both Sheehan and Scanlon departed the company.

In October 2020, according to the Private Equity Stakeholder Project, H. I. G. sold most of the CIS subsidiaries to Atar Capital. Three months later, CIS filed for bankruptcy. Two of the remaining affiliates, South Bay and Futures Behavioral Therapy Center, were bought out of bankruptcy by Centerbridge Partners for $39.5 million. Unsurprisingly, H. I. G. has not paid any price for the harmful effects on kids and the collapse of CIS. To the contrary, the PE firm continues to acquire health care companies.[66]

Trumpet Behavioral Health

Assisting children and adults with ASD in eight states by 2019, Trumpet Behavioral Health has obtained PE financing since it was established. One of its cofounders, Lani Fritts, told me that his background was in management rather than behavioral health. However, after a few years working in a technology company, he decided he wanted to do something more mission-oriented, and he and Chris Miller explored health care services. At the time, reimbursement of ABA services through commercial insurance had become more common, piquing their interest in autism.[67] In 2008, they met with two proprietors who were engaged in ABA research and consulting for school systems in Southern California and who were ready to retire and cash in on their businesses.[68] In 2009, through loan financing from three minority investors (HCP & Co., GrowthWorks, and Peterson Partners), Fritts and Miller merged the two companies and began the expansion process, beginning with six locations in Northern California and Hawaii. From that time on, they transformed Trumpet into a service model for ASD facilities.[69]

By 2017, the two cofounders were barraged with solicitations from PE firms, and they sold the chain to MTS Health Investors (later rebranded as WindRose Health Investors) in March of that year. The PE firm appointed as CEO Ned Carlson, a person with no background in autism therapy; rather, his expertise is in "technology-enabled service markets" and "providing intelligent claims routing, re-pricing optimization, cost containment and data analysis to healthcare payers."[70] That did not bode well for the future quality of Trumpet's services to vulnerable children.

Lani Fritts left the company and took a few years off. He said that during that time he received phone calls from various investors in the field. He eventually chose TPG Capital because he sensed that one of its senior advisors, Dr. Fred Cohen, was interested in building and scaling a high-quality company, especially because he had a daughter with ASD.[71] In 2019, TPG, along with Viola Ventures, launched a new platform, Kadiant, with Fritts as its CEO. The company's goal, similar to others in the autism market, is to consolidate existing businesses and expand its footprint geographically.[72] By the end of 2019 they had acquired at least eight places.

Camelot Education

Spun out of Camelot System of Care, Camelot Education operates residential educational facilities for students with disciplinary problems or who are at risk for not graduating, along with therapeutic day schools for youngsters with ASD, learning disabilities, emotional disorders, and orthopedic impairments. Contracting with school districts and charter schools, the organization serves kids in kindergarten through high school. As of 2019, there were roughly thirty-two residential places across six states; in addition, there were seven therapeutic day schools in Illinois and one in Philadelphia (grades 9–12). In a 2011 LBO, the Riverside Company acquired Camelot Education from Charterhouse Group (which had bought Camelot System of Care in 2006) for an estimated $100 million.[73] Todd Bock, its president, is a former executive with the Brown Schools, a troubled company under whose care at least five children died from restraints between 1988 and 2003.[74]

Camelot Education has a scandalous history. The residential schools have been accused by students and their parents of undue disciplinary actions, including beatings. In Philadelphia, Teach for America instructors observed "choke-holds, employees pinning students down with a knee in their back, and 'body slamming.' "[75] Teach for America's executive director, who visited on several occasions, noticed that staff and administrators "verbally berated students." At the Paramount Academy in Reading, Pennsylvania, parents also complained of abusive behavior, such as the use of excessive force in restraining children.[76] In addition, Camelot carried out full-body searches, even in its schools that did not have behaviorally challenged students.[77]

Molly Hensley-Clancy, a reporter for BuzzFeed News, argues that Camelot "has made a growing business out of taking in troubled kids at sharp discounts compared to publicly run schools, allowing the districts to slash costs—and, at times, to improve their own metrics by shunting off their lowest-performing students."[78] In New Jersey, Camelot promised to operate its Millville school for only $8,000 per pupil, as compared to the $15,000 the district had been spending. Indeed, cost savings is Camelot's chief marketing tool. Its employees tend to be untrained and underpaid, sometimes dramatically so, allowing it to offer bargain prices. Yet despite the accusations of beatings, aggression, and body slamming, Camelot has sustained its growth and experiences few government inspections.[79]

Riverside Company is not daunted by the transgressions: the schools are worth millions to its PE owner. For example, Camelot's contract with Philadelphia is valued at $10 million annually.[80] In Chicago, the company raked in $50 million from 2014 to 2017.[81] The financiers pocket the money, and the students—including those with autism—are given short shrift.

Some school districts are fighting back. In Houston, the school board voted unanimously in 2017 to rescind its $8.6 million contract after newspaper accounts of the abuses.[82] Camelot also lost a $6.4 million annual contract in Georgia's Muscogee County School District by a single vote; one of the slashed programs was for a therapeutic day school.[83] Elsewhere, Camelot continues its operations as a PE portfolio company, providing outsized profits to its owner.

Rebecca School

Another controversial array of schools for children with special needs is MetSchools, a New York City education management company founded by Michael Koffler in 1985.[84] MetSchools's first facility, Sunshine Developmental School, was followed by several others, including Aaron School and Rebecca School. The latter was established specifically for children with ASD and other neurodevelopmental delays.[85] Both of these places experienced their first PE investment when they were spun out of MetSchools and sold to Veronis Suhler Stevenson in 2010.

According to one source, "New York City's open checkbook for autism is at the heart of the business plan for the Rebecca School, the latest in New York City's fastest-growing chain of for-profit educational institutions."[86] Koffler, who has a degree in business administration and accounting, streamlined operations at the school by such means as assigning staff to two or more autistic children at a time, rather than the more accepted, evidence-based one-on-one ratio. As part of his business plan, Koffler facilitates parent suits against New York City for the $72,500 annual tuition. Given federal entitlements for such children, the city tends to settle. Koffler expects Rebecca School to gross more than $14 million annually from ongoing city and state revenue streams.[87] Not only are Rebecca School and others of its ilk enriching PE owners and top management, but they are appropriating resources from the revenue-starved New York City school system.

As with many PE purchases, after building up its financial value and magnifying its gains, in 2018 Veronis Suhler Stevenson sold both Rebecca School and Aaron School to Sequel Youth and Family Services, a portfolio company of Altamont Capital Partners.[88] Now it is Altamont's turn to milk them.

Bellwether Behavioral Health (originally Au Clair School, rebranded as AdvoServ in 1997 and rebranded as Bellwether in 2017)

Serving developmentally challenged adolescents and adults, mostly individuals with ASD, Bellwether Behavioral Health provided group homes and day centers. Much of its funding was through public school districts and Medicaid waivers.[89] Established in 1969 as the Au Clair School for autistic children by Kenneth and Claire Mazik, the Delaware-based company was entangled in allegations of abuse for decades. According to a 1997 account in the *New York Times* and other reports, the establishment was accused of whipping a disabled boy, hitting children with plastic bats, the consistent use of mechanical restraints, and allowing living quarters to reek of urine and feces.[90] Au Clair School was renamed AdvoServ in 1997.

Despite horrific conditions, AdvoServ was presumably raking in sufficient revenue to attract GI Partners at the end of 2009. The company grew, and the abuse continued unabated; there was a rash of complaints against AdvoServ, especially concerning its routine use of mechanical restraints and the resultant injuries. Ex-workers also said they saw children beaten as part of their treatment.[91] In response, the place was rebranded again in 2017, this time as Bellwether Behavioral Health.

Notwithstanding the abuse accusations, the company became Florida's largest provider of group homes for people with autism and other intellectual and developmental disabilities. It dipped heavily into the taxpayer well: the state's outlays amounted to $23.9 million in 2013 for its Medicaid-eligible adults alone. Overall, Bellwether received about $75 million annually from the welfare medicine program.[92] In addition, money poured in from the Delaware Department of Education, $300,000 per month for seventeen students in AdvoServ's residential care facilities.[93]

By 2015, it was time for the PE to unload the asset, which was purchased by Wellspring Capital Management in an SBO that added $120.4 million in debt. Despite the sale, new scathing reports surfaced: there were residents suffering from dehydration and abuse; medicine

mix-ups; untrained and unsupervised frontline workers; understaffing; sorely inadequate generic patient plans and treatment, if any;
and neglect, scalding, and sexual assaults. A disability rights group
cited fourteen state abuse investigations at Florida facilities in 2015
and twenty-eight more in 2016.[94] A *Tampa Bay Times* investigation exposed a 2017 rat infestation and an incident where two staff members
"taunted, ridiculed, and humiliated a resident and then locked him in
a shower, naked, for four hours."[95] The following year, Florida's Agency
for Persons with Disabilities announced that "conditions are so dire
that residents face 'a substantial probability' of 'death or serious harm'
under current management."[96] In fact, there had been two deaths of
children with autism at AdvoServ care homes.[97]

State agencies in New York, Delaware, and Florida stopped referring individuals to these facilities or paying for their care in 2017;
New Jersey officials held out longer, despite allegations by prior Bellwether employees that "once Wellspring purchased Bellwether, the
firm began to cut costs by cutting administrators and home staff and
hiring less-educated workers."[98] New Jersey's Division of Developmental Disabilities subsequently conducted a series of surprise visits
at Bellwether homes and found inadequate staffing, falsified documents, missing pill bottles, rooms that smelled of urine and rotting
wood, and the use of restraints for extended periods.[99]

Finally, after a moratorium on admissions, in May 2019 New Jersey
revoked the company's license, displacing 460 residents. Incredibly,
Bellwether demanded state funds for their transition, claiming its financial situation was precarious; the company was $83.5 million in
debt and soon filed for bankruptcy.[100] The PE, as usual, faced no consequences, and simply wiped Bellwether's name from its website's previous portfolio ownership list.

The Whirlwind Buyouts

As autism treatment companies continue to turn huge profits, ever
more PE firms jump into the business, characteristically acquiring
places from founder-owners.

Centria Healthcare

The largest homecare service for children with ASD in Michigan, Centria Healthcare also operates in several other states.[101] In 2016, seven years after its founding, the business had become sufficiently valuable to draw the attention of PE. Medicaid costs in Michigan for ASD services increased from $5.6 million in 2012 to $187 million in 2018; the previous year, Centria had billed $29 million for such care in Detroit alone.[102] Capricorn Healthcare (rebranded Martis Capital) bought the establishment.

Sadly, the company's moneymaking know-how was accompanied by mistreatment of the vulnerable children in its charge. Centria had a history of deficiencies in the years prior to its purchase, which apparently did not give Martis pause. For example, one Michigan county, which had regularly cited a Centria center for poor patient care, inadequately trained staff, and billing offenses, eventually put it on probation. Centria then lost contracts in two Michigan counties, as well as an $8 million grant from the Michigan Economic Development Corporation; it had initially obtained the funding after threatening to leave the state.[103]

In 2017, the Detroit Free Press executed a full-scale investigation into complaints by former workers. Reporters found that Centria violated patient privacy and hired unqualified workers to treat children with ASD; there were more than a hundred substantiated allegations of abuse, neglect, and use of unwarranted force. The journalists even located a tape that captured an employee abusing a youngster; she had bruises on her chest, neck, and arms. Centria also was alleged to be engaged in a Medicaid fraud scheme that targeted indigent and minority communities. Among other questionable practices, the company charged for services that never occurred, depriving children with ASD of much-needed help. The company wages aggressive patient recruitment as well, and places enormous pressure on supervisors to augment their billing hours.[104]

One of the journalists observes that these serious, manifold wrongdoings are "unlikely to hinder the rapidly expanding health care behemoth, which serves 2,300 autistic children in eight states and plans to grow to 20,000 children in the coming years."[105] Notably, the *Detroit Free Press* reports never mention Martis Capital as complicit in the litany of Centria transgressions. In fact, the chain continued to flourish as a Martis Capital portfolio company until it was sold to Thomas H. Lee Partners at the end of 2019; Centria Healthcare was valued at $415 million.[106]

Family Treatment Network

Family Treatment Network, based in Franklin, Tennessee, is a platform established by Pharos Capital Group. Formed in 2016, FTN is a behavioral health services business—mostly ABA treatments for children in residential therapy clinics, day schools, and community outpatient programs. From the beginning, Pharos's intention was to achieve a national footprint for the portfolio company.

FTN soon acquired Logan River Academy, a treatment center for adolescents with autism, PTSD, substance abuse, and depression.[107] In my view, this was a curious investment since in 2013, Logan had been accused of cruel treatment toward its residents, warehousing kids, and extremely harsh disciplinary measures. For instance, students were subjected to harsh time-out periods even for slight infractions; they had to sit straight and not move, avoid looking at anyone, and remain silent. Such punishment could persist for nearly a day. Several parents had petitioned to shut down the academy.[108] Regardless, the PE house backed the acquisition, and Logan became an affiliate of FTN. To make matters worse, the two disreputable founders were kept on. Perhaps Pharos was seduced by the hefty revenue flow: $7,500–$8,900 per child each month.

In 2018, FTN picked up the pace, acquiring several companies offering ABA therapy. Behavior Care Specialists, purchased in January, added four states to the platform: South Dakota, Iowa, Minnesota, and Wyoming. Five months later, Pharos's portfolio company added CCMC School, an affiliate of Connecticut Children's Medical Center, which focuses on special education for children who require intensive intervention for behavioral, emotional, and learning challenges. Renaming it Solterra Academy, FTN aimed to expand its therapies to include the more revenue-generating ABA techniques.[109] By the end of the year, FTN signed on ABA of North Texas, an outpatient autism provider; the chain now operated in seven states.[110] What will be the consequences for kids with autism spectrum disorders as Pharos endeavors to reach its national geographic goal for Family Treatment Network?

Center for Autism and Related Disorders

CARD, an autism treatment company that offers services at homes, schools, and community sites, is an example of an already mature company (established in 1990) snatched by one of the largest PE firms, Blackstone Group. Under its founder, Dr. Doreen Granpeesheh, CARD had expanded to more than 239 locations in thirty-three states at the time of the 2018 PE purchase. Most important, Granpeesheh is a leading expert in autism treatment. Among other achievements, she is a clinical psychologist and behavior analyst, has authored *Evidence-Based Treatment for Children with Autism: The CARD Model*, produced the documentary film *Recovered: Journeys through the Autism Spectrum and Back*, and is the recipient of numerous awards. She also founded Autism Care Today, a nonprofit organization that provides grants to individuals and families in need of resources and treatment. Now, for roughly $600 million (the largest autism LBO to date),[111] CARD is in the hands of financiers whose sole goal is outsized earnings for themselves and their limited partners.

Blue Sprig Pediatrics, Inc.

Another long-established, giant PE shop has hopped aboard the autism moneymaking bandwagon. Launched by KKR as a platform for ASD therapy in 2017, Blue Sprig is among the smaller but expanding health care companies that the PE intends to build up through its strategic growth fund.[112] Soon after its LBO, Blue Sprig acquired the Shape of

Behavior (2018), followed by Verbal Behavior Consulting (2019), Tangible Difference Learning Center (2019), and West Texas Autism Center (2019). Each of these investments had previously been directed by its autism-knowledgeable founder. For example, Dr. Domonique Randall, who instituted the Shape of Behavior, has studied ASD and worked hands-on with children having the condition since 1996. After establishing the company in 2000, she implemented a professional training school. Similarly, Amanda Ralston, creator of Verbal Behavior Consulting, has two decades of experience with ASD; she also lectures and conducts public workshops. Dr. Melissa Richardson worked with special education children in public schools prior to launching West Texas Autism Center. Dr. Michael Conteh, a behavioral analyst, launched Tangible Difference in 2005 and has been involved with assisting children with ASD since then.

Now these chains are controlled by Blue Sprig's CEO, Keith Jones, whose expertise, according to his self-description, is a "proven ability to bring rapid bottom line growth to multi-site, multi-state and international businesses."[113] By the end of 2019, KKR's portfolio company had bought ASD centers in seven states. In early 2020, it acquired Florida Autism Center from Shore Capital Partners, thus positioning Blue Sprig as one of the five largest US providers of services for the disorder. And its rapacious takeovers were just beginning.[114]

And There Are More

The gold rush in the autism treatment industry, often for quick bucks, since the second decade of the twenty-first century includes a panoply of additional places. Petra Capital Partners, Altos Health Management, and MMC Health Services bought Alternative Behavior Strategies in an $11.6 million deal in 2017 that placed $3 million of debt on the business.[115] That year, Baird Capital and Vista Verde Group purchased Homefront Learning (rebranded as Hopebridge), which operated in Indiana and Kentucky. Via PE-financed buyouts, Hopebridge added locations in Ohio and Georgia. Valued at roughly $255 million, less than two years later it experienced an SBO by Arsenal Capital Partners.[116]

The financialization of ASD continues. For example, in 2018 MBF Healthcare Partners established Acorn Health, based in Coral Gables, Florida, a new platform formed through two acquisitions. The goal is to grow services in Michigan, Florida, and Virginia.[117] Also in 2018, DW Healthcare Partners acquired California Psychcare and rebranded the enterprise as 360 Behavioral Health. Ten months later, TA Associates invested as well.[118] Abry Partners obtained Lighthouse Autism Center, a place with five treatment centers in Michigan and Indiana.[119] Action Behavior Centers, which treats children with ASD throughout Texas, is the winner in autism services flipping: NexPhase Capital, which procured the chain in October 2018, placed it on the market eleven months later.[120] Comprehensive Educational Services (ACES), operating in six states, was sold to General Atlantic in 2020. Founded in 1996 by Kristin Farmer—an expert in autism treatment—ACES has two representatives from General Atlantic on its board of directors to help steer the ship.[121]

Concluding Remarks

The ASD sector has been especially alluring to the PE industry because it is ripe for consolidation, lacks clinical standardization in its evidence-based ABA treatment, remains vulnerable to cost-saving measures, boasts a considerable and steady revenue flow from public and commercial sources, and most important, has proven to be extremely lucrative. Founder-owners, many of whom are experts in the field and dedicated to assisting children with the disorder, are increasingly succumbing to aggressive sales tactics, high valuations for their businesses, and for some, the aspiration to meet needs through growth; there is a dearth of facilities relative to demand. They are being replaced by the PE titans.

As I have shown, the PE-owned chains, for the most part, have not paid sufficient attention to the requirements of their young clients with ASD. Intent on scaling the businesses and extracting value for personal gain, the shops sanction, or indeed foster, the deterioration of care. The PE response to wrongdoings by their portfolio companies has been, in many cases, to rebrand them, with the expectation that they can whitewash the financial fraud and individual harm perpetrated on vulnerable youngsters.

The burst of activity in the autism sector feeds the PE industry but draws down essential resources meant to care for children and adults with ASD. PE ownership has not added to refining the quality of treatment, research, or affordability. To the contrary, it appears that the quality of care suffers while the ongoing consolidation and monopolization could allow PE-backed companies to boost prices for already costly services.

9 |

Hijacking an Industry

Medical Ambulances and Emergency Air Transport

GROUND EMERGENCY medical services (EMS) is a relatively young industry. In earlier years it was mostly either hospital-based, part of fire departments, or the duty of city and county governments. One of the bigger companies today, Rural/Metro, began in 1948 as a private fire protection company.[1] Since the 1990s, localities have increasingly outsourced their EMS functions to private, for-profit companies in an attempt—often misguided—to economize.[2]

The US ground ambulance landscape is still dotted with scores of small, volunteer stations that operate only one or two transport vehicles. At the other end is American Medical Response (AMR), the foremost private business (now a subsidiary of Global Medical Response) and several relatively smaller ones, such as Acadia, Falck A/S, and Rural/Metro, until the latter was acquired by AMR. In 2017, commercial establishments accounted for roughly 20 percent of providers.[3]

With an aging population that uses ambulance services at a 150 percent higher rate than the rest of society, and greater insurance coverage because of the Affordable Care Act, the commercial value of the sector has been rising. There are payers everywhere: public programs (Medicare and Medicaid), private insurance, and out-of-pocket customers who generally have no choice of company or price.

Consequently, private equity firms have shown considerable and growing interest. In 2011, the PE firms CD&R and Warburg Pincus purchased two of the leading ambulance companies, Emergency Medical Services Corporation (EMS) and Rural/Metro, respectively. One knowledgeable observer notes that this was "a game-changer for EMS service in this country."[4] PE control over the industry has grown enormously since then as GPs have scaled and consolidated average-size and substantial enterprises alike.

As usual, what has been valuable for PE shops has not benefited the public commensurately. According to a *New York Times* report, PE ownership of ground ambulances has fostered worsening response times; more aggressive billing procedures and lawsuits; fewer (and often inadequate) supplies at hand, including medicine; ambulance and equipment shortages and breakdowns; and greater pressure to use emergency vehicles rather than equally viable but less expensive alternatives.[5] As I discuss below, customers also have been beset by steep out-of-pocket fees. Workers have suffered too, particularly with cost-cutting that has reduced the companies' pension obligations.

Commercial ownership apparently has led to greater service disparities among neighborhoods as well. According to a study by Dr. Renee Hsia and colleagues, people who experience heart attacks in low-income areas wait four minutes longer for ambulances than those in more affluent ones. She concludes that differential wait times could be due to a number of factors, including the shift from publicly funded to privately owned firms.[6] Critically, the evidence suggests that delays in ambulance response times can seriously affect mortality rates: a report published in the *British Medical Journal* concludes that attaining a five-minute ambulance response time "could almost double the survival rate for cardiac arrest."[7]

Whir, Whoosh, and Dollar Signs: Air Medical Transport

Emergency air medical transport has even larger private equity ownership today than ground ambulances do and far greater problematic financial and service issues.[8] Prior to the twenty-first century, most providers had been hospital-based, nearly all of them nonprofit. Medicare subsequently raised reimbursement rates sharply, thereby attracting commercial interest and an explosion of independent, community-based companies. The industry morphed from relying on fixed contracts through hospitals, with set fees, to a situation in which operators are paid directly by insurers, public programs, and customers only when services are utilized; there is no control over prices.[9]

Witnessing the phenomenal growth of Air Methods Corporation, GPs turned their attention to the airlift industry in 2002 for the first time.[10] Apparently the sector had become well matched to their investment yardstick, and they viewed it as simply waiting for them to turn on the spigot. Certainly, the massive rise in Medicare fees, including a 50 percent premium for helicopter emergency medical services (HEMS), had aroused PE interest. But the surge in demand played a significant role too. Henry H. Perritt, an expert in the field, argues that we now have an enhanced ability to treat life-threatening conditions that require immediate care. He contends that the closure of more and more rural hospitals and the growth in specialized hospitals and trauma centers have created further opportunities for HEMS. In addition, there is a mounting need for organ transport services.[11]

There is no certificate-of-need requirement for the industry, which permits an uncontrolled expansion of facilities.[12] The PE houses took advantage of the situation, and between 2012 and 2017, 100 new bases materialized in the most financially rewarding areas. A glut in emergency service helicopters arose as well, climbing from roughly 350 in 1997 to 1,045 in 2016.[13] Just as accommodating to the PE industry, the Airline Deregulation Act of 1978 prohibits states from regulating air carrier rates, including those for medical helicopters. As a result, companies charge exorbitant fees for emergency services, and given the condition of victims, they are obviously in no position to shop around or negotiate the amount, even if there is more than one local carrier. A 2016 ABC News investigation "found a hard-edged air ambulance industry, free to set any price it wants, often leaving the very people it saved facing financial ruin with bills of more than $40,000 for a short flight."[14]

Individuals and families are hard-hit by such expenses, especially since insurers pay only the in-network charge. Yet two-thirds of all HEMS operators in 2017 were out-of-network for their clients, rendering them responsible for the remainder of bloated bills.[15] As Susannah Luthi reports, "Surprise charges for various medical flights from the past four years ranged from $26,000 to nearly $534,000—although the latter number is a major outlier. Most charges fell between $30,000 and $88,000, with the average hovering around $60,000." She recounts the tale of an insured patient who was transported eighty-four miles, invoiced $66,000, and wound up paying $50,000 out-of-pocket to Valley Med Flight; the insurance company offered a reimbursement of just $16,000.[16] These inflated bills generally are unforeseen, leaving families to struggle financially, remortgage their homes, endure garnished wages, or even declare bankruptcy. Indeed, Consumers Union in 2017 detected a substantial upsurge in the number of people facing such devastating situations because of emergency flights.[17]

Huge, unanticipated medical bills are an immense problem for individuals requiring emergency ground transportation as well; fully 85 percent of rides to the ER entail an out-of-network tab. Since the patient is at the mercy of the ambulance company, as Eileen Appelbaum and Rosemary Batt put it, "the result is another perfect opportunity for surprise medical bills, and a perfect target for unscrupulous investment funds."[18]

A few states endeavored to restrict such balance billing, but they inevitably faced a lawsuit by the companies, which won each time; judges consistently ruled that these state enactments violate the Airline Deregulation Act, which prohibits them from regulating routes or payments.[19] Finally, in the summer of 2019, Congress indicated that it was ready to take action against surprise medical bills, but as discussed above, the focus was on physician staffing, which had been perpetrating the same egregious pricing practices (see chapter 4). The proposed legislation sought to implement parity between in-network and out-of-network charges for hospital doctor services, or limit them to 125 percent of Medicare's fee. Only the Senate version of the bill included a provision that extended the regulation to medevac aircraft.[20] Lobbyists against the legislation cropped up in hordes, including PE representatives of ground and air transport firms.[21] Ultimately, a bill was enacted at the end of 2020 that will protect patients against surprise bills from medical air transports but not from ground ambulances, beginning in 2022. Arbitration details between insurers and the medical transports are a work in progress (see chapter 4).

Overpricing is not the only concern related to PE ownership of HEMS. There are questions about the quality of services as well. Perritt observes that national and local governments have enacted few meaningful requirements as to the type of aircraft, kind of equipment that should be carried, maintenance, or level of pilot training. Nor is there effective oversight of the industry by the Federal Aviation Administration, Medicare, Medicaid, or any other federal or state regulators. Therefore, it is the HEMS operators themselves that make basic decisions, and "that opens up a fairly wide set of opportunities for cost cutting. . . . It is also true that operators can cut costs by reducing expenditures on safety."[22]

Despite safety issues, light single-engine helicopters account for a significant percentage of the US industry, especially among PE-owned businesses, and the share is growing. In 2015, for example, Air Methods reported that 61 percent of its helicopters were single-engine.[23] Greater profitability appears to be the main consideration: a company can reduce fixed costs by purchasing and operating less expensive but more dangerous single-engine transports. First, twin-engine aircraft entail higher maintenance expenditures. Second, single-engine HEMS helicopters tend to be certified only for visual flight rules and not instrument flight rules (IFR) because the latter requires an autopilot system or at least two pilots on board. According to Perritt, the upshot is that with IFR capability, one is more protected from unexpectedly hazardous weather. He adds that autopilots "provide a considerable measure of safety enhancement."[24] Third, night operations are less risky with autopilots since, in certain environments, pilots cannot visually detect mountains, other obstacles, or landing sites.[25] Significantly, the rest of the industrialized world has stricter criteria for emergency aircraft; France, for example, mandates that companies employ twin-engine helicopters.[26]

Another means for PE houses to cut costs is to replace fleets and other equipment less frequently, something that is tempting given their short ownership time frames. Curtailing pilot training also can assist the bottom line, even though it is a recipe for more errors and accidents. And despite visual flight rule minimums, there may be pressure for pilots to fly when the forecast indicates "temporary" or the "probability of" perilous conditions, even though pilots generally have the final say. High helicopter utilization is one of the key components of profitability.[27] There is no financial incentive to provide the safest, most comfortable, and best possible service since current and future customers cannot choose their operator when they are in dire need of assistance. At the same time, Medicare reimbursement rates—and I dare say all payer fees—are also not dependent on providing the safest equipment or high levels of pilot and medical personnel training.[28]

PE firms engage in other improper endeavors to enrich themselves. In certain regions, the growth of both HEMS locations and the number of helicopters, for example, has led to the dogged acquisition of competitors. In addition, in places where there is more than one transport business, the firms aggressively seek individuals to airlift, grabbing customers from each other; one observer of this phenomenon describes it as "the wild west."[29] A number of establishments derive substantial revenue from annual affiliation fees, and they can use forceful tactics to secure them. Air Evac Lifeteam, for instance, charges $85 per year, collecting $255 million in 2018. There is a catch, however: memberships are valid only for the association you join; if you need emergency assistance, any one of a number of medevac firms could show up. North Dakota insurance commissioner Jon Godfread told NPR, "Too often, the company responding to a patient's call for help is not the one the patient signed up with. . . . North Dakota has nine different air ambulance operators that respond to calls, and patients have no control over which will be called." He described these fees as just "another loophole that air ambulance companies use to essentially exploit our consumers."[30]

The three largest air medical transports today control two-thirds of the industry; two of them are PE portfolio companies (Air Medical Group Holdings since 2004 and Air Methods since 2017). They increasingly mingle their business with ground EMS, and Air Medical Group Holdings merged with the leading provider of land services, American Medical Response.

The Emergency Rescue Giant: Global Medical Response
American Medical Response (formerly Emergency Medical Services Corporation / Envision Healthcare Holdings)

The juggernaut in the ground ambulance sector, AMR provides emergency vehicles and wheelchair transports; it also serves as a standby for concerts, athletic events, parades, and conventions. Established in 1992 by Paul Verrochi through the consolidation of four regional ambulance companies, AMR was placed on the New York Stock Exchange later that year; it raised $23.7 million in the IPO. By the end of 1995, AMR had acquired fifty-eight ambulance providers, many of them from privatizing municipal and county operations.[31] AMR was purchased in 1997 by Laidlaw International for $1.2 billion "as part of Laidlaw's own aggressive acquisition plan in the transportation industry."[32] It was then merged with Medtrans, also owned by Laidlaw: the united business, which assumed the AMR name, was now the largest ambulance company in the nation.[33]

Next, Onex Partners, AMR's first PE owner, took it and another subsidiary of Laidlaw (EmCare) private in a 2004 LBO for $980 million. Onex combined the two into a new corporation, Emergency Medical Services (EMS), with AMR as its ambulance division. The following year, the PE shop placed EMS on the NYSE, securing $113.4 million through the IPO, and soon sold some of its shares.

In 2011, the corporation was taken private once more, this time by Clayton, Dubilier & Rice (CD&R) for $3.2 billion, including $878 million in debt; Onex sold its remaining 30 percent stake.[34] According to Kevin Conway, vice chair of CD&R, Onex had earned eight times its money since the initial buyout.[35] After another two years of acquisitions via CD&R, EMS—now renamed Envision Healthcare—was placed yet again on the NYSE. In 2014, CD&R sold a quantity of shares for $838.8 million, and later that year some more for $935 million. Another PE shop had drained mega-bucks from emergency medical transports.

As a division of EMS/Envision, AMR continuously expanded and consolidated, acquiring medical ambulance businesses nearly every year, as well as an occasional air medical or nonemergency ground transport enterprise.[36] One of its most consequential buyouts, discussed below, was Rural/Metro, purchased in 2015.[37] The now beefed-up AMR was far too alluring to escape the eye of one of the foremost private equity firms, KKR, which already owned Air Medical Group Holdings. In March 2018, KKR took Envision's AMR division private for $2.4 billion in a highly leveraged buyout, loading it with $2.1 billion in debt.[38] AMR had again become a PE portfolio company. Shortly thereafter, KKR united its two giants under the name Global Medical Response, which serves more than 5 million people per year across forty-six states.

Rural/Metro Corporation

One of the oldest commercial ambulance businesses, Rural/Metro was founded in 1948 by Lou Witzeman as a subscription firefighting service in his Scottsdale, Arizona, neighborhood; in 1969, it spread into ambulances and wheelchair van assistance. In 1978, Witzeman sold slightly more than 60 percent of the company to his employees for $1 million. The firm prospered throughout the 1980s as it entered into ever more contracts with localities across several states and amassed numerous establishments in the sector; by the end of the 1980s, Rural/Metro served people in fifty communities.[39]

In 1993, the corporation went public through an IPO on the NASDAQ, and a few months later experienced a second public offering, amounting to $22 million and $19 million, respectively. Rural/Metro continued its avid procurements, and more than seventy entities were added to the firm through 1998. Despite its ongoing, rapid expansion, it had a stellar reputation. For example, in 1996, "the company was declared Private Ambulance Provider of the Year by The Texas Department of Health, for the quality of its care and the community services the company performed. It also received the American Ambulance Association's Community Partnership Award."[40]

Not all was well, however. In 2002, Scottsdale firefighters sued both Rural/Metro and its accounting firm, Arthur Andersen, for covering up the real financial situation of the chain, which adversely affected its workers' retirement assets.[41] Rural/Metro also had to pay $5.4 million to settle a 2009 whistleblower suit brought by a former employee in Alabama. The federal government, along with officials in four other states—Kentucky, Tennessee, Ohio, and Indiana—substantiated a complaint that the company had been billing Medicare and Medicaid for transporting dialysis patients, though the services either were not provided or were medically unnecessary.[42]

Nevertheless, poised to be a foremost private sector ambulance and fire protection provider, Rural/Metro stood out as a prize catch for the PE industry. In a 2011 public-to-private LBO, Warburg Pincus took it over; the $728 million deal included $525 million in debt financing (72 percent of the total buyout). In next to no time, the PE portfolio company bought two regional ambulance operators, Pacific Ambulance and Bowers Ambulance, adding another $108 million in debt.[43] Rural/Metro did not fare well under Warburg Pincus's ownership: the mounting liabilities were unsustainable, and it filed for Chapter 11 in August 2013, less than two years after the PE shop had purchased it. Warburg Pincus exited the business, none the worse for wear.

After receiving capital from Oaktree Capital Management, which also procured the distressed company's bonds (presumably at a fire sale price), Rural/Metro emerged from bankruptcy in December 2013. Only two short years later, it was taken over by American Medical Response via Onex for $620 million; Oaktree sold its 40 percent stake, raking in huge profits from the chain's insolvency.[44] Now, it was the turn of subsequent PE firms to bleed it, but under a new trademark.

Air Medical Group Holdings

Unlike the others, AMGH originated as a PE-owned platform in 2004. Created by Brockway Moran and Partners and MVP Capital Partners, the establishment has been through the PE mill ever since. It also has had its share of questionable practices, starting with the LBO and recapitalization of Air Evac Lifeteam that first year.[45] According to *New York Times* reporter Barry Meier, "if one company exemplifies the industry growth, as well as its excesses and problems, it may be Air Evac Lifeteam." Under Brockway Moran's ownership it was blasted for numerous egregious practices, such as performing unnecessary, expensive medical transports; engaging in hard-hitting drives for memberships; and lowering expenses "by buying single-engine helicopters and retro-fitting them as medical aircraft."[46] Air Evac Lifeteam also was accused by the US government of Medicare and Medicaid billing fraud. Regardless, the enterprise kept growing, along with its acquirer, AMGH.[47]

After a gluttonous six years of pushing memberships, obtaining ever more providers, developing bases in additional states, and expanding debt, Brockway Moran was ready to capture the monetary gains. AMGH was sold in 2010 to Bain Capital and Millpond Equity Partners in a $1.01 billion transaction that added $545 million in new liabilities to the company. During its five-year ownership, Bain was equally aggressive, doubling the size of AMGH and increasing its earnings tenfold. The PE firm also augmented lines of service with personal and chartered air transportation.[48] At the midpoint, Bain grabbed a $200 million dividend recap for itself by means of an unsecured loan on the chain.

One of the more substantial AMGH buyouts via Bain was REACH Air Medical Services, purchased for $244 million at the end of 2012. Afterward, REACH operated as a major Bain platform for fueling AMGH's expansion.[49] Two other large purchases, both in 2014, were Airmed International (formerly Medjet International) and Lifeguard Ambulance Service, which provided the business with abundant ground vehicles.

The financiers were well prepared to sell by 2015: AMGH was the second largest air medical transport in the United States, with roughly 16 percent of the sector's total revenues. It was fully equipped with a fleet of widely spread helicopters, airplanes, and ground ambulances. Consequently, the corporation faced its third LBO by another notorious PE firm, KKR, for $2.09 billion, including $1.38 billion in debt.[50] Like Bain, KKR was not shy about scaling and consolidating AMGH. The shop drove REACH's control even further with the purchase of one of its competitors, CALSTAR Air Medical Services, in 2016, and then Sierra Lifeflight in 2017.

Another far-reaching investment the following year, Air Medical Resource Group (formerly Eagle Air Med) already held eleven affiliates.[51] In short order, Air Medical was rebranded as Guardian Flight, LLC.[52] Concomitantly, AMGH via KKR acquired Transplant Transportation Services, which ships organs and medical cargo by means of ground vehicles and aircraft. By the summer of 2017, KKR had become the largest owner of medical air and ground transportation in the nation.[53]

But the PE firm was not played out: as discussed above, the most consequential LBO was the 2018 buyout of American Medical Response, the massive emergency ambulance provider, and subsequent merger with AMGH—now under the umbrella of Global Medical Response. And KKR's AMGH is still expanding.[54]

A Ground Transport Liquidates: Transcare Ambulance

One commercial ambulance company that went into bankruptcy (in this case, twice), Transcare Ambulance, had been one of the largest ground emergency operations in the mid-Atlantic states, serving areas in New York, Pennsylvania, Maryland, and Washington, DC.[55] Launched in 1993, the enterprise was first acquired by Hampshire Equity Partners at the beginning of 1997. The PE firm initiated an expansive series of acquisitions, especially Metropolitan Ambulance (New York City) in 1999 for $42 million, and then landed Transcare in bankruptcy court a few years later.

In 2003, Patriarch Partners and two other investors purchased the insolvent company through three Zohar funds that were managed by Lynn Tilton, founding partner of Patriarch; Zohar lent money to distressed firms that were afterward run by Tilton, including Transcare. After thirteen years in Patriarch's portfolio and with millions in additional debt, Transcare abruptly filed for bankruptcy again in 2016. Tilton faced several charges related to the business, especially her appropriation of $2.8 million from Transcare the year before it failed. Just as important, a former CFO told the Wall Street Journal, "The company was using every spare dollar it had to pay management fees and interest to Patriarch."[56]

The New York Times opened an investigation of Transcare, including a review of its internal memos. The reporters discovered that during 2015 it had not paid most invoices; curtailed purchases of lifesaving drugs and other supplies; neglected to disburse wages on time; and failed to keep ambulances and other emergency vehicles in good repair, so they regularly broke down or ran out of fuel. They added, "Employees were encouraged to replenish supplies from hospital emergency rooms."[57]

In the wake of the bankruptcy, more than 1,700 employees lost their jobs, and some did not even receive their last paycheck. They also were deprived of retirement benefits. Tilton refused to pay, claiming that Patriarch was not the workers' employer. New York City, meanwhile, suffered a loss of critical ambulance services in the Bronx and Manhattan; officials had to make do with vehicles and crews brought in from other boroughs, resulting in overextended and exhausted medics.[58] The Transcare debacle and eventual liquidation underscore the drawbacks of PE ownership of public services, especially the heavy debt the shops place on the enterprises.

Air Methods: The Air Rescue Kingpin

Accounting for more than 25 percent of all air ambulance revenues by 2021, Air Methods has made its appearance as a PE portfolio company. Set up in 1980 by Roy Morgan, the Colorado-based Air Methods initially possessed only one helicopter and contracted with a single hospital.[59] In due course, Air Methods was placed on the NASDAQ through a 1987 IPO, becoming one of only two publicly traded air ambulance companies at the time. Fully thirty years later (2017), in a public-to-private LBO, American Securities bought the company for $2.5 billion.

During Air Methods's NASDAQ years, its CEO, George Belsey, restructured the financially ailing enterprise, cut staff sharply, sold off aircraft, and embarked on a series of buyouts. One of its early purchases was Mercy Air Service in 1997, whose stock then was used as collateral for the acquisition of Helicopter Services, Inc. Mercy also served as a platform for further buyouts, including Area Rescue Consortium of Hospitals, a nonprofit organization, and Metro Air Services, owner of Flight for Life.[60]

Air Methods grew prodigiously through the first decades of the twenty-first century, including the addition of ground ambulances, air tourism, and aircraft maintenance and refurbishment services, but left a mixed record along the way. Like other air medical transports, the company acquired independent, community-based providers as well as those attached to specific hospitals. Periodically, Air Methods has served as an exit for various PE shops in the industry. The most noteworthy is Omniflight Helicopters, a company with a hundred medical air vehicles and seventy-two bases in eighteen states. At the time of its buyout in 2011, Omniflight had undergone two previous PE LBOs.[61]

According to one source, Air Methods was farsighted, investing in equipment, aircraft, and training, at times even to the detriment of immediate earnings. Wall Street applauded the speed of its expansion: "In 2002, the company was named number 30 on the 'America's Fastest Growing Small Companies' list in the July–August issue of *Fortune Small Business Magazine*. Air Methods was also profiled in *Business Week* as one of the magazine's 'Hot Growth Companies,' listing it as 57th."[62] To avoid competition, it bought its rivals when feasible. Rocky Mountain Helicopters, equivalent in size to Air Methods and bought in 2002, was one of its most striking purchases since it had been a major competitor.[63]

Consequently, customers received inordinately high bills for Air Methods's emergency services. The enormously successful enterprise forcefully boosted fees an average of 283 percent between 2007 and 2016, from $13,000 to $49,800; the comparable rates during that time span for similar enterprises were only 10 percent. Air Methods was especially hard-hitting in its collection tactics as well. An ABC News investigation uncovered countless lawsuits against clients who owed money on their inflated bills; the company sought to garnish salaries or obtain payment through other oppressive means.[64]

By the end of 2015, one of its largest shareholders, J. Daniel Plants (founder of Voce Capital Management), goaded the publicly traded Air Methods into seeking a PE owner.[65] This wasn't the first rodeo for Plants: his website states that Voce "selectively uses public activism to enhance its returns and has repeatedly generated significant outcomes using this approach, including the sale of multiple portfolio companies, large returns of capital, substantial changes to corporate strategies and corporate governance reforms."[66] Indeed, Voce instigated a director election proxy fight in 2017, and just prior to the vote American Securities took Air Methods private for $2.5 billion, including debt of more than $900 million. Shareholders, including Plants, received an 11 percent premium on their stock.[67] American Securities, which invests in everything from dental practices and school buses to specialty chemicals, had no particular interest in emergency air services; rather, it was attracted by the company's great cash flow and strong profit margins.[68] The PE took firm charge of Air Methods, placing three of its executives on the five-member board of directors.

Metro Aviation: Not for Sale

One of the top air medical transports, Metro Aviation, has remained a private corporation under long-term family proprietorship. Established in 1982 in Shreveport, Louisiana, its founder, CEO, and president, Mike Stanberry, spoke to me about some downsides of PE ownership. He voiced concern that because GPs seek a steep return on their equity, they push for greater flight volume than a non-PE company, such as his, does. He said that if they do not run sufficient flights to generate maximum earnings, they might close or relocate the business. This could cause psychological pressure on pilots for whom it is essential to maintain jobs where they live. In addition, Stanberry stated that all of his clients are in-network; he does not do any balance billing.[69] Nor does his company push memberships, like many of the others, because, as his director of communications told NPR, they "aren't right for patients."[70]

Stanberry commented about the differences in Metro Aviation's fleet. He said that 90 percent of his transports are twin-engine as compared to companies under PE ownership, in which 95 percent use the less expensive, single-engine helicopters. He explained that one can use single-engine aircraft safely, but the pilot must take longer trips to go around hazards.[71] Of course, extended flight time could adversely affect traumatized patients, who require the quickest possible medical attention.

I was somewhat surprised by his response when I questioned him about oversight of the industry. Despite the problems, Stanberry feels that the Federal Aviation Administration and other government entities are already too involved and that what is needed are more self-imposed regulations. Finally, I asked whether he has received any offers from PE firms. "The company is not for sale," he said firmly.

Concluding Remarks

Since the 1990s, ground and air medical transport has shifted from small, nonprofit players to commercial enterprises, and since the early years of the twenty-first century, they have increasingly been taken over by private equity firms. Accordingly, emergency services have endured unrestrained scaling and consolidation, especially in the air rescue sector, leading to the dominance of a few big guns. There are few government controls over the sector as to fees, response time, balance billing, level of personnel training, and type, quantity, or quality of transport vehicles and medical equipment. Nor is this a free-market situation where buyers are capable of shopping around and purchasing the finest service at the best price.

The evidence suggests that given its financial model, PE control over lifesaving services collides head-on with the needs of seriously ill or injured individuals and their families. As a 2016 *New York Times* headline implies: what happens "when you dial 911 and Wall Street answers"?[72] Among the multitude of adverse consequences, medical transportation has become overly expensive, engages in abusive billing practices, and cuts corners, with potentially compromised standards of quality and safety. Taxpayers pay much of the tab, along with beleaguered consumers who at times forfeit their homes, savings, credit ratings, or a portion of future wages. Vital emergency services themselves are also at risk: the bottom could fall out of these highly leveraged enterprises owing to an economic downturn, reduced Medicare reimbursement rates, or any other financial setback. Certainly, bankruptcy is not unknown to the PE-owned segments of the industry.

Infiltrating Our Health Care System

MY JOURNEY into the secretive world of private equity has cracked it open only enough to peek into its impact on US health care. For the most part, the industry is not accountable to anyone. Unlike companies traded on the stock exchanges, PE financial disclosure to the Securities and Exchange Commission is not only limited but also unavailable to the public. PE firms acquire countless small to medium-size businesses from founders of autism, alcohol, drug, and eating disorder treatment centers; dentists; specialty physicians; and the like, who generally have to sign nondisparagement clauses as well as nondisclosure agreements. That, too, seals off vital information both about PE's financial maneuverings and the consequences for the enterprises it buys, including the effects on workers, clients, and communities. I attempted to interview former owners who sold their businesses to a PE shop, and relatively few of them were willing to share their experience, especially if the outcome was disquieting. With only some exceptions, those founders who agreed to talk to me either were cautious in their responses or requested anonymity. Only one PE general partner I contacted responded at all, and in that case consented only if I kept his remarks and the shop itself nameless.

Through my research I noticed that investigations of commercial entities, including profit levels and quality of care, often fail to set apart PE-owned companies, also limiting our knowledge about their undertakings. In newspaper, government, and academic inquiries into corporate misdeeds, private equity involvement tends to be disregarded or not even recognized in the first place. Even PitchBook and PE Hub, two places that dig deeply into PE daily activities, which I relied on for much of my data, frequently cannot acquire certain details on transactions, especially the exact cost of acquisitions or if and how often a firm captures dividend recaps for itself. PE is a tight-lipped community that even advises the hundreds of individuals at conferences for business students that the words of invited speakers and panelists are "off the record."

As shown in this book, in some cases a PE firm attempts to obfuscate its ownership of facilities by labeling each of them individually, rather than with the chain's corporate name. For example, a person seeking treatment for glaucoma, one of the leading causes of blindness, might visit a shop run by EyeCare Services Partners or Eyecare Partners without any knowledge that they are PE-owned; the chains operate under thirty-two and twenty separate brand names, respectively. Anyone wary of dental care from portfolio company Smile Brands would have to recognize at least eight different business names as its affiliates (see chapter 5). Heartland Dental's 840 practices are under the cover of discrete identities as well.

Even more, when the wrongdoings of one of their businesses are exposed, the GPs are likely to sweep the problem under the rug by rebranding it. With the intention of wiping the slate clean before unloading it, in 2018 Onex changed the name of ResCare—a homecare company with a horrific history of patient neglect, severe understaffing, failure to adequately train or supervise frontline workers, violations of the federal Fair Labor Standards Act, and fraudulent billing practices—to BrightSpring Health Services. Evercare Hospice, another place with a sordid history, soon became Optum Palliative and Hospice Care after its purchase by Formation Capital and Audax Group. Similar attempts to mask transgressions include drug and alcohol rehabilitation enterprises Camp Recovery Center (now Mirror Lake Recovery Center) and Colonial Management Group (now New Season). At times, a PE house will expunge the offending name entirely from its website, as in the case of Castlewood, which was retitled Alsana by the Riverside Company. Abracadabra. The establishments get fresh starts and the private equity owners move on, leaving devastated clients, families, and employees in their wake.

The Latest Pot of Gold: Health Services

The PE industry is attracted to the health sector, nearly always acquiring flourishing places, and interest in the domain has accelerated since 2017. The financiers invested in a few segments during the mid-1990s, including ophthalmology and dental service organizations, but these proved disastrous. In the early years of the twenty-first century, GPs tentatively entered businesses treating substance abuse, eating disorders, and autism, along with those providing emergency medical services, and these niches have become hot commodities since then. Other areas, including dermatology, gastroenterology, fertility therapies, and home health care, first drew PE attention by the second decade of the twenty-first century and spiked shortly thereafter. Orthopedics, urology, and hospice caught private equity's eye several years later, and they are expected to skyrocket as well.

What all these domains have in common is the opportunity for strong earnings. Though intense competition has elevated their valuations and concomitant debt levels, PE shops have been cashing out at lucrative rates of return. The substance abuse tragedy has engendered one of the most financially rewarding spaces for them, as have the frail elderly and ill people at the end of life. GPs that invested in Camp Recovery Center in 2002, for example, earned more than three times their equity investment only three years later. The treatment of girls and others with life-threatening eating disorders can earn clinics financial margins of up to 20–30 percent. Eating Recovery Center, valued at $1.2 million in 2010, was worth $550 million or more nine years later. Families struggling to assist their children on the autism spectrum, too, are enriching the financiers. Invo Healthcare Associates, purchased in 2013 by Post Capital Partners, "earned" 6.5 times its investment when it was sold four years later, not counting the minority share that Post retained. MyTherapyCompany/Stepping Stones Group netted Shore Capital Partners and other PE investors a 700 percent return in a correspondingly short time frame.

It became clear to me as I studied various health-related services that PE firms will go wherever the money is; addicts, children with ASD, dying elders, people with eating disorders, and accident victims are all mere commodities to be squeezed for financial gain. Therefore, a typical portfolio may contain Len the Plumber, a sewer system, cosmetics, and a clothing concern, together with a nursing home chain, jail facilities, and fertility centers. Even PE houses that specialize in health services are not committed to any particular niche, only to the potential for an inordinate return on their investment.

The Evidence Is In

Despite its penchant for privacy, the PE industry is not shy about taking advantage of taxpayer dollars to subsidize its holdings. The home health, hospice, and dialysis subsectors, for example, are reliant on Medicare and Medicaid for the bulk of their revenues. Drug and alcohol rehabilitation, autism therapy, and physician practices are also highly dependent on these programs for a portion, if not the lion's share, of their income. There is clearly something amiss when financial firms can take control of health services and use federal and state money to fund them, but don't have to answer to the public.

It is especially questionable when GPs impose measures that harm clients and workers. Quality of care under PE ownership has suffered to varying extents in every health-related area that I studied. In nearly all of them, the shops are preying on vulnerable people. And the PE owners rarely if ever face repercussions. Frequently, a portfolio company continues to flourish financially in tandem with abhorrent conditions. What is more, despite substandard and even abusive practices, a business is often kicked to the next owner, generally at a high rate of return for the PE titans.

To be sure, as this inquiry has made clear, the PE playbook, although endlessly adaptable, has only one primary goal—to garner as much money as possible from investments. Return on investment is the paramount principle on which the industry is based, and GPs will do whatever they can to maximize their yields, regardless of the consequences. Thus, despite the prohibition against the corporate practice of medicine (CPOM), PE firms are ultimately in charge of the physician practices they purchase; doctors may render decisions regarding patient care but only within tightly controlled financial targets. Where profits—and, in the case of PE, outsized profits—trump medical needs, physicians may be pushed to speed up services, with bonuses and an equity stake in the practice as incentives. Some ongoing trends in the profession may be vastly augmented, including a greater but dubious use of unsupervised physician extenders for procedures they are not qualified to perform. As a case in point, studies have shown that in dermatology these assistants are liable to carry out unnecessary procedures and miss potentially cancerous lesions. PE-owned Bedside Dermatology, a subsidiary of the largest chain in the United States (Advanced Dermatology and Cosmetic Surgery), sends out paraprofessionals in mobile clinics without supervising doctors, churning out second-rate services.

A year-long study on corporate medicine by the American Medical Association was presented at its 2019 annual meeting. The AMA's concerns center on a rise in costs and service volume, the drawbacks of internal referrals, and the misuse of physician extenders, especially by PE firms. Nonetheless, the report notes not only that doctors should "have the right to enter into whatever contractual arrangements they deem desirable and necessary," but that there is "a lack of empirical evidence regarding the impact of these practice models [corporate investors] on physicians, medical practices, and the costs and quality of care."[1] Apparently, the AMA is willing to ignore the inconvenient realities of past and current harms perpetrated by PE-owned ophthalmology and dermatology chains and in fields such as dentistry, home health care, and rehabilitation centers. It also failed to address the ill effects on newly minted and non-owner practitioners and on the medical specialties overall. I have read several documents by authors and have spoken to individuals who equivocate on the effects of PE ownership on health enterprises, claiming that they need more data. Likewise, there are observers who are taking a wait-and-see approach to the latest rounds of health investments. Notwithstanding this hesitation, appalling transgressions have already been verified.

Investigations into quite a few large-scale dental service organizations (DSOs), all reliant on Medicaid, found them exploiting their patients, mostly children. These problems include excessive sedation and the use of straitjackets to quicken the pace; performance of unneeded procedures, such as baby tooth root canals; inferior care more generally; and charging for treatments that were not performed. Several of these DSOs have been tossed from PE shop to PE shop, each siphoning off public dollars that were meant to serve our neediest youngsters.

In substance abuse rehab centers, few addicted individuals receive help based on evidence-based care. Moreover, supplementary services that are financially unrewarding for the GPs but vital for the long-term recovery of their clients, such as psychosocial supports, are generally not offered or else truncated to the bare minimum. Nearly half of rehab recipients suffer from comorbidities that require medical supervision, but physicians and psychiatrists are conspicuous by their absence. In places such as Camp Recovery Center, there have been rampant abusive practices that put patients at risk. In fact, the vast majority of alcohol and drug rehab businesses purchased by PE firms in the first decade of the twenty-first century engaged in disreputable practices to various degrees in order to pump up PE earnings, including Acadia Healthcare, New Season, and Foundations Recovery Network. Girls requiring eating disorder assistance also have been subjected to questionable regimens, and sometimes, as in the case of Castlewood/Alsana, they have been psychologically abused.

Homecare, too, has its share of bad PE actors who are either complicit in the wrongdoings or ignore them. Despite its ignominious history, ResCare enriched Onex by millions when the PE firm pocketed dividend recaps and then sold the chain to KKR for $1 billion in 2019. The quality of care in places like Aveanna worsened under PE pressure to meet financial goals; some children died. Bain Capital, its owner, is doing fine. Dying individuals in hospice have suffered the consequences of patient disregard as the type and extent of end-of-life services have declined under PE control. Not only is neglect prevalent, but illegal recruitment can prevent clients from receiving Medicare-funded curative remedies.

Second-rate services are widespread among PE-owned firms treating children with ASD. The most evidence-based technique, ABA, lacks clinical standardization; to enhance earnings, companies can—and do—water down complex, costly techniques, training, and supervision. Moreover, PE firms, such as the fast-growing Stepping Stones Group, have increasingly replaced founding clinician-owners, who were committed to the needs of children affected by ASD, with specialists in finance and management. This subsector has experienced numerous instances of acute misconduct, including but not limited to Camelot Education, Rebecca School, Bellwether Behavioral Health, and Centria. In the latter case, despite more than a hundred validated allegations of neglect and the use of unwarranted force on youngsters, the chain turned out to be a valuable asset for its PE owners. Equally repugnant behavior forced Bellwether into bankruptcy, but its owner, Wellspring Capital Management, merely wiped the chain's name from its website.

PE ownership of ground and air emergency transit is disturbing in numerous ways. For one, surprise-billing practices, at least in the past, left many people in crisis situations with unnecessarily enormous bills that may put their economic well-being in jeopardy. The data suggest that health and safety may be compromised as well because of the use of more dangerous aircraft and less pilot and medical staff training. In some cases, PE-owned ambulances have been shown to have worse response times, fewer supplies, and shoddier vehicles than public-sector emergency transports have.

Poor people are especially hard-hit by PE moneymaking ploys. In some areas, the financiers either eschew welfare medicine patients entirely or whip them through a Medicaid mill, like some PE-held dental practices and drug rehabilitation centers. Another PE strategy after taking over a health agency is to change its payer mix to dispense with or lower the number of Medicaid participants. Homecare portfolio companies, for instance, are less interested in caring for high-maintenance Medicaid-funded customers because they are not sufficiently profitable. PE-controlled eating disorder facilities generally do not accept Medicaid participants at all, leaving academic centers to care for the low-reimbursement clients, who are often the sickest.

The Enablers

As limited partners (LPs), public pension funds are complicit in PE buyouts, providing the lion's share of equity for investments—along with endowments, institutional accounts, foundations, and wealthy families. The shops themselves are sparing with their own money and rely to a great extent on LP capital. Yet workers tend to be treated as disposable commodities in PE-owned enterprises, and particular deals may be especially at odds with the interests of the state and local fund beneficiaries themselves. For instance, jobs, retirement obligations, and other benefits may be placed at risk by the worker funds that financed a company's leveraged buyouts in the first place. John Tozzi points out that several states have laws curbing balance billing but simultaneously have their public employee pension assets invested in enterprises engaging in the practices they have banned, including Envision.[2] LPs have no direct say in investments and do not even receive insider information on transactions.

Founder-owners are joining in: they are offered lucrative incentives, including a stake in future buyouts, to sell their establishment. The high valuations today are proving too enticing for some people to hold out. But for a number of them, it turns out to be a Faustian bargain as they lose independence and control over their business. PE shops promise to take over only the bureaucratic tasks, but in reality they keep tight control over the monetary and, indirectly, clinical aspects, especially through representatives on the board of directors. And they set rigid performance targets, can sell the place at any time, and have the power to fire the top team—including the founders—whenever they don't meet the PE firm's financial objectives.

But money is not the only reason small proprietors are willing to off-load their agencies or practices, including those that were built with loving care for their clients. From my discussions with founder-owners, insurance companies are the elephant in the room; nearly all of them, from dermatologists and dentists to ASD treatment providers, told me that the actions of commercial insurers caused them constant anguish and excessive time, rendering it challenging to maintain their business. Despite parity laws, for example, insurance companies resist paying for eating disorder treatments, or they drop children with ASD at will.

In addition, PE may be the only option for individuals of retirement age since younger professionals nowadays, especially in medicine and dentistry, are burdened with such huge school debt that they cannot afford to purchase a practice. Owners of autism treatment centers, home health agencies, and other health services indicate that apart from private equity there are few avenues for selling their business, and they would otherwise just have to close shop. A few prior owners indicated that they were pressured to take on PE partners because they could not obtain capital anywhere else; banks are reluctant to lend to small firms. On the other hand, bankers have been relatively liberal with PE debt, spurring on mega-investments through low-interest, covenant-lite loans and refinancing opportunities.

Federal and state political officials have been mostly responsible for aiding and abetting the financiers: the entrance and timing of PE into all health segments have been galvanized by government policies over the decades. The statutes have always affected investors' interest in home health care, for instance. Beginning in the 1980s, Congress allowed commercial players, and now private equity, to enter the previously nonprofit field. The push for at-home assistance in lieu of institutional facilities for both long-term and post-acute services released a sufficient flow of money to lure a flood of PE shops to enter the scene. The Bipartisan Budget Act of 2018, which revamped the homecare reimbursement model once again, has triggered even more PE acquisitions and consolidation of the market.

End-of-life care, authorized for payment under Medicare through the 1982 Tax Equity and Fiscal Responsibility Act, also opened the money spigot that is satisfying the voracious appetite of GPs. The Social Security Amendments of 1973 spurred the for-profit dialysis industry—and PE involvement—by allowing people of any age with kidney disease to receive Medicare-funded treatment. The PE industry flocked to dentistry as states added these services to their Medicaid plans. Unquestionably, PE ownership of air medical transport has been facilitated by the Airline Deregulation Act, which prohibits states from regulating air carrier charges, including emergency medical helicopters. A massive rise in Medicare fees for such services enticed the shops as well.

Furthermore, political leaders have unwittingly colluded by not providing sufficient vital services, thus inviting PE to fill the gap. This undoubtedly has been the case with substance abuse and eating disorder treatments for which the need is far greater than the supply of public-sector or nonprofit providers. Federal officials aroused GP interest by mandating that insurers cover behavioral and mental health benefits equivalently to physical conditions (the Mental Health Parity and Addiction Equity Act). Other legislation also generated big bucks for PE to take advantage of, whether through government programs or commercial insurers: the Affordable Care Act, Comprehensive Addiction and Recovery Act, 21st Century Cures Act, and Opioid Crisis Response Act. None of these bills extends the number of community-run treatment centers to any great extent.

Similarly, government has provided limited options relative to the demand for treatment of children with autism spectrum disorders. The void has been filled by PE firms that were stirred up by the Individuals with Disabilities Education Act's mandate that school districts offer free and appropriate public educational services for all disabled children, including those with autism, and grant access to government-funded early ABA programs for infants and toddlers under age three. The Combating Autism / Autism CARES Act, the Affordable Care Act, and state requirements that commercial insurers cover ABA as a benefit in their plans also sparked the movement of PE into the area.

At the same time, political officials have not instituted sufficient or effective regulations, nor have they enforced those in place, allowing PE firms to exploit desperate people requiring health and caring services. In fact, it is the very dearth of external controls that draws PE to a niche in the first place. Dialysis, for instance, is a free-for-all that has made possible profitable but unsafe conditions for patients with failing kidneys. Home health agencies are heavily reimbursed by Medicare and Medicaid while lacking close scrutiny of how well they take care of their frail charges. PE efficiency measures, such as reduced staff training, cutbacks in wages and benefits, and low-quality services, stay under the radar of public scrutiny. PE firms are given free rein in the hospice industry, where they prey on people at the end of life and their families.

In the drug and alcohol rehabilitation, eating disorders treatment, and autism therapy industries, there is a paucity of government guidelines and oversight, and providers have few, if any, other standards that they must meet. PE firms are essentially given carte blanche to offer treatments based on what brings them the greatest financial returns in the shortest period, rather than meeting the specific needs of their customers. In air medical transport, there are few meaningful government requirements as to the type of aircraft, kind of equipment, extent of maintenance, or level of pilot training. Nor is there any certificate-of-need constraints on the number of service localities, leading to disconcerting practices at times.

Commodification of Health Services: The PE Toolkit

Beginning in the 1980s, the United States increasingly shifted from small, frequently nonprofit health businesses to larger commercial entities, even before private equity entered the picture. Physician practices, for example, were steadily purchased by hospital health systems. Nevertheless, a significant number of subsectors, especially those responsible for vulnerable populations, remained in the hands of founder-owners who were mission-driven to varying extents. PE firms take over commercial as well as nonprofit places, transforming them into moneymaking machines. And the number of such acquisitions, whether as add-ons or new platforms, is skyrocketing.

Debra Satz in her celebrated book on the moral limits of markets asks whether there are some things that should not be bought and sold.[3] Other scholars, too, argue that the United States should eschew the commercialization of certain products and services. Health care is high on the noxious market scale since it is, among other factors, fundamental for individuals and society at large; the stakes are far higher when you are dealing with people's lives, safety, and overall well-being. Nor do free-market conditions exist since the average patient is incapable of shopping around for high-quality services at the best prices. These problems epitomize a market failure: consumers tend to be unaware of costs, may be too sick or incapacitated to find out, and for a variety of reasons also may be powerless to choose among providers.

Private equity strategies, however, raise additional, possibly more troublesome questions about the commodification of medical and health services. Unlike large hospital health systems, for example, when PE firms purchase specialty medical practices, they put nonmedical owners in charge, potentially threatening physicians' autonomy over patient care. And efficiencies in a manufacturing production line that maximize profits can be harmful in a doctor's office or operating room. Patients' welfare should always come above all else. The evidence suggests, however, that given its financial model, PE control over lifesaving services—whether emergency medical transport or dialysis—collides head-on with the requirements of seriously ill or injured individuals.

The PE playbook inevitably entails placing outsized earnings first and foremost, and using whatever schemes are necessary to maximize

ROI. As discussed throughout this book, one tactic is leveraged buy-outs—a mainstay of PE financial wizardry—which necessitates loading mostly thriving companies with huge debt. Millions in liabilities are placed on physician and dental practices; autism, alcohol, drug, and eating disorder treatment centers; homecare agencies; and emergency transport enterprises, which drain their cash flow for repayment. These debts also engender cost-cutting strategies, generally resulting in worsening services. I maintain that it would take a magician to regularly pay down the immense debts, pay GPs their extensive fees and carried interest, and also provide affordable, high-quality health care.

Persistently high leverages in health segments do not augur well for indispensable caring businesses if conditions deteriorate into a recession, if other unanticipated interruptions in the economy occur (see below on COVID-19), or if they encounter sharp payment reductions or other financial setbacks. Over the decades, a number of extremely leveraged medical and health service enterprises have been ushered into bankruptcy, even without a calamitous event in the larger society. Geoff Lieberthal, a partner at Lee Equity Partners, bluntly stated that he worries the physician buyouts "will end badly."[4] Yet, as previous cases of Chapter 11 filings show, PE owners tend to remain largely unscathed while patients, workers, and communities pay the price. Can we afford mass insolvencies of physician offices when there already is a shortage of doctors and nurses? What about homecare, emergency medical transit, or other places serving at-risk individuals? The liquidation of Beatrice Companies and Toys "R" Us is far different than depriving individuals with kidney failure of dialysis treatments or dermatology patients of cancer therapies.

In conjunction with leveraged buyouts, GPs consolidate health areas through a buy-and-build strategy that involves creating new platforms or attaching acquisitions to established ones. PE shops seek niches that are highly fragmented, with the intention of scaling them into local, regional, or national chains. They push everyone and everything out of their way with smooth talk and promises of riches. At times, the procurements are so fast that the platform becomes a train wreck: it can't integrate the add-ons effectively.

In the second decade of the twenty-first century, the buying spree intensified in spaces such as homecare and hospice, including some mega-deals (Kindred Healthcare, Aveanna Healthcare, BrightSpring Health Services/ResCare, Encompass Health, Elara Caring). PE already has captured nearly half of all urgent care centers and two-thirds of the largest air medical transports (Air Methods and Air Medical Group Holdings). Correspondingly, it has amalgamated the leading ground ambulance company (American Medical Response) with Air Medical Group Holdings, forming an emergency rescue behemoth, Global Medical Response. And the far-reaching mergers have led to even greater debt for health-related portfolio chains. When KKR took Envision's American Medical Response division private, for example, it placed $2.1 billion in liabilities on the establishment.

The consolidations have not engendered any advantages for the beneficiaries of services. As chains emerge or enlarge, they boost prices for clients and public programs, seizing a significant portion of the gains for themselves. By the same token, when they are the only game in town, consumer choice is curtailed, even if the only option is low-quality care, for example in the case of dialysis centers. Because of their monopoly power, the PE-owned dialysis chains have successfully lobbied against strict regulations. Concentrated holdings have empowered other PE-backed companies to push against controls that threaten their financial well-being.

Despite the benefits touted by the PE industry—greater efficiency, an increased supply of limited services, and enhanced bargaining power with insurance companies—clients and employees are inevitably shortchanged. Yes, PE firms have augmented the availability of help for children with ASD, people with addiction or eating disorders, and elders in need of at-home assistance, but more has not meant sound, high-quality care. Greater efficiency in health care, at least under PE ownership, often translates into measures that undermine services, such as curtailed training of frontline workers and overuse of less qualified, unsupervised paraprofessionals; fosters an assembly line approach to patient care; and streamlines or eliminates investments in research, technologies, and capital equipment. Moreover, any improvements in insurer reimbursement rates tend to benefit the PE owners and not consumers or taxpayers.

The Eye Is Always on Exit

Short-term commitments to their portfolio companies underline and reinforce private equity's unwillingness to invest substantially in anything other than acquisitions and mergers. The short time frames also create incentives to economize on the frontline labor force and patient care alike. What services the business actually performs and its long-term viability are of little importance except for its ability to increase ROI; a GP's single-minded concern is to prime an enterprise for a high-value resale, and the sooner the better. Sales prior to the end of the usual PE hold period, roughly six years, ultimately yield a greater internal rate of return for the PE shop and its LPs.

As this book has made clear, serial leveraged buyouts are prevalent in health sectors, and these are ongoing. Aspen Dental Management, the largest but troubled dental management chain, has encountered four LBOs since 1997 and most likely is being prepared for a fifth, as is Smile Brands, which has an equally long PE turnover history. ReachOut Healthcare America was sold after three years of buying companies, two of them rivals. These are places with such scandalous conditions that they should have been shut down, not be enriching one PE firm after another.

Other examples of quick flips in the health sector abound, as I have detailed. After its first LBO, Forefront Dermatology changed hands eighteen months later; U.S. Dermatology Partners was transferred after only seventeen months and then again two years later. Home-care examples include Elara Caring and Abode Healthcare, which each dealt with three PE owners in ten years and slightly more than eight, respectively. In the ED market, Eating Recovery Center faced serial ownership by three PE firms in nine years, while Remuda Ranch / Meadows Ranch was tossed from PE to PE four times from 2001 to 2016. Likewise, the hospice provider Curo underwent three LBOs in eight years.

In seemingly never-ending scaling as they pass through multiple PE shops, health enterprises are subjected to financial piracy by each one. The PE titans soak up, like sponges, essential private and public money meant for at-risk individuals. Through myriad fees, intermittent dividend recaps, and oversized gains on investment from sales, extracted from their portfolio companies, a series of PE firms wrests every penny they can prior to relinquishing the businesses to the next buyer. Multiple rounds of refinancing, which bleed even more cash, add to their overall returns.

Full Steam Ahead

Despite the prospect of a recession, PE deals continue to flourish: in 2019 there were 5,133 transactions amounting to $678 billion. Elevated buyout costs persisted, along with growth in median deal size to more than $250 million. LPs, especially public pension funds, earmarked greater percentages of their total assets to the industry. CalPERS (the largest US public-sector pension fund), for instance, in 2020 targeted 8 percent of its $385 billion in assets for private equity, with the possibility of raising the percentage in coming years.[5]

GPs also increasingly turn to the less regulated private debt market that, by the end of 2019, had accumulated reserves of $276.5 billion; in that year, direct lenders—mostly PE firms—raised $74.5 billion, up from slightly less than $4 billion in 2009.[6] In other words, private equity's heavily leveraged loans are progressively financed through its own secretive industry, and with laxer terms and even less monitoring. According to Sebastien Canderle, a PE and venture capital advisor, roughly half of leveraged loans today are secured through non-bank lenders, and fully 80 percent of all LBOs are covenant-lite.[7]

The private equity industry is on a sugar high, having accumulated an unprecedented amount of committed dry powder. In North America alone, it secured $300 billion during 2019, an increase of 26 percent from 2018, reaching $1 trillion; total assets under management worldwide amounted to a staggering $4.5 trillion.[8] The shops continue to raise ever-larger funds, with even more unprecedented

sums envisioned for the rest of the 2020s. Fifteen mega-vehicles—
$5 billion and over—accounted for slightly more than half of the cap-
ital raised in 2019. Blackstone captured $26 billion, the highest sum
in PE history. Vista Equity Partners, Thoma Bravo, and Green Equity
Investors brought in more than $15 billion each.

Then the Coronavirus Arrived

Few GPs had substantially revamped their tactics because of the looming economic downturn, but COVID-19 forced them to do so; during
March 2020 the stock market crashed, losing 20 percent or more of
its overall value. Even though it subsequently rebounded, portfolio
companies were now at risk. As PitchBook researchers put it: "Because
PE is in many ways a leveraged bet on future economic growth, current portfolio companies will likely experience serious economic
carnage stemming from the COVID-19 fallout."[9]

Consequently, the financiers concentrated much of their attention
on protecting certain debt-loaded businesses from sinking by inject-
ing capital through such means as drawing down revolving lines of
credit, recapitalizations, subscription credit lines (temporarily using
LP commitments as security instead of actually calling in their capital), fund-level leveraged debt, preferred equity (secured by assets), or
resorting to the earnings of investment sales.[10] PE firms have proven
quite parsimonious with their own money over the decades so rescu-
ing their portfolio companies with assets derived primarily from their
LPs or with borrowed money corresponds to their modus operandi.[11]
The industry, particularly shops without an established LP base, also
faced considerable but temporary reductions in fundraising; delayed
exits because of reduced pricing levels; a slowdown in acquisitions and
mergers; and suppressed ROIs, especially in vintages 2012–2017.[12]

As would be expected, the pandemic affected various sectors of the
economy differently. In health markets, many providers struggled
with a dearth of customers because of state shelter-in-place mandates
or a barrage of cancellations from individuals who were adhering
to social distancing guidelines. Steadily drained of cash to cover

operating expenses, an increasing number of places downsized or furloughed staff, cutting hours and reducing pay and benefits. PE-owned places indubitably encountered difficulties in servicing their onerous debt, and as the outbreak of coronavirus continued, countless bankruptcies followed. For example, KKR's Envision Healthcare suffered declining revenues as potential patients deferred elective surgeries and steered clear of emergency rooms. Miriam Gottfried, a reporter for the *Wall Street Journal*, writes that prices on Envision bonds depreciated to "a level normally seen in companies in danger of bankruptcy."[13]

PE most likely will engage in slash-and-burn tactics in certain portfolio companies as the economic downturn lingers or if it develops into a recession. Canderle argues that highly distressed PE-held businesses, mostly with covenant-lite loans, could "defer payments to suppliers, reduce the quality of services to clients, cut salaries and employee benefits, renegotiate rental payments with landlords, delay R&D spend[ing], reschedule debt maturities, all in a bid to survive and enable their owners to continue charging commissions." Despite the distressed financial condition of their properties, PE firms have continued to collect their lucrative management fees. He warns that they could operate "for years in aimless, zombie-like mode," triggering "widespread economic paralysis."[14]

Equally important, if currently independent small and medium-size health businesses—from physician and dental practices to autism treatment and drug/alcohol rehabilitation centers—sustain revenue losses for an extended period of time, a large number of them will be more open to takeovers by PE firms but now at depressed valuations. For example, a survey of physician practices in Massachusetts indicated that more than 20 percent were "mulling consolidating with other practices, joining hospitals or health systems, or selling their practice."[15] The PE shops, of course, are like lurking lions, ready to pounce on their prey and gobble them up. Ultimately, the pandemic most likely will be a boon to the PE industry, hastening its consolidation goals.

One should never underestimate the PE industry's creativity and flexibility as it capitalizes on the pandemic and the financial turmoil it has wrought.[16] As Anton Levy, copresident and managing director at General Atlantic, pointed out: "recessions create opportunities."[17] The subgroup of PE that invests in financially troubled companies is experiencing increased market prospects for special situations, distressed, and opportunistic deals at huge discounts; these firms netted outsized returns during the 2008 economic crisis.[18] Bruce Flatt, CEO of Brookfield Asset Management, even enthuses that the pandemic created "one of the greatest environments possibly to buy distressed debt that may have ever been in existence."[19] The cash-rich traditional buyout shops are joining in but typically targeting strong places that are struggling only for the short term.[20] Ultra-low interest rates, which the Federal Reserve dropped to nearly zero in March 2020, buttressed their hard-nosed profiteering at a time of hardship in the larger society.

PE firms also are equipped to purchase stock in publicly traded companies through private investments in public equity, taking advantage of collapsed share prices.[21] A number of struggling companies, such as the Cheesecake Factory and Expedia Group, were forced to resort to private equity for rescue financing, but at a steep price: the shops generally collect huge dividends on the preferred stock they purchase, and eventually gain an equity stake in the business. Crystal Tse and Liana Baker, reporters for Bloomberg News, write, "It's gotten so popular that the bidding for slices of distressed companies can resemble a heated takeover battle, with as many as 20 private equity firms clamoring for a piece of one deal."[22]

The PE industry also benefited, albeit to a limited extent, from the national response to COVID-19. In mid-April 2020, PE-held home health and hospice agencies obtained a portion of the $50 billion in grants allocated specifically for health care providers (the Provider Relief Fund) under the Coronavirus Aid, Relief, and Economic Security (CARES) Act; they could use the money for just about anything since there were "no strings attached."[23] Certain portfolio companies also initially secured loans from the Federal Reserve's middle-market business lending program, which lacked substantial restrictions as well; they were subsequently cut out because of harsh political backlash.[24] In addition, certain establishments were able to tap into the government's accelerated and advance Medicare payments, which distributed billions to eligible providers, including home health agencies, hospitals, physician offices, and durable medical suppliers.

Characteristically, GPs lobbied vigorously through the American Investment Council (AIC) for other pieces of the $2.3 trillion CARES disaster relief, which at first prevented PE-owned companies from qualifying.[25] For example, the shops initially were explicitly excluded from the $660 billion Paycheck Protection Program (PPP), run by the Small Business Administration and the Treasury Department, because they are primarily engaged in investment and speculation. But the PE industry successfully pressed its case with Congress, and it was soon allowed to benefit from the bailout loans. However, the affiliate rule, which commingles the revenue and employee count of portfolio companies in a PE firm's fund, rendered it challenging for individual businesses to take advantage of PPP and other CARES Act opportunities.[26]

Regardless of these hurdles, roughly 2,500 PE-controlled entities circumvented the regulations, each receiving $150,000 or more in potentially forgivable loans; nearly half of the businesses collected more than $1 million.[27] For example, some dental practices, which are indirectly owned through dental services organizations, availed themselves of the cash. Reporter Heather Perlberg found that nearly all of Aspen Dental Management's offices (owned by American Securities and Candescent Partners) applied for and were accepted for PPP loans.[28] As discussed above, the serially PE-held chain has a scandalous history of abusive behavior.

Perlberg writes that several PE-owned physician practices also benefited, including Oliver Street Dermatology of U.S. Dermatology Partners (Abry Partners), New Jersey Urology (Prospect Hill Growth Partners), and Eyecare Partners (Gauge Capital); they received $5 million–$10 million, $2 million–$5 million, and $2 million–$5 million, respectively.[29] In other industry sectors, eleven of Riverside's portfolio companies received loans totaling between $28.4 million and $59 million, and thirty-one companies owned by Main Street Capital Corporation got loans worth between $38.4 million and $88.4 million.[30]

The AIC was particularly successful in ensuring that the industry could partake in the Federal Reserve's subsequent $600 billion Main Street Lending Program, although the preponderance of PE-owned companies exceeded the program's debt limit. PE's appeal for more taxpayer money was supported by the Institutional Limited Partners Association, which lobbies on behalf of public pension funds. The association's major concerns are employment and especially the potential for appreciably lower earnings on its PE investments, which would adversely affect public employee retirement benefits.[31]

Unexpectedly, several Democrats, anxious about a reduction of jobs in their districts, pushed for greater PE access to the national largesse. Bethany Mclean points out that because PE is so inextricably interwoven with the US economy, "its losses, to a remarkable degree, will belong to all of us. . . . Like the big banks in 2008, private equity is holding us all hostage." Has private equity become, as she suggests, too big to fail?[32] The industry employs approximately 9 million people at more than 35,000 US businesses. And public pension funds are highly dependent on PE investment earnings to fund a portion of the retirement benefits for as many as 19 million workers.

Despite trillions in committed capital already under management, PE firms intend to dig deeper into the US economy by capturing the untapped reserves of *private* pension funds as well. GPs and the AIC have been salivating for years at the prospect of snaring more workers' retirement assets.[33] Up until now, fearing lawsuits alleging violation of their fiduciary duty under the Employee Retirement Income Security Act, administrators of corporate programs shied away from these risky investments. But under the guise of spurring an economy devastated by the COVID-19 pandemic, and with Trump's mandate to "remove barriers" to growth, the US Labor Department issued a guidance letter in May 2020 permitting managers of defined contribution programs to add PE to their plan offerings. The directive allows GPs potential access to more than $6.2 trillion in 401(k) plans and $2.5 trillion in IRA accounts.[34]

Even Vanguard Group, the largest provider of mutual funds and the second largest of exchange-traded vehicles, with $6.2 trillion in assets, is opening its doors to PE shops. In February 2020, Vanguard announced that it was teaming up with HarbourVest to expand its platform by providing institutional clients access to stakes in private equity investments. Antoine Gara, a reporter for *Forbes*, suggests that this step "is a watershed, which will continue to push private equity buyouts into the center of the financial world."[35] Vanguard plans to eventually allow individual savers to have access as well.

The PE industry also anticipates spreading its reach markedly, especially expanding the type, magnitude, and range of its health investments. The US medical system and its related businesses are brimming with dollars that will steadily climb to $6.19 trillion and consume nearly 20 percent of the GDP toward the end of the 2030s.[36] In their ongoing foray into health services, PE titans are like northern snakeheads, voracious, fast-growing, and invasive fish with sharp dagger-like teeth, which overwhelm their environment.

Where Do We Go from Here?

Private equity is not going away anytime soon, but the nation must severely limit its spread. Most important, loopholes in the US tax code undergird the entire PE industry. Carried interest, the main source of outsized earnings for GPs, is assessed at the far lower capital gains rate rather than as income. Interest paid on leveraged buyouts is tax deductible, engendering excessive debt on portfolio companies. The Stop Wall Street Looting Act would be a start in that it considers carried interest as personal earnings, strictly limits the deductibility of interest payments, and places levies on monitoring and transaction fees. The Carried Interest Fairness Act of 2021, introduced by Bill Pascrell (the Democratic chair of the Oversight Subcommittee of the House Ways and Means Committee), would tax carried-interest gains as ordinary income (as high as 37 percent) rather than at the capital gains rate (15–20 percent).[37] Undoubtedly, if the United States eliminates the industry's tax advantages, it can put a powerful chokehold on the PE industry's advancement.

Among other stark and in my view indispensable PE-related provisions, the Stop Wall Street Looting Act would render GPs partly liable for the debt placed on their portfolio companies; curb dividend recaps within a year of an LBO; assist workers in capturing their back pay, severance, and pensions in cases of bankruptcy while restraining executive payoffs; and require far greater disclosure to the Securities and Exchange Commission.[38] I propose that it should also extend the unveiling of private equity's secret maneuvers to include its private lending business, and all information must be publicly available. At a minimum, regulators should be able to access data on the extent of PE firms' holdings, financial engineering, and dividend recaps; the terms and scope of their loans; and other vital, currently concealed material, exposing the industry's most aggressive and exploitive behaviors.

To control the excesses of PE shops and the loading of portfolio companies with unsustainable debt, the US government must enact and strengthen banking and lending laws. Among other issues, financial institutions and private direct-lending funds should be prevented from doling out weakly supervised, covenant-lite loans that heighten the odds of bankruptcy. We must also place upper limits on the allowable debt for portfolio companies. When investee businesses go belly-up, they leave others to bear the costs. Equally critical, political officials should reexamine the federal laws and rules that allow PE shops to dodge financial responsibility for repaying the heavy debts they impose on their acquired firms. The Stop Wall Street Looting Act would render GPs partially liable, but in my view they should be held fully accountable for such irresponsible financial piracy. In addition, the nation must prohibit the draining of vulnerable establishments via dividend recaps, not just limit the practice to within a year of an LBO. The declawed Securities and Exchange Commission, Federal Reserve Board, Consumer Financial Protection Bureau, and Internal Revenue Service— at least when it comes to private equity—require stronger mandates, tougher supervision, and real consequences for perpetrators.

In other areas, stringent regulations, enforcement, and penalties for the mostly unfettered PE industry would check the damage it does to clients and workers alike. In particular, the shell entities that own physician and dental practices—physician practice management companies, and dental service organizations, respectively—violate the CPOM doctrine and should be banned; they are only camouflages for PE control. Criminal charges and penalties for GPs for instigating and abetting any mistreatment of individuals by their portfolio companies surely would capture their attention.

PE's buy-and-build strategy, commonplace in health sectors, often generates local, regional, or national monopolies. Indeed, as I have shown throughout this book, consolidation and control are the goals of this approach. In the process, PE firms may acquire their portfolio company's competitors to corner the horizontal market, and its suppliers, including testing labs, to expand vertically. How do these pursuits evade the three federal antitrust laws: the Sherman Act, the Federal Trade Commission Act, and the Clayton Act? Together, among other objectives, these statutes prohibit monopoly dominance of an industry or sector by one corporation while cutting out the competition; anticompetitive acquisitions and mergers; acquiring market share through exclusionary or predatory practices; price rigging; and discriminatory prices, services, and allowances in dealings between merchants.

However, under the Hart-Scott-Rodino Antitrust Improvements Act of 1976 (amending the Clayton Act), only large companies must file a report alerting the Federal Trade Commission and the US Department of Justice of impending acquisitions and mergers. Private equity add-ons in health care are often low enough to slip under the transaction threshold—$94 million in 2020—thereby eluding scrutiny by regulators. Evidently, the United States must tighten the antitrust laws that the PE industry is sidestepping, sometimes legally, and just as important, put teeth into additional regulatory bodies and more fully fund them, especially the FTC and the Department of Justice's Antitrust Division.

Finally, the nation must starve the beast by fortifying and enforcing breach-of-fiduciary-duty regulations on executives and trustees, including those managing public pension funds. To be sure, there are growing questions as to whether the risks of PE are worth the extra returns or even whether its yields outperform public stocks.[39] Correspondingly, the federal government should reverse its unsound decision on opening PE access to the trillions in company 401(k) plans and individual IRA accounts.

Clearly, with seemingly unlimited capital at its disposal—more than $1.5 trillion in dry powder by 2022 and the potential for trillions more in new investor money—the private equity industry presently has carte blanche to drain value from ever more companies and leave everyone else with the bill. Indeed, even in the midst of the COVID-19 pandemic, Blackstone jumped on Ancestry, a genealogy corporation, in a $4.7 billion deal; the PE behemoth now has the ability to capitalize on vast amounts of DNA, hereditary material of incalculable value. Only a radical transformation of the US tax laws, financial system, and regulatory bodies will truly stop PE from gaming the system and looting everything of value.

Selected Private Equity Firms Buying
Health Care Businesses

Name	Health Subsectors (covered in this book)	Overall Investment Sectors (as identified on each PE firm's website)
Abry Partners	dermatology, dentistry, autism disorders	health care IT services, business, communications, information services, insurance services, media & entertainment
Advent International Corporation	home health care	business & financial services, health care, industrial, retail, consumer & leisure, technology
Altamont Capital Partners	autism disorders	business services, consumer, financial services, health care, industrial, retail & franchising
Altaris Capital Partners	home health care	health care
Altos Health Management (acquired by MMC Health Services)	autism disorders	health care
American Securities	dentistry, emergency medical transport	consumer, health care, industrial, power & energy, services
Amulet Capital Partners	gastroenterology	health care
Apax Partners (merged with Saunders Karp & Megrue)	home health care	tech & telco, services, health care, consumer
APG Partners	dentistry	health care
Apollo Global Management (publicly traded)	substance abuse, therapy staffing	financial services, business services, consumer services, chemicals, natural resources, consumer & retail, leisure, manufacturing & industrial, media, telecom & technology
aPriori Capital Partners	substance abuse	health care, retail & consumer, energy, business services, certain industrial sectors
Arcapita, Inc.	dentistry	senior living, industrial logistics / warehousing services, retail / consumer services
Ares Capital Corporation (publicly traded)	dentistry	diversified
Arsenal Capital Partners	autism disorders	specialty industrial, health care

Name	Health Subsectors (covered in this book)	Overall Investment Sectors (as identified on each PE firm's website)
A. S. F. Co-Investment Partners	dentistry	out of business
Atlantic Street Capital Management	orthopedics	diversified
Atlas Partners	eye care	diversified
Audax Group	dermatology, orthopedics, gastroenterology, urology, reproductive medicine, dentistry, hospice, home health care	business services, health care, industrial technology, consumer products & services
Bain Capital	renal care, home health care, substance abuse, emergency medical transport, hospitals	consumer, financial & business services, health care, industrial, technology
Baird Capital	autism disorders	health care, technology & services, industrial solutions
Beecken Petty O'Keefe & Company	medical staffing	health care, medical products, IT
BelHealth Investment Partners	home health care, substance abuse, dermatology, physician staffing	health care
Beringea	homecare	health care, clean technology, consumer, media, business services, technology
Black Canyon Capital (out of business)	dentistry	business services, consumer & retail, health care, restaurant, industrial products & services, media & environment, niche manufacturing
Blackstone Group (publicly traded)	medical staffing, autism disorders	diversified
Blue Ox Healthcare Partners	substance abuse	health care
Blue Sea Capital	urgent care, eye care	aerospace & defense, health care, industrial growth
Blue Wolf Capital	home health care	health care, forest & building products, energy services, niche manufacturing & distribution, industrial & engineering
Bow River Capital Partners	orthopedics	diversified
BPEA Private Equity	autism disorders, urgent care	health care
Brentwood Associates	dentistry, urgent care	business services, consumer
Brockway Moran & Partners	urgent care, emergency medical transport	consumer, industrial, services
Brown Brothers Harriman Capital Partners	home health care	diversified
C3 Capital	substance abuse, orthopedics	chemicals, consumer products, business services, distribution, niche manufacturing

Caltius Structured Capital	substance abuse	business / professional services, consumer services, consumer products, financial services, health care services, specialty manufacturing, specialty staffing, tech-enabled services
Cambria Group	substance abuse	business services, consumer products & services, health care, industrial products, manufacturing, retail
Candescent Partners	dentistry, orthopedics, eye care	health care, software, business & technology-enabled services, consumer products & services
Capital Resource Partners	dentistry, substance abuse	software & informational services, proprietary industrial products & services, business services, consumer products & services, health care services, products & technology
Capital Southwest	orthopedics	diversified
Capstar Partners	home health care, hospice	diversified
Carlyle Group (publicly traded)	dentistry, home health care, hospice, eating disorders	diversified
Catalyst Group	home health care	diversified
CCMP Capital	eating disorders	consumer, industrial, health care
Celerity Partners	substance abuse	health care, contract manufacturing, energy services, infrastructure & environmental services, transportation & logistics
Centerbridge Partners	renal care	consumer, financial services, health care, industrial, real estate, technology, media & telecom
Centre Partners	eye care, eating disorders, home health care	consumer, health care, business services, industrial, energy, cable / media, financial services
Charterhouse Group	autism disorders	consumer, health care, industrial, services
CHL Medical Partners	drug abuse	health care
Clayton, Dubilier & Rice (CD&R)	physician staffing, emergency medical transport	consumer / retail, health care, industrial, services
Constitution Capital Partners	home health care	diversified
Cornerstone Equity Investors	medical staffing, home health care	real estate, professional services, technology, logistics & transportation, consumer products
Court Square Capital Partners	dentistry	business services, general industrial, health care, technology & telecommunications
Cressey & Company	dermatology, renal care, home health care, hospice	health care & health care IT
DW Healthcare Partners	autism disorders, renal care	health care

Name	Health Subsectors (covered in this book)	Overall Investment Sectors (as identified on each PE firm's website)
EOS Partners	home health care	consumer, energy & energy services, financial services, health care services, transportation & logistics, business services / other, marketing services & media
Eureka Capital Partners	home health care	industrial, health care, business services, consumer
FFL Partners	eye care, dentistry, substance abuse, autism disorders, urgent care	business services, consumer, financial services, industrial, health care
Five Arrows Capital Partners (PE arm of Rothschild & Co.)	autism disorders	health care, business services, data & software, technology-enabled services
Flexpoint Ford	substance abuse, eye care	financial services, health care
Formation Capital	home health care, hospice	seniors housing & care, post-acute & health care, real estate investments
Frazier Healthcare Partners	orthopedics, gastroenterology, home health care, hospice, dermatology, renal care	health care
Freeman Spogli & Co.	dentistry, renal care	consumer services & products, consumer health care, e-commerce, multiunit rental, restaurants, retail services, distribution
Frontenac Company	substance abuse	services, consumer, industrial
Fulcrum Equity Partners	substance abuse	health care services, health care IT, software & software-as-a-service, tech-enabled services
Gauge Capital	eye care, primary care	food safety, health care, technology
Gemini Investors	home health care, substance abuse, dentistry	business services, consumer products & services, health care, later-stage technology, manufacturing & distribution, waste & recycling
General Atlantic	autism disorders, urgent care	consumer, financial services, health care, technology
GI Partners	autism disorders	health care, IT infrastructure, services, software
Golden Gate Capital	autism disorders	consumer, financial services, industrial, software, information systems, tech-enabled services
Great Point Partners	surgical assistant staffing, autism disorders	health care
Greenridge Investment Partners	substance abuse	business services, education & training, enterprise software & technology services, health care services (limited exposure to Medicare & Medicaid), media & communications

Gryphon Investors	dentistry, autism disorders, dermatology	business services, consumer products & services, industrial growth, software
GTCR Private Equity	home health care, dermatology	financial services & technology, health care, technology, media & telecommunications, growth business services
Halifax Group	home health care, substance abuse, autism disorders	franchising, health & wellness, outsourced business services
Hampshire Equity Partners	ground ambulance	diversified
Harvest Partners	dermatology, eye care, dentistry	business services, consumer products & services, industrial services, manufacturing & distribution, health care
HCP & Co.	autism disorders	business services, consumer products, education, health care services
HealthView Capital Partners	home health care, hospice	health care service delivery, patient-driven outcomes, health care information services
Heritage Group	home health care	health care
H. I. G. Capital	hospice, substance abuse, autism disorders, eye care	diversified
H. I. G. Growth Partners	substance abuse	technology-enabled services, internet & digital marketing services, cloud & data software, consumer e-commerce, health care, industrial technologies
Highland Capital Partners	home health care, hospice	consumer & enterprise technology, enterprise software, health technology, next-generation infrastructure, robotics, real estate technology, digital media & marketing
Housatonic Partners	substance abuse	technology, business services, communications, health care
ICG Enterprise Trust	home health care	diversified
J. H. Whitney & Company	home health care	consumer, health care, specialty manufacturing
JLL Partners	dentistry	health care, industrial, business services
Jordan Company	autism disorders, home health care	consumer & health care, energy, industrial, tactical opportunities, telecom, technology & utility, transportation & logistics
J. W. Childs Associates (renamed Prospect Hill Growth Partners)	urology	consumer products & services, health care
KarpReilly	home health care	branded consumer products, digitally native brands, food & beverage, restaurants, retail

Name	Health Subsectors (covered in this book)	Overall Investment Sectors (as identified on each PE firm's website)
KKR	physician staffing, emergency medical transport, dentistry, home health care, substance abuse, autism disorders, health information, hospitals	diversified
Kohlberg & Company	orthopedics, substance abuse, eating disorders	industrial manufacturing, consumer products, business services, health care services, financial services
Lee Equity Partners	reproductive medicine, home health care, eating disorders, substance abuse	diversified
Leonard Green & Partners	renal care, dentistry	business services, consumer products / retail, consumer services, distribution, health care services, industrial, other
Levine Leichtman Capital Partners (LLCP)	home health care, eating disorders	consumer, education, health care, light manufacturing, services
Linden Capital Partners	orthopedics, dentistry, substance abuse	health care
Linsalata Capital Partners	home health care	diversified
Littlejohn & Company	dentistry	diversified
LLR Partners	autism, dermatology, eye care, substance abuse	business services, education, financial technology, health care, human resources technology, industrial, security, software
Lorient Capital	orthopedics	health care
Lunsford Capital	eating disorders, nursing homes, real estate	health care, technology, entertainment, real estate
Madison Dearborn Partners	physician staffing	basic industries, business & government, software & services, financial & transaction services, health care, telecom, media & technological services
Mammoth Equity Partners	substance abuse	health care, business process outsourcing, pharmaceutical services, light manufacturing, distribution
Martis Capital (rebranded from Capricorn Healthcare)	autism disorders	services & outsourcing, IT, consumer & wellness, products & diagnostics
MBF Healthcare Partners	autism disorders	health care
Milestone Partners	autism disorders, medical staffing	financial services, tech-driven manufacturing, tech-enabled solutions
Millpond Equity Partners	emergency medical transport	business services
Morgan Stanley Investment Management	dentistry, reproductive medicine	diversified

MVP Capital Partners	emergency medical transport	media, renewable energy, technology, telecom towers
Nautic Partners	eating disorders, home health care, primary care	health care, industrial, services
New Mainstream Capital (publicly traded)	dermatology, dentistry, eye care, medical staffing, urology	business services, health care services
New Mountain Capital	dentistry	education, health care, software, business services, logistics, specialty chemicals, federal services, financial services & insurance, environmental services
NexPhase Capital	home health care, autism disorders	consumer, health care, software & services
North Castle Partners	substance abuse	beauty & personal care, fitness, food & beverage, home / leisure, specialty nutrition, sports, outdoor recreation & active living, sustainable living, wellness & consumer-driven health care
Northwestern Mutual Capital	home health care	diversified
Oak Hill Capital Partners	home health care	services, industrial, media & communications, consumer, retail & distribution
Oaktree Capital Management	emergency medical transport	diversified
OMERS Private Equity	dentistry, dermatology	business services, health care, industrial, consumer, software
One Equity Partners	home health care	industrial, health care, technology
Onex Partners (publicly traded)	physician staffing, home health care, emergency medical transport	consumer & retail, financial services, health care, industrial, services
Ontario Teachers' Pension Plan	dentistry	industrial & business services, energy & power, financial services, consumer & retail, health care, technology, media & telecommunications
Paladin Healthcare Capital	hospitals	health care
Palladium Equity Partners	home health care	consumer, services, industrial, health care
Partners Group	eye care	health care, consumer, media & telecom, IT, industrial, infrastructure / energy & utilities, financial services & business services, real estate
Patriarch Partners	emergency medical transport	automotive & aerospace, beauty, consumer, fashion, home, industrial, manufacturing, services, tech
Pauschine Cook Capital Management	home health care	health care services, business services, education & training, environmental services, industrial manufacturing, specialty chemicals

Name	Health Subsectors (covered in this book)	Overall Investment Sectors (as identified on each PE firm's website)
Peterson Partners	autism disorders	business services, health care, retail / consumer, software & internet
Petra Capital Partners	autism disorders, substance abuse	business services, health care, technology-enabled services
Pharos Capital Group	home health care, autism disorders, dermatology	health care
Pimlico Capital	renal care	business & technology, communications, health care
Post Capital Partners	autism disorders, home health care, eating disorders	business services, environmental & industrial services, security services, education services, health care, data / information services, financial information services, niche manufacturing & distribution, transportation & logistics, consumer products & services
Prairie Capital	dermatology, eating disorders	business services, consumer, education, health care, industrial, technology
Prospect Partners	eating disorders, substance abuse	diversified
Quad-C Management	dentistry, eye care	business & consumer services, health care, industrial, specialty distribution, transportation & logistics
Resolute Capital Partners	autism disorders, dermatology, orthopedics	energy, commercial real estate, technology & software
Revelstoke Capital Partners	orthopedics, renal care, substance abuse, physician staffing, eye care, urgent care	health care
Ridgemont Equity Partners	home health care	business & industrial services, energy & sustainable strategies, health care, tech & telecom
Riverside Company	home health care, dentistry, substance abuse, eating disorders, autism disorders	business services, consumer brands, education & training, franchisers, health care, software & IT, specialty manufacturing
Roark Capital Group	dentistry	franchise / multiunit restaurant & food, health & wellness, retail health care, business services
Safanad	home health care	health care, education
Sentinel Capital Partners	dentistry, home health care	aerospace / defense, business services, consumer, distribution, food / restaurants, franchising, health care, industrial
Sheridan Capital Partners	dentistry	health care
Shore Capital Partners	eye care, dentistry, autism disorders, urgent care	health care, food & beverage

Stellus Capital Management	eating disorders	aerospace & defense, business services, consumer products, distribution, education, financial services, health care, manufacturing, media & entertainment, restaurants & retail, software & technology, telecommunications
Sterling Partners	dermatology, eye care, substance abuse	consumer, education, business services, financial services & technology, health care services, industrial services & maintenance
Summit Partners	renal care, dentistry, hospice, physician staffing	technology, health care, life sciences, growth products & services, financial services, consumer
Sverica Capital Management	reproductive medicine	technology, business services, health care, high-value industrial
TA Associates	autism disorders	business services, consumer, financial services, health care, technology
Tailwind Capital	dentistry, home health care	health care, business services, industrial services
Thoma Bravo	eating disorders	software, technology
Thomas H. Lee Partners	home health care, hospice, autism disorders	financial services, health care, consumer, technology & business solutions
TowerBrook Capital Partners	home health care, physician staffing	consumer, financial services, health care & health care services, industrial, telecommunications, media & education
TPG Capital	urgent care, home health, hospice, autism disorders, nurse staffing	consumer & retail, financial services, health care, internet & digital media, industrial services, real estate, natural resources & energy, technology
Trimaran Capital Partners	autism disorders	energy, infrastructure, telecom / media, technology, consumer products & services, manufacturing
Trinity Hunt Partners	home health care, substance abuse, eating disorders	business, health care, consumer services
Valor Equity Partners	dentistry	diversified
Varsity Healthcare Partners	dermatology, eye care, orthopedics, gastroenterology, home health care, emergency staffing	health care
Veronis Suhler Stevenson	autism disorders	business services, health care—IT & services, information, education
Vestar Capital Partners	eating disorders, oncology, hospitals	consumer services, health care services, business & technology services
Vicente Capital Partners	dermatology	diversified

Name	Health Subsectors (covered in this book)	Overall Investment Sectors (as identified on each PE firm's website)
Vista Verde Group	autism disorders, dentistry	technology, health care
Vistria Group	substance abuse	health care, education, financial services
W Capital Partners	home health care	software, financial technology & services, business services & industrial, health care, education technology, e-commerce & consumer, media
Warburg Pincus	urgent care, emergency medical transport	consumer, energy, financial services, health care, industrial & business services, real estate, technology, media & telecommunications
Warwick Capital Group	substance abuse	health care, IT, niche manufacturing, business services, payment processing, value-added resale, specialty finance, contract management, government services, distribution & logistics
Waud Capital Partners	eye care, substance abuse, eating disorders, gastroenterology	health care services, business & technology services
Webster Equity Partners (rebranded from Webster Capital Management)	home health care, substance abuse, eating disorders, medical staffing	health care
Wellspring Capital Management	home health care, autism disorders	general industrial, business services, health care services, packaging, distribution, consumer / restaurants
Welsh, Carson, Anderson and Stowe (WCAS)	urgent care, home health care, hospice, dentistry, dermatology, renal care, physician staffing	health care, technology
West Street Capital Partners (PE division of Goldman Sachs)	eye care	diversified
Wicks Group	autism disorders	business, consumer, education
WindRose Health Investors (rebranded from MTS Health Investors)	reproductive medicine, substance abuse, autism disorders	health care
Yukon Partners	substance abuse	automotive, consumer products, industrial manufacturing, building products, food & beverages, specialty manufacturing, business services, health care products & services, transportation & logistics

ABA	applied behavior analysis
ASD	autism spectrum disorders
AUM	assets under management
CMS	Centers for Medicare and Medicaid Services
CPOM	corporate practice of medicine
DSO	dental service organization
EBITDA	earnings before interest, taxes, depreciation, and amortization
ED	eating disorders
EMS	emergency medical services
ER	emergency room
EV	enterprise value
GAO	Government Accountability Office
GI	gastrointestinal
GP	general partner
HCBS	home- and community-based services
HEMS	helicopter emergency medical services
HHA	home health agency
IPO	initial public offering
IRR	internal rate of return
IT	information technology
IVF	in vitro fertilization
LBO	leveraged buyout
LP	limited partner
LTC	long-term care
MA	Medicare Advantage
NYSE	New York Stock Exchange
PACE	programs of all-inclusive care for the elderly
PE	private equity
PIPE	private investment in public equity
PPMC	physician practice management company
PPS	prospective payment system
R&D	research and development

RBT	registered behavior technician
REIT	real estate investment trust
ROI	return on investment
SBO	secondary buyout
SEC	Securities and Exchange Commission
UCC	urgent care center

alternative investments. Assets that are not a traditional investment type (cash, stocks, bonds), including private equity, hedge funds, commodities, real estate, and venture capital.

arbitrage. When an investor profits from simultaneously buying and selling a commodity or asset through different platforms, exchanges, or locations so as to cash in on the price differential.

balance billing. When a provider bills a patient for the difference between its charge and the amount paid by the insurance company. This is not allowed when physicians, hospitals, or other health care providers participate in the patient's insurance network.

board-certified behavior analyst. A person certified in applied behavior analysis (ABA).

bridge loan. Temporary, limited amount of financing until a long-term debt or equity investment can be secured.

carried interest. A general partner's share of the capital gains from a fund, usually 20 percent.

cash flow. The amount of money generated or spent on operations, capital investments, and financing activities for a specific period.

Chapter 11. The section of the US Bankruptcy Code that outlines the process for asset reorganization.

club deal. When two or more private equity firms join to pursue a deal.

collateralized loan obligations. Security backed by a pool of loans that are sold to investors in various slices with different interest rates reflecting their different degrees of risk.

corporate practice of medicine doctrine. Prohibits corporations from practicing medicine or employing a physician to provide professional medical services.

covenant. A legally binding promise by the borrowing company that certain activities will or will not take place, thereby protecting lenders from debtors defaulting on their financial obligations. Some covenants are checked regularly while others are only tested upon the occurrence of a specific event.

covenant-lite. Borrower-friendly loans that place fewer restrictions than traditional covenants and have fewer safeguards for banks and other institutions that finance PE transactions.

distressed debt investing. Acquiring stakes in the bank loans of troubled companies to generate returns through a potential appreciation of the debt or a subsequent right to the business upon resale.

distressed investment. An investment made in a company experiencing liquidity, capitalization, or underperformance issues.

dividend recapitalization. A financial restructuring of a private equity–owned company whereby the company takes on additional debt to pay a special dividend to the PE owners.

dry powder. Total amount of capital from limited partners that PE funds have available for investments but have not deployed yet.

EBITDA. A common PE metric used to value buyouts. A multiple of EBITDA is often used to describe the sale price of a company.

enterprise value. A measure of a company's aggregate value, including debt, less any cash or cash equivalents it holds.

financial buyer. An investor interested primarily in the return achieved from buying and selling companies.

general partner. A private equity firm that manages all aspects of a fund.

growth equity investment. When an investor gives a mature company capital it can use to expand or restructure in exchange for equity (usually a minority stake).

hard cap. Maximum fund size as stated by fund managers in a limited partnership agreement, although they often surpass these limits.

hedge fund. An investment company that pools the assets of clients to invest in various types of opportunities, often using complex strategies to boost profits. These funds are more liquid than private equity investments and more open-ended in that clients can redeem their money at any time.

high-yield bond. See junk bond.

home- and community-based services. Opportunities for Medicaid beneficiaries to receive services in their home or community rather than in an institution.

hurdle rate. A carried interest provision that investors will receive a certain percentage return before the GP is entitled to receive any carried interest.

initial public offering. The first time a company's stock is available to the public.

inorganic growth. Growth from acquisitions and mergers rather than an increase in a company's own business activities.

internal rate of return. Dominant measure used by the PE industry to measure a fund's performance, on average, over time.

investment bank. A financial organization that advises companies and governments on fundraising activities; advises companies on merger and acquisition activities; and acts as manager of a company's initial (or later) public offering, debt issuance, and other complex financial transactions.

junk bond. Debt that is not backed up with any collateral and has a greater risk of default than most other bonds but is compensated with higher interest rates.

leveraged buyout. Use of above-average debt to finance the purchase of investment assets.

limited partner. An entity that commits capital to a general partner's fund.

management buyout. A buyout that a company's management team leads or participates in.

management fee. A fixed charge by a PE firm to cover expenses for overseeing an acquisition.

management services organization. An entity designed to help physicians with the nonmedical administration work involved in running a practice.

managing director/partner. The most senior member of a private equity firm and the ultimate decision-maker.

Medicare Advantage. A type of health insurance plan that provides Medicare benefits through a private-sector health insurer.

mezzanine financing. A form of junior unsecured debt or preferred equity raised in the private institutional market, usually for leveraged buyouts.

middle-market company. A company with an enterprise value of $25 million–$1 billion.

multiple arbitrage. Investment gains achieved by increasing the sales multiple relative to the original investment multiple without making any operational improvement.

nondisclosure agreement. A legal contract that restricts access of third parties to information shared between the signatories.

organic growth. Growth resulting from expanding an organization's output, customer base, and new products, along with engaging in internal activities that increase revenue.

patient-driven groupings model. An approach for reimbursing home health agencies that relies on thirty-day payment periods.

physician practice management company. A firm that provides non-clinical business administration services to private practices.

platform company. Private equity–backed company that is used as the base for acquisitions.

portfolio company. A company that a PE firm invests in and holds in its fund.

post-acute care. The range of continued medical and other services, either at home or in a specialized facility, that support an individual's continued recovery from injury or illness following a hospitalization.

preferred stock. A senior form of equity that provides shareholders with certain preferential rights relative to common equity shareholders.

private equity. Alternative market that provides financial backing and makes investments in companies through a variety of strategies, including leveraged buyouts and growth capital.

private equity fund. A vehicle for enabling pooled investments by several investors in equity and equity-related securities of companies.

private investment in public equity. Private sale of shares of a publicly listed company to selected investors.

prospective payment system. A method of reimbursement in which Medicare payment is made based on a predetermined, fixed amount.

rate of return. Net gain or loss of an investment over a specified time, quantified as a percentage of the investment's initial cost.

recapitalization. An investment strategy that involves restructuring a company's debt and equity mix.

refinancing. Paying off existing debt with new debt.

return on investment. A measure of the amount of gain relative to the investment cost, often expressed as a percentage and calculated as net profit divided by cost of investment.

reverse merger / reverse takeover. When a private company acquires a public company.

revolving credit. A line of bank credit that a company can draw on as needed to fund its working capital needs.

roll-up. The process of acquiring and merging multiple smaller firms in the same industry and consolidating them into an increasingly larger company.

secondary buyout. The purchase by a private equity firm of majority ownership in a company from another private equity firm.

senior debt. Higher-level liens that must be repaid first in case of default by or liquidation of the issuer.

service debt. The process of paying off debt.

strategic investor. Usually a large, established company that makes an investment in a business for its technology, products, or services.

take private. The acquisition of a publicly listed company and its subsequent delisting. Also referred to as a public-to-private transaction.

target company. The entity purchased by a PE firm.

tranche. One of several related securities that are part of the same transaction.

valuation multiple. An expression of the market value of a company relative to a key statistic driving that value.

value-based care. A health care delivery model in which providers, including hospitals and physicians, are paid based on patient health outcomes.

venture capital. A type of investing that focuses on start-ups and early-stage companies with long-term, high-growth potential.

vintage year. Date when a fund is closed to additional capital and starts investing.

zombie company. A firm that received its first capital investment long ago, is not growing or is growing very slowly, has barely enough cash flow to keep operating, and has no clear path to liquidity (being sold or having an IPO).

zombie fund. A private equity fund that is beyond the original fund term (ten to twelve years), is long past its investment period, and has few remaining portfolio companies that have not been exited. It may hold on to these enterprises to continue collecting management fees.

Sources: Zeisberger, Prahl, and White, *Mastering Private Equity;* "Venture Capital, Private Equity."

Introduction. Hiding in Plain Sight

1. This book targets private equity firms, excluding other alternative investments such as venture capital and hedge funds.

2. Aschoff, "Ban Private Equity."

3. For example, in early May 2020, J. Crew and Neiman Marcus filed for Chapter 11 largely because they could not sustain their inordinate debt loads, especially when faced with the loss of sales during the COVID-19 pandemic. In 2011, J. Crew had been taken private by TPG Capital and Leonard Green & Partners for $3 billion, and in early 2020 it had $1.7 billion in liabilities. In 2013, Ares Capital and the Canadian Pension Plan Investment Board had acquired Neiman Marcus from TPG Capital and Warburg Pincus in a $6 billion leveraged buyout; at the time of its bankruptcy the company was saddled with $5.1 billion in debt. Dowd, "11 Big Things."

4. Throughout this book, the terms "shop" and "house" are used interchangeably for a PE firm.

5. Harvey, *Brief History*.

6. Harvey, *Brief History*, 3.

7. Brown, *Undoing the Demos*.

8. Lebow, "Trumpism."

9. Wharton School, Twenty-Fifth Conference.

10. The Business Roundtable is an association of chief executive officers of leading US companies. Gelles and Yaffe-Bellany, "Shareholder Value."

11. Harvey, *Brief History*, 174.

12. Brown, *Undoing the Demos*.

13. Brown, *Undoing the Demos*.

14. Kelly, "Everything Is Private Equity Now," 13.

15. Quoted in Kelly, "Everything Is Private Equity Now," 13.

16. Limited partners also include university endowments, wealthy families or individuals, and foundations.

17. Former Pennsylvania treasurer Joe Torsella, who sits on the boards of the state's two employee pension funds, has suggested that "private equity managers are mostly running a grift"; he tweeted that they too often "buy companies, load them with debt, and pay themselves off in secret while decimating a firm and a community" (@JoeTorsella, Aug. 26, 2019). Nevertheless, Pennsylvania pension funds' investment in private equity amounted to $12 billion in 2019. Cited in Institutional Investor, "Private Equity Managers."

18. Harvey, *Brief History*, 32.

19. Kelly, *New Tycoons*, xxi.

20. As a result, throughout this book all speakers at the conference remain anonymous. Wharton School, Twenty-Fifth Conference.

21. Appelbaum and Batt, *Private Equity at Work*.

22. Bluth, "GoFundMe CEO."

23. According to Frakt, until 1980, US health spending both per capita and as a percentage of GDP was about the same as other industrialized nations. Frakt, "Medical Mystery."

24. Burrough and Helyar, *Barbarians at the Gate*, 544.

25. Canderle, *Debt Trap*, 18.

26. Bernstein, keynote speaker, Rocco Tressolini Lectureship.

27. Financial covenants are contractual mandates as to what a debtor can and cannot do. Their main purpose is to protect lenders from default. Covenant-lite loans place fewer restrictions on borrowers and have fewer safeguards for banks and other institutions that finance PE transactions.

28. A platform company serves as the base for subsequent PE acquisitions and organic growth in a specific market niche.

Chapter 1. Who Even Are They?

1. In 2020, the eight largest US-based PE houses were Blackstone Group ($571 billion in total assets under management, AUM); Neuberger Berman Group, LLC ($356 billion in AUM); Apollo Global Management, Inc. ($331 billion in AUM); Carlyle Group ($224 billion in AUM); Kohlberg Kravis Roberts, now KKR ($218 billion in AUM); Bain Capital ($105 billion in AUM); Warburg Pincus (more than $58 billion in AUM); and Vista Equity Partners (more than $52 billion in AUM). Such shops have various types of holdings (i.e., real estate, credit, hedge funds), but the most predominant form is private equity. For example, PE represents 32 percent, 23 percent, 38 percent, and 62 percent of the total assets held by Blackstone, Apollo, Carlyle, and Bain, respectively. Kolakowski, "World's Top Ten Private Equity Firms." Further, Josh Kosman, author of *The Buyout of America*, reminds me that because they only put down a small percentage of equity in leveraged buyouts, maybe 30 percent, their buying power is greatly magnified. Kosman, email, May 3, 2020.

2. Ivory, Protess, and Bennett, "When You Dial 911," A1.

3. Middle-market vehicles are expanding steadily. The average middle-market fund reached more than $1 billion for the first time in 2019. Fernyhough, Davis, and Klees, "US PE Middle Market Report."

4. The "vintage year" is the date when a fund is closed to additional capital investment.

5. To correspond to the actual timeline that funds have closed since the 2008 Great Recession, a few PE firms have lengthened the period for up to fifteen years. Devine, "USPE Breakdown."

6. The typical hurdle rate is 8 percent of the IRR (internal rate of return). The PE owner must achieve the established hurdle rate to receive its full carried interest in the portfolio company.

7. Targets are the companies purchased by the PE firm.

8. One of the GPs at the Wharton School conference impassively noted that PE just goes wherever potential investments are.

9. Kosman, *Buyout of America*.

10. Beginning in the 1980s, permissible debt for a deal reached as high as 85–95 percent; from 1993 through 2002, creditors insisted on equity amounting to at least 40 percent of a transaction's value, which slipped to 30 percent by early 2007. Vaughan, Robbins, and Rudsenske, "Private Equity Investment"; Cordeiro, "US PE Breakdown"; Kosman, *Buyout of America*.

11. Nowadays, the collateralized loan obligations management business, which is composed mainly of large PE firms, buys more than 60 percent of all US leveraged loans.

12. Canderle, *Debt Trap*, 478.

13. Canderle, *Debt Trap*, 214.

14. Fernyhough, Davis, and Klees, "US PE Middle Market Report."

15. Jeremy Lynch, partner, Trilantic North America, panel on state of PE, Columbia Business School, Twenty-Fifth Conference.

16. Peggy Koenig, chair, Abry Partners, first afternoon fireside chat, Columbia Business School, Twenty-Fifth Conference.

17. Kelly, "Everything Is Private Equity Now." Multiple arbitrage is a means of increasing EV without providing any operational enhancements.

18. The *PitchBook* platform defines the "middle market" as US-based companies acquired through buyouts between $25 million and $1 billion.

19. Provident Healthcare Partners, "Private Equity Investment in Gastroenterology."

20. Gelfer, Hanson, and Klees, "Addictive Dealmaking."

21. For example, PE managers can blend down the overall purchase price of a platform company acquired at a high valuation by tacking on small-scale businesses with much lower valuations.

22. Kosman, email, May 3, 2020.

23. Cox and Klees, "Measuring SBOs Effect."

24. Since the turn of the twenty-first century, there are 50 percent fewer publicly traded corporations. Knauth, "PE Fundraising Remains Resilient."

25. Today, PE has accumulated more than $1.5 trillion of dry powder, which is money committed by its investors but not yet deployed.

26. The evidence indicates that third and fourth buyouts were 20 percent and 8 percent, respectively, of all SBOs in 2017. That year, there were 761 companies undergoing a third buyout; 55 companies, a fourth buyout; and 14 companies, a fifth buyout. Gelfer and Klees, "Echo Buyouts"; Lightbrown, "SBOs and Beyond."

27. Espinoza, "Private Equity Plays Risky Game"; Lykken, "Making a Case for SBO"; Gelfer and Klees, "Echo Buyouts"; Hoffman, "How Four Private-Equity Firms Cleaned Up."

28. Carey and Morris, *King of Capital*, 169.

29. Wharton School, Twenty-Fifth Conference.

30. Wharton School, Twenty-Fifth Conference.

31. Wharton School, Twenty-Fifth Conference.

32. BDO, "Tenth Annual Private Equity Perspective Survey."

33. Major players in direct lending are KKR, Blackstone Group, Carlyle Group, Apollo Global Management, and Ares Capital.

34. Gottfried and Ensign, "New Business Banker."

35. W. Blake Holden, partner, Warburg Pincus, luncheon learn session, Columbia Business School, Twenty-Fifth Conference.

36. As of 2020, there were seven PE firms that were publicly traded: KKR, founded in 1976; Blackstone Group, founded in 1985; Carlyle Group, founded in 1987; Apollo Global Management, founded in 1990; Oaktree Capital, founded in 1995; Ares Capital, founded in 1997; and Main Street Capital Corporation, founded in 1997.

37. These PE firms include Leonard Green & Partners, Silver Lake, Golub Capital BDC, Francisco Partners, Accel-KKR, and HGGC. Beltran, "Investcorp's Maniscalco."

38. Corkery and Protess, "How the Twinkie." Equilar provides comprehensive data on executives and board members of public companies.

39. Pearlstein, "$786 Million Question."

40. Perlberg, Metcalf, and Willmer, "Private Equity Poised."

41. Gelfer and Klees, "Echo Buyouts."

42. Kelly, "Everything Is Private Equity Now," 17.

43. At times, these can be limited through bank covenants.

44. Fernyhough and Beck, "US PE Breakdown"; Taub, "Coming Downturn."

45. BDO, "Tenth Annual Private Equity Perspective Survey."

46. Lewis, "Sycamore Set to Take $1B out of Staples."

47. Lewis, "5 PE-Backed Retail Deals."

48. Beltran, "Leonard Green Gets Its Money Back."

49. Quoted in Idzelis, "Most Aggressive Buyout Firms."

50. Kelly, "Everything Is Private Equity Now."

51. Median holding periods over the years: 2008, 3.8 years; 2009, 3.9 years; 2010, 5.7; 2011, 4.8; 2012, 5.5; 2013, 5.8; 2014, 6.3; 2015, 3.6; 2016, 4.2; 2017, 6.7; 2018, 5.2; and 2019, 4.9. Murphy and Jain, "Global Healthcare"; Lykken, "PE Firms Aren't Keeping Portfolio Companies."

52. There is a six-month lockup period before PE firms, former employees, and current executives are legally allowed to sell their shares.

53. Fernyhough, Davis, and Klees, "US PE Middle Market Report."

54. At the same time, the two PEs had to pay shareholders a $16 million settlement in a lawsuit alleging inside knowledge. Kelly, New Tycoons, 142. In 2020, J. Crew filed for Chapter 11 protection.

55. Appelbaum and Batt, Private Equity at Work.

56. Lewis, "PE-Backed Distressed Exits."

57. Though the Pension Benefit Guaranty Corporation will assume pension commitments for insolvent companies, it is generally not for the full amounts due. Eileen Appelbaum and Rosemary Batt report that from 2003 to 2012, employees and retirees forfeited more than $650 million because of bankrupt PE-controlled enterprises. Appelbaum and Batt, Private Equity at Work.

58. Quotes in Idzelis, "Watch Out for This Ballooning Pool."

59. Weitemeyer, "Ninety-Nine PE-Backed Companies."

60. Monk, "Having Skin in the Game."

61. In the early 1950s, 96 percent of pension fund investments were in bonds and other safe securities; by 2016, 73 percent of their capital had moved to publicly traded equities, private equity, venture capital, and hedge funds. Foltin et al., "Public Pension Underfunding."

62. Through the Oregon Investment Council, the state was among the first to dedicate sizable capital to PE firms. During 2018, it allocated roughly $17.9 billion of its $76 billion pension plan and common school assets to the shops. Kelly, *New Tycoons*; Knauth, "Oregon Defends Paying PE Fees." Also among the earliest and most prominent public pension investors are the California Public Employees' Retirement System (CalPERS); the California State Teachers' Retirement System; the Pennsylvania Public School Employees' Retirement System; and the Washington State Investment Board. CalPERS, for example, averaged $3 billion a year in PE commitments between 2011 and 2017; by the end of 2019 it had $27.6 billion in private equity investments, or nearly 8 percent of its total assets ($355.8 billion). Appelbaum and Batt, *Private Equity at Work*; Kosman, *Buyout of America*; Knauth, "CalPers Committed $1 Bln."

PE commitments of other top state and local investors include the New York State Common Retirement Fund ($6.3 billion in 2018); the Virginia Retirement System ($4.5 billion in 2017–2018); the Employees Retirement System of Texas (earmarked $1 billion for 2019 and $5.6 billion over the next five years); the Teachers' Retirement System of the State of Illinois ($6.3 billion in 2019); the New Jersey pension system (with a statutory cap of 12 percent for its $78 billion system, it plans to allocate $500 million–$700 million in 2019 but more than $1 billion per year from 2020 to 2025); the San Francisco Employees' Retirement System ($4.4 billion in 2019); the Pennsylvania Public School Employees' Retirement System ($8.4 billion, or 14.6 percent of its total assets); the Pennsylvania State Employees' Retirement System ($3.9 billion, or 14.5 percent of its total assets); and the Public School and Education Employee Retirement Systems of Missouri ($4.8 billion, or 10.8 percent of its total assets).

63. Wharton School, Twenty-Fifth Conference.

64. Marham, "LP Perspectives Survey."

65. At a minimum, they count on 12 percent or more annually on their investment. Covert, "You Buy It, You Break It." It has been noted that "PE funds returned more than 13% annualized, compared with about 9% for an equivalent investment in the S&P 500," but there is skepticism among scholars about whether the PE industry is gaming rate of return calculations. Kelly, "Everything Is Private Equity Now," 3.

66. Krouse, "State and Local Pension Woes."

67. Foltin et al., "Public Pension Underfunding." In 2016, states across the nation had a total of $1.4 trillion in funding deficits. Loughead, "How Well-Funded Are Pension Plans."

68. As stated in Foltin et al., "Public Pension Underfunding."

69. Appelbaum and Batt, *Private Equity at Work*.

70. Wharton School, Twenty-Fifth Conference.

71. Marham, "LP Perspectives Survey."

72. Carey and Morris, *King of Capital*; Appelbaum and Batt, *Private Equity at Work*.

73. The IRR is the dominant measure of overall PE fund performance in the PE industry. It measures how much the capital appreciated on average over the time it was invested.

74. "Private equity funds returned 17.3 percent in the 12 months through June 2017, according to Preqin. That compares with 13.4 percent annual gains

over the three years and 15.4 percent for the five years through last June." Idzelis, "Everything about Private Equity Reeks," 5. Several GPs acknowledge that returns likely will be declining, according to luncheon keynote speaker Greg Mondre of Silver Lake. Wharton School, Twenty-Fifth Conference.

75. Wharton School, Twenty-Fifth Conference.

76. Grant, "LPs Grow Uneasy"; Mitchell, "LPs Would Like More Vigorous Defense."

77. Carey and Morris, *King of Capital*, 226.

78. Haas and Pagani, "How PE Operation Teams."

79. Burrough and Helyar, *Barbarians at the Gate*.

80. Kosman, *Buyout of America*; Kelly, *New Tycoons*.

81. Kosman, *Buyout of America*.

82. Kelly, *New Tycoons*, 46.

83. Appelbaum and Batt, *Private Equity at Work*, 73.

84. Lykken, "How US Tax Reform"; Fernyhough and Klees, "IRS & IRRs."

85. Lykken, "How US Tax Reform."

86. Lewis, "Q&A."

87. Kosman, *Buyout of America*, 93.

88. Kosman, *Buyout of America*; Foroohar, *Makers and Takers*.

89. Kosman, *Buyout of America*.

90. Private Equity Stakeholder Project, "Private Equity."

91. Nolan, "Worker Person's Guide."

Chapter 2. The Emergence of the Alternative Asset Class

1. For example, Kohlberg Kravis Roberts's (KKR) first fund in 1976 only totaled $25 million. Carey and Morris, *King of Capital*.

2. Appelbaum and Batt, *Private Equity at Work*.

3. Canderle, *Private Equity's Public Distress*; Kosman, *Buyout of America*.

4. In March 1989, Milken was indicted for nearly a hundred counts of racketeering and securities fraud.

5. Bruck, *Predators' Ball*.

6. Burrough and Helyar, *Barbarians at the Gate*, 86. By 1987, according to Bruck, Drexel's revenues swelled to $4 billion, rendering it the most profitable investment banking firm in the United States. At the same time, its questionable practices were being scrutinized by Congress. In 1984–1985, thirty bills dealing with regulating takeovers had been introduced, but not one passed, and President Ronald Reagan threated to veto any such bill if it were enacted. In fact, the SEC and the President's Council of Economic Advisers, in its 1985 annual report, lauded these acquisitions, including the hefty debt, as fostering efficiency and imposing discipline on companies. Drexel and the investment banks had assembled a huge lobbying team, including the Alliance for Capital Access, to oppose any limits on takeovers and junk-bond financing. Bruck, *Predators' Ball*.

7. Bruck, *Predators' Ball*.

8. Anchor had been a leading manufacturer of low-cost glass tableware and was the second largest producer of glass containers in the United States. The company employed at least 20 percent of the town's population and many

thousands more elsewhere. The following paragraphs about Anchor and the town of Lancaster are based on Alexander's account in *Glass House*.

9. Cerberus renamed the combined companies Global Home Products, LLC.

10. In 2013, Global Home was merged with the flatware brand Oneida and renamed EveryWare Global.

11. Monomoy merged EveryWare with another company, ROI, before the IPO.

12. Carey and Morris, *King of Capital*.

13. Kosman, *Buyout of America*, 29.

14. Carey and Morris, *King of Capital*; Anders, *Merchants of Debt*; Sterngold, "Shaking Billions."

15. Anders, *Merchants of Death*; US Government Accountability Office, *Case Studies*.

16. Faludi, "Safeway LBO," 3.

17. Faludi, "Safeway LBO"; Anders, *Merchants of Debt*; US Government Accountability Office, *Case Studies*; Kelly, *New Tycoons*.

18. The company produced popular baked goods and other food product lines—Oreos, Ritz Crackers, Fig Newtons, Chips Ahoy!, Life Savers candy, Premium Saltine Crackers, Barnum's Animal Crackers, Lorna Doone, Mallomars, Shredded Wheat cereal, Canada Dry soft drinks, Fleischmann's margarine, and Del Monte foods—along with Winston and Salem cigarettes.

19. Burrough and Helyar, *Barbarians at the Gate*.

20. Sellers, "New Siege."

21. For instance, the chair of R. J. Reynolds Tobacco, Edward A. Horrigan, reaped $45.7 million; the chief executive officer of RJR Nabisco, F. Ross Johnson, $53 million; Drexel Burnham Lambert, $227 million; Merrill Lynch, $109 million; Morgan Stanley, $25 million; and a syndicate of 200 banks, $325 million. Burrough and Helyar, *Barbarians at the Gate*.

22. Burrough and Helyar, *Barbarians at the Gate*.

23. Canderle, *Private Equity's Public Distress*; Appelbaum and Batt, *Private Equity at Work*; Anders, *Merchants of Debt*.

24. Burrough and Helyar, *Barbarians at the Gate*.

25. Because of low-interest conditions, investors were seeking higher rates than were available from stocks and bonds.

26. Kosman, *Buyout of America*.

27. Carey and Morris, *King of Capital*, 105.

28. Carey and Morris, *King of Capital*.

29. Kosman, *Buyout of America*, 89.

30. Kosman, *Buyout of America*.

31. The banks had only limited risk because they were converting nearly all their investments into collateralized loan obligations, which contained slices of debt from up to 200 different loans. By mid-2007, these funds had amassed $270 billion from such loans. Kosman, *Buyout of America*.

32. Moreover, because of the tech bubble crash, venture capital was far less appealing, and public pension managers who wanted high returns in the alternative market turned to private equity to a greater degree. Kosman, *Buyout of America*.

33. Canderle, *Private Equity's Public Distress*.

34. These multibillion-dollar acquisitions included Hertz (by Carlyle Group and two other PE houses in 2005) for $14.4 billion, where interest payments grew by 80 percent as a result, and Dunkin' Brands, which owns Dunkin' Donuts and Baskin-Robbins (by Carlyle Group and Bain Capital in 2010) for $2.4 billion. Dunkin' Brands incurred a $2.4 billion debt from the takeover and needed another $1.25 billion to pay the two PE firms a dividend recap. Canderle, *Private Equity's Public Distress*; Carey and Morris, *King of Capital*; Taibbi, "Greed and Debt."

35. Kosman, *Buyout of America*, 112.

36. Appelbaum and Batt, *Private Equity at Work*, 100.

37. Espinoza, "Private Equity Plays Risky Game."

38. Kosman, *Buyout of America*; Kelly, *New Tycoons*.

39. Carey and Morris, *King of Capital*; Appelbaum and Batt, *Private Equity at Work*.

40. Aschoff, "Ban Private Equity."

41. Lykken, "Consequences of PEs Fundraising"; Fernyhough and Beck, "US PE Breakdown," 1–14.

42. For example, Apollo's ninth flagship fund in 2017, totaling $24.7 billion, was the largest vehicle ever up to that time. Lykken, "PE Firms Look to VC-Backed Companies." Blackstone Group, KKR, and Carlyle Group are also regularly raising mega-funds: Carlyle closed its seventh vehicle at $18.5 billion and Blackstone its eighth at more than $22 billion. Lewis, "US PE Middle Market"; Dowd, "Carlyle Closes New Mega-Fund." TPG amassed at least $14 billion for its eighth buyout fund. Willmer and Perlberg, "TPG Joins Apollo, Blackstone."

43. Wharton School, Twenty-Fifth Conference.

44. SC&H Capital, "How Private Equity Is Helping."

45. Wharton School, Twenty-Fifth Conference.

46. Fernyhough and Beck, "US PE Breakdown."

47. In PE parlance, companies with valuations of a billion dollars and more are "unicorns." The largest—Blackstone's leveraged buyout of Thomson Reuters (renamed Refinitiv)—amounted to an astounding $20 billion. Espinoza, "Private Equity Plays Risky Game." Other mega-buyouts include KKR's takeover of Envision Healthcare for $9.9 billion; Dr Pepper Snapple, which was soon merged with Keurig Green Mountain, for $21 billion; BMC Software for $8.3 billion; Sonic Drive-In for $1.6 billion; and Buffalo Wild Wings for $2.9 billion. Typically, mega-deals include more than one firm since it is too risky to put a significant percentage of a fund's capital into one deal. Fernyhough and Beck, "US PE Breakdown."

48. Kevin Conway, vice chair, CD&R, second morningside chat, Columbia Business School, Twenty-Fifth Conference.

49. Fernyhough and Beck, "US PE Breakdown." EBITDA is used by PE to measure companies' overall financial performance.

50. Christopoulos, managing director, CVC, panel on state of PE, Columbia Business School, Twenty-Fifth Conference.

51. Wharton School, Twenty-Fifth Conference.

52. Gottfried and Tracy, "Risky Deals Return."

53. Kelly, "Everything Is Private Equity Now."

54. Lewis, "Sycamore Set to Take $1B"; Lewis, "PE Firms Keep Deploying."

55. Dayen, "Will the Tax Act."

56. Cited in Covert, "You Buy It, You Break It."

57. Weitemeyer, "Retail Leads Long List."

58. Butler-Young, "Private Equity Pumped Billions"; Gustafson, "Payless ShoeSource Files."

59. Lewis, "5 PE-Backed Retail Deals"; Lewis, "Retail Roundup."

60. In March 2019, the Children's Place, Gymboree's rival, bought the brand for $76 million, and Gap Inc. acquired its Janie and Jack clothing line for $35 million. The following year, the Children's Place announced it was closing roughly a third of its locations by 2021.

61. Toys "R" Us was the last surviving toy chain. KB Toys, the fifth largest toy retailer in the United States, filed for bankruptcy in 2004. It had been acquired in 2000 by Bain Capital in a leveraged buyout for $303 million, 88 percent in borrowed money. KB's financial liabilities rose even higher when sixteen months later the PE firm put the chain in $83 million more debt to pay itself a dividend recap. Ultimately, Bain earned a return of roughly 370 percent on the now insolvent enterprise. Kosman, *Buyout of America*; Taibbi, "Greed and Debt."

62. Berfield et al., "Tears 'R' Us"; Covert, "You Buy It, You Break It."

63. Dayen, "Toys 'R' US Workers"; Morgenson and Rizzo, "Who Killed Toys 'R' Us?"; Lewis, "Congress Confronts Bain Capital"; Weissman, "Toys 'R' US."

64. Lewis, "Congress Confronts Bain Capital"; Berfield et al., "Tears 'R' Us."

65. Covert, "You Buy It, You Break It," 6.

66. Lewis, "Bain Capital, KKR"; Hirsch and Thomas, "Life after Liquidation."

67. Sweethearts are said to have been consumed by soldiers as early as the Civil War and also during World War II.

68. Lewis, "Private Equity Deprives World."

69. Lewis, "5 PE-Backed Retail Deals."

70. Idzelis, "Buyout Firms."

71. Lykken, "Next Financial Crisis."

72. Taub, "Coming Downturn."

73. Christopoulos, Columbia Business School, Twenty-Fifth Conference.

74. Wharton School, Twenty-Fifth Conference.

75. Bush served from 1998 through 2003.

76. Asmail, "Investing in War," 4; Kelly, *New Tycoons*. Similarly, Veritas Capital hires numerous notable military leaders; the PE firm has received $2.2 billion in defense contracts on behalf of its portfolio companies.

77. Barr, "Baker to Retire."

78. Naomi Klein, "James Baker's Double Life."

79. Asmail, "Investing in War."

80. Roumeliotis, "Carlyle Group Hires." Other former government officials with ties to Carlyle include Office of Management and Budget (OMB) director Richard Darman; Clinton chief of staff Thomas F. McLarty; and Securities and Exchange Commission chair Arthur Levitt.

81. Their prior government positions: Kissinger, secretary of state and national security advisor under Richard Nixon and secretary of state under Gerald Ford, 1973–1977; Rumsfeld, secretary of defense and chief of staff under

Gerald Ford, 1975–1977, and secretary of defense in 2001–2006 under George W. Bush; Shultz, secretary of state under Ronald Reagan, 1982–1989; Powell, chair of the Joint Chiefs of Staff under George H. W. Bush, 1989–1993, and secretary of state under George W. Bush, 2001–2005; Gingrich, speaker of the US House of Representatives, 1995–1999.

82. Geithner had been secretary of the treasury under Barack Obama in 2009–2013. Previously he had been CEO of the International Monetary Fund and the Federal Reserve Bank. Husyar, "Tim Geithner."

83. Additional examples of the PE-government revolving door include former president Bill Clinton (advisor for Yucaipa Companies); Federico Peña, secretary of energy and secretary of transportation under Clinton (Vestar Capital Partners); William Simon, secretary of the treasury under Nixon and Ford (founder of Wesray Capital Corporation); David Stockman, OMB director under Reagan (cofounded the failed Heartland Industrial Partners); John Snow, secretary of the treasury under George W. Bush (chair of Cerberus Capital Management); Nicholas Brady, secretary of the treasury under G. H. W. Bush and Reagan (started Darby Overseas Investments); Joe Lieberman, US senator (chair of the executive board, Victory Park Capital); Nancy-Ann DeParle, assistant to the president, deputy chief of staff for policy, counselor to the president, and director of the White House Office of Health Reform under Obama (cofounded Consonance Capital Partners); Erskine Bowles, White House chief of staff under Clinton (cofounded Carousel Capital); Al Gore, US vice president (cofounded Generation Investment Management); Evan Bayh, US senator (Apollo Global Management); Dan Quayle, US vice president (chair of Cerberus Capital Management and Cerberus Global Investments); Leon Panetta, director of OMB and chief of staff under Clinton and CIA director and secretary of defense under Obama (advisor at Cerberus); Thomas Scully, administrator of the federal Centers for Medicare and Medicaid Services under George W. Bush (general partner at Welsh, Carson, Anderson and Stowe); Paul Ryan, speaker of the House of Representatives, 2015–2019 (senior advisor at Seidler Equity Partners); Deval Patrick, governor of Massachusetts, 2007–2015 (co-head of impact investing at Bain until he departed to run for president); and Rahm Emanuel, Obama's chief of staff and two-term mayor of Chicago (senior counselor at Centerview Partners).

84. Lipton and Vogel, "Biden Aides' Ties to Consulting."

85. Center for Responsive Politics cited in Protess, Silver-Greenberg, and Abrams, "How Private Equity Found Power." Campaign contributions include money for candidates, leadership PACs, political parties, congressional committees, and outside spending groups. The donations are from individuals in each organization. As to campaign contributions and lobbying, KKR gave $980.6 million and $1.2 million, respectively; Warburg Pincus, $0.9 million and $0.7 million; Apollo Global Management, $1.1 million and $1.3 million; Bain Capital, $9 million and $30,000; TPG, $2.2 million and $1.3 million.

86. Donmoyer, "Baucus Drops."

87. Perlberg and Bain, "Private Equity Wields More Power."

88. Confessore, "Too Rich for Conflicts." Other Trump appointees included Wilbur Ross, secretary of commerce (founder of WL Ross and Co., acquired by

Invesco); Kenneth Juster, deputy assistant to the president for international economic affairs and deputy director of the National Economic Council (partner at Warburg Pincus); William Hagerty, ambassador to Japan (cofounder of Hagerty Peterson); Thomas Barrack, chair of Trump's inauguration committee and economic and national security advisor (founder of Colony NorthStar); and Betsy DeVos, secretary of education (cofounder of the Windquest Group).

89. Protess, Silver-Greenberg, and Abrams, "How Private Equity Found Power," 1.

90. Lewis, "Elizabeth Warren Proposes Legislation"; Editorial, "Private Equity Must Be Less Private."

91. Witkowsky, "Holding PE Partners Liable."

92. Witkowsky, "Editor's Letter."

93. Another powerful lobbying group is the Association for Corporate Growth. Doctor Patient Unity, which represents large PE-owned physician practices and ER staffing companies, has devoted more than $28 million to ads to squash the Stop Wall Street Looting Act. Gustafsson, Seervai, and Blumenthal, "Role of Private Equity."

94. Lewis, "Private Equity's Campaign Funding."

Chapter 3. Consolidating Health Care

1. I'm referring to Burrough and Helyar, *Barbarians at the Gate*.

2. Edmands, managing partner, Consonance Capital Partners, panel on health care, Columbia Business School, Twenty-Fifth Conference.

3. BDO, "Healthcare's Consolidation Funnel."

4. Since 2016, the leading health fund final closes include WCAS ($3.33 billion in 2016, $3.5 billion in 2018); Linden Capital Partners ($1.5 billion in 2018); Cressey & Company ($995 million in 2018); Webster Capital ($875 million in 2018); Water Street Healthcare Partners ($863 million in 2018); Five Arrows Capital Partners ($655 million in 2018); and Frazier Healthcare Partners ($525 million in 2016). Pringle, "WCAS, Linden, Cressey."

5. Witkowsky, "Larger Funds."

6. Vaughan, Robbins, and Rudsenske, "Private Equity Investment."

7. Appelbaum and Batt, *Private Equity at Work*, suggest that from 2000 to 2012, 12 percent of the leveraged buyouts were in health care.

8. After assuming HCA's $11.7 billion previous debt and adding $16 billion more for the acquisition, the LBO by the three PE firms doubled the amount of money owed; they put down only $4.6 billion (12 percent) in cash. Mullenkamp, "HCA Pays Owners"; Kosman, *Buyout of America*; Creswell and Abelson, "Giant Hospital Chain Is Blazing"; Dowd, "This Day In Buyout History."

9. Creswell and Abelson, "Giant Hospital Chain Is Blazing."

10. Creswell and Abelson, "Giant Hospital Chain Is Blazing."

11. McCue and Thompson, "Impact of HCA's Leveraged Buyout."

12. Meyer, "Healthcare Lawyers Tout Surge."

13. Sunshine, managing director, Blackstone Group, panel on health care, Columbia Business School, Twenty-Fifth Conference.

14. Witkowsky, "Deal of the Year Awards."

15. Becker et al., "15 Private Equity in Healthcare."

16. From September 2016 to September 2017, offices of health practitioners other than physicians and dentists took second place, with an 82.5 percent return; offices of dentists, third place, with an 81.3 percent return; offices of physicians, fifth place, with a 68.5 percent return; home health care services, sixth place, with a 65.9 percent return; outpatient care centers, seventh place, with a 65.1 percent return; and personal care services, eighth place, with a 63.7 percent return. The overall average return on equity for that period was 38 percent. Flynn, "Home Health Care."

17. Medicare and Medicaid are expected to grow 7.5 percent and 5.5 percent, respectively, annually by 2030.

18. Certain founders are seeking capital to enhance their business but are reluctant to relinquish majority control. In a growth equity fund, the PE not only takes a minority stake but generally does not add new debt straightaway or otherwise impose sizable debt on the target. For other founders, especially owners nearing retirement age, an LBO will offer substantial cash in exchange for surrendering power over their business.

19. Lykken, "Inside PE's Record-Breaking Push"; DJl Consulting, "Dynamics Driving Dealmaking."

20. Brentwood Capital Advisors, "Healthcare Services Middle-Market Update," 3Q2018. In order to compete with corporate buyers awash in capital and that do not have to sell their acquisitions within a given time frame, a few PE firms are setting up longer-life funds without exit deadlines. KKR, for example, has amassed $9.5 billion for this type of portfolio; it is seeking businesses with recurring revenue, such as dental chains with consistent customers.

21. Edmands, Columbia Business School, Twenty-Fifth, Conference.

22. Murphy and Jain, "Global Healthcare."

23. Quoted in Gamble, "Is Private Equity Helping."

24. Quoted in Kacik, "Monopolized Healthcare Market." The investigation was conducted by researchers from the Center for Health Policy at Brookings Institution and Carnegie Mellon University's Heinz College.

25. Gondi and Song, "Potential Implications."

26. Appelbaum, "How Private Equity Makes You Sicker."

27. Galston, "Perils of Corporate Concentration," 3.

28. Rothstein, "How One Hospital's Bankruptcy Shows."

29. Appelbaum, "How Private Equity Makes You Sicker."

30. Kacik, "Monopolized Healthcare Market."

31. Cited in Kacik, "Healthcare Credit Ratings Dip."

32. Koenig, chair, Abry Partners, first afternoon fireside chat, Columbia Business School, Twenty-Fifth Conference.

33. Edmands, Columbia Business School, Twenty-Fifth Conference.

34. Amin, managing partner, Madryn Asset Management, panel on health care, Columbia Business School, Twenty-Fifth Conference.

35. Kraft, "Physician Practice Management Companies," 55.

36. St. Christopher's Hospital for Children was subsequently saved from liquidation. In December 2019, Tower Health and Drexel University acquired the 188-bed facility for $50 million and restored its not-for-profit status.

37. George, "City Councilwoman Introduces"; Rush, "Hahnemann University Hospital's Inner Turmoil."

38. George, "City Councilwoman Introduces"; Rush, "Hahnemann University Hospital's Inner Turmoil"; Rothstein, "How One Hospital's Bankruptcy Shows"; Picchi, "Private Equity Rushed"; DePillis, "Rich Investors."

39. Appelbaum, "How Private Equity Makes You Sicker."

40. George, "City Councilwoman Introduces."

41. At least one observer argues that 21st Century's problems stemmed from reimbursement issues and lawsuits by the former founder and the executive team. Perhaps. But it was also drowning in debt. Pringle, "21st Century Oncology."

42. Pringle, "21st Century Oncology."

43. In 2012, KKR had bought a 45 percent stake in GenesisCare for $380 million, sold its shares in 2016 to China Resources and Macquarie Capital, and then reinvested in 2019 for a 20 percent stake. The company's doctors and management still hold significant shares.

44. Willmer, "Wall Street Corners Cancer Care."

45. Becker et al., "15 Private Equity in Healthcare."

46. Surgery Partners acquired National Surgical Healthcare from Irving Place Capital for approximately $760 million, partially funded via Bain Capital.

47. KKR has been on a mega-buyout shopping spree and has become a powerhouse in several health industries. At the end of 2017, in a $1.4 billion take-private (with Walgreens Boots Alliance as minority stakeholder), it acquired PharMerica, a leading provider of institutional pharmacy and specialty home infusion and oncology services. Two years later, KKR acquired for $1.32 billion BrightSpring Health Services, a major homecare company, and merged the two entities. In 2017, it also bought WebMD (a respected go-to internet health information provider since 1996) for $2.8 billion, and Nature's Bounty (nutritional supplements) for $3 billion.

48. One competitor, TeamHealth, was taken private by Blackstone in early 2017 for $6.1 billion. Another provider of physician hospital services, Sound Physicians, was acquired in 2018 for $2.2 billion through an LBO club deal consisting of Athyrium Capital Management, Summit Partners, Silversmith Capital Partners, and Revelstoke Capital Partners. Sound Physicians initially had received PE development capital from TowerBrook Capital Partners in 2007 and was acquired by Fresenius Medical Care, a public company, seven years later.

49. Kincaid, "Envision Healthcare."

50. The combined companies consist of regional health systems, community hospitals, physician practices, outpatient centers, and post-acute care facilities. In 2017, LifePoint had formed a partnership with LHC Group to purchase and share ownership of home health and hospice services. They are continuing to expand jointly in these buyouts. McDermott and Palasota, "Visiting the Home Health Marketplace."

51. See www.LifePoint Health.com.

52. In 2017, Kindred at Home served 570,000 patients daily in forty-one states.

53. One division held Kindred's long-term care hospitals and inpatient rehab facilities, the second its at-home operations.

54. Curo had 245 locations in twenty-two states at the time of its purchase by Kindred.

55. For example, Platinum Equity acquired the thirty-five-year-old company LifeScan; according to the latter's website, fully 20 million people depend on its OneTouch products to manage their diabetes. Because it is awash in debt from the LBO, it is most likely that any forthcoming cash will be used to pay off the money owed—nearly $1.8 billion—rather than research new or better products. See www.lifescan.com.

56. The range of health-related acquisitions is broad. Examples of company buyouts by PE include Paragon Bioservices, Inc. (gene therapy manufacturing), Comprehensive Pharmacy Services (outsourced pharmacy services), Crystal Tip (disposable air/water syringe tips), AdaptHealth (distributor of oxygen therapy products and other durable medical equipment), Collagen Matrix (tissue repair and regenerative medicine), Press Ganey Associates (surveys for hospitals to measure patient satisfaction and quality of care), Nelipak Healthcare Packaging (thermoformed packaging products), Mini Pharmacy Enterprises (diabetic supplies), HealthChannels (medical scribe services), Center for Diagnostic Imaging (diagnostic imaging), Reliant Rehabilitation (contract therapy services), MultiPlan (health cost management services), Cotiviti (health risk assessment and data analytics), Convey Health Solutions (enrollment and billing), Equian (health insurance claim management), Zelis Healthcare (health care claims, cost management, and payments), and Symplr (health care credentialing).

57. Such investments consist of hospitals and boarding kennels (VetCor, Southern Veterinary Partners, PetVet), nonclinical business services to veterinarians and hospitals (Heartland Veterinary Partners), assistance to veterinarians in selling their practice (Veterinary Practice Partners), and online advice on animal care (FirstVet). In addition to health, there is a vastly increasing PE market for animal toys, carriers, bedding, grooming, and especially food products.

58. Examples of PE-backed all-natural products and vitamins include Zarbee's Naturals (vitamins and cough syrup), Juice Plus (dietary supplements), and Nature's Bounty (nutritional supplements).

59. Phalippou, *Private Equity Laid Bare*.

Chapter 4. It's between Me and My Doctor?

1. In 2017, there were more than 200,000 physician groups, which earned more than $265 billion in revenues. Kacik, "For the First Time Ever"; Kaufman, Hall, and Associates, "Industry Flash Report."

2. Kacik, "For the First Time Ever"; Kaufman, Hall, and Associates, "Industry Flash Report"; Kacik, "Health Systems Driving Prices Higher."

3. Meyer, "Medical Group Deals."

4. These insurers include UnitedHealth Group's Optum Care, Centene, Humana, and Athenahealth.

5. Court, "Doctor's Offices."

6. Pazanowski, "Private Equity Investment."

7. LaMantia, "Physician Practices Increasingly Turn."

8. Bill Brown of A2B Advisors quoted in Meyer, "Concerns Grow."

9. In 2017, Medicare covered 58.4 million elderly and disabled people at a cost of $710 billion.

10. Jain, Murphy, and Martin, "Why Private Equity Loves Retail Healthcare."

11. Harbin, "Private Equity Buyouts"; Smith, "Private Equity Flouts State Regulations."

12. Aprill, "Private Equity Investment in Orthopedics."

13. Another lure is that upon selling the practice, the proceeds are taxed as capital gains and not at the higher rate on salary.

14. Harbin, "Private Equity Buyouts"; Meyer, "Specialty Physician Groups."

15. Wharton School, Twenty-Fifth Conference.

16. See, for example, Fred and Scheid, "Physician Burnout."

17. Meyer, "Concerns Grow."

18. Epprecht, "Corporate Practice of Medicine Laws."

19. PPMCs are also referred to as management services organizations.

20. Smith, "Private Equity Flouts State Regulations."

21. Vaughan, Robbins, and Rudsenske, "Private Equity Investment."

22. According to a 2020 study by the Association of American Medical Colleges, the shortage in physicians will reach between 54,000 and 139,000 nationwide by 2033. These figures include between 21,400 and 55,200 primary care doctors and between 33,700 and 86,700 specialists. Christ, "Physician Shortage."

23. Court, "Doctor's Offices"; Kacik, "Advanced Practice and Nurse Practitioners."

24. Harbin, "Private Equity Buyouts."

25. Smith, "Private Equity Flouts State Regulations."

26. Court, "Doctor's Offices"; Solo Building Blogs, "Private Equity and Ophthalmology"; Harbin, "Private Equity Buyouts."

27. Investigators have found that physician market concentration is associated with higher fees, whether the market is consolidated by hospital systems, insurance companies, or PE. However, state and federal antitrust officials have less ability to inspect PE deals because they tend to be off their radar screen. Meyer, "Medical Group Deals."

28. Carey interview.

29. Morris, "Comment: Guest Expert," 29. Privia Health is a national physician organization focused on value-based health care.

30. Kronemyer, "6 Concerns."

31. Tan et al., "Trends in Private Equity Acquisition"; Bundy, "Dermatology Market." Dermatologists represent only 1 percent of US doctors but 15 percent of PE physician practice acquisitions. Kronemyer, "6 Concerns."

32. Bundy, "Dermatology Market"; Resnick, "Dermatology Practice Consolidation."

33. Bundy, "Dermatology Market"; Resnick, "Dermatology Practice Consolidation."

34. Bundy, "Dermatology Market."

35. Quoted in Bundy, "Dermatology Market."

36. Wernli, Rothstein, Jampel, and Evans all in Margosian, "Pulling Back the Curtain," 35.

37. Resnick, "Dermatology Practice Consolidation."

38. Resnick in Kronemyer, "6 Concerns."

39. Konda and Francis, "Corporatization and the Rise of Private Equity," parts 1 and 2.

40. Konda et al., "Future Considerations for Clinical Dermatology."

41. Hafner, "Why Private Equity Is Furious."

42. Hafner and Palmer, "Skin Cancers Rise."

43. Court, "Doctor's Offices."

44. Court, "Doctor's Offices."

45. Mostaghimi interview.

46. Mostaghimi interview.

47. Meyer, "Specialty Physician Groups."

48. Quoted in Meyer, "Concerns Grow."

49. Quoted in Kronemyer, "6 Concerns."

50. Mostaghimi interview.

51. Anonymous, owner of dermatology practice, interview. The following quotes are all from this interview.

52. Court, "Doctor's Offices"; Margosian, "Pulling Back the Curtain."

53. As of 2017, the management group served more than 4 million patients. It had 192 physicians, 124 physician assistants, and more than 180 locations in thirteen states. Hafner and Palmer, "Skin Cancers Rise."

54. Hafner and Palmer, "Skin Cancers Rise."

55. Bedside Dermatology was founded by CEO Steven K. Grekin and is located in Warren, Michigan.

56. Hafner and Palmer, "Skin Cancers Rise."

57. Dr. Kenneth Katz, president of Forefront, in 2001 had taken charge of his father's sole clinic in Manitowoc, Wisconsin.

58. Margosian, "Skin in the Game."

59. Penfund at the time became a minority investor as well.

60. Zarling, "Forefront Dermatology."

61. https://www.indeed.com/cmp/forefront-dermatology/reviews.

62. https://www.yelp.com/biz/forefront-dermatology-grand-rapids.

63. Eagle Private Capital and Harbert Credit Solutions invested as minority partners in 2013, and Brookside Mezzanine Partners, Resolute Capital Partners, Bay Capital Investment Partners, Providence, and Spring Capital Partners invested as minority partners in 2014.

64. The company was renamed in 2017 to reflect its unified brand.

65. Brooks interview. The following information is from this interview.

66. QDP, too, is based in Brentwood, Tennessee. The company was founded in 2013 by William Southwick and Susan Brownie and as of 2019 was operating in five states. In December 2017, Granite Growth Health Partners bought out Apple Tree's share.

67. These LBOs include Cumberland Skin Surgery and Dermatology (August 2017), Bain Dermatology (May 2018), Zitelli and Brodland Dermatology (September 2018), and Barrett and Geiss Dermatology (December 2018).

68. Located in Linthicum Heights, Maryland, AAD was founded in 1980 by Robert Handwerger, Richard Pfau, and Angela Peterman. It was formerly known as M. Eugene Tudino MD.

69. https://www.indeed.com/cmp/anne-arundel-dermatology/reviews.

70. Parr, "DermOne to Close Six Locations on Friday"; Parr, "DermOne Brand."

71. Riverchase Dermatology and Cosmetic Surgery—formerly known as Naples Center for Dermatology and Cosmetic Surgery—was first recapitalized by Prairie Capital and GMB Mezzanine Capital in January 2013. Nearly four years later (October 2016), the company was purchased by GTCR Private Equity in an SBO for $33 million. Since 2017, Riverchase and GTCR have been on a buying spree; the business now has thirty-seven locations in Florida. Enhanced Equity Fund, which acquired West Dermatology at the end of 2014, has since purchased dermatology practices in California, Nevada, and Arizona. The PE firm cashed in on its investment when West Dermatology was purchased by Sun Capital Partners in early 2020. CI Capital Partners became the owner of Epiphany Dermatology in June 2016, at which time the company operated seven clinics in Central Texas. By the end of 2018, the PE firm and Epiphany had picked up fourteen practices in New Mexico, Texas, Oklahoma, Arizona, Colorado, Iowa, Minnesota, and Missouri. Chicago Pacific Founders bought Pinnacle Dermatology in January 2017. It acquired no fewer than fourteen dermatology practices in a little more than two years and is poised to take control over many more. For example, in June 2018 the company received $75 million in debt financing from AllianceBernstein Private Credit Investors to support multiple add-ons and future growth. Two PE firms, Welsh, Carson, Anderson and Stowe and Riata Capital Group, launched the holding company Select Dermatology, which acquired its first specialty practice, Mindful Dermatology (Texas), in May 2018. In July 2018, BelHealth Investment Partners created the platform NavaDerm Partners through the merger and recapitalization of four dermatology groups (two each in New York and New Jersey). Its goal is to be the foremost brand in the northeastern United States.

Other PE shops participating in dermatology leveraged buyouts include Tonka Bay Equity Partners and Clearwater Equity Group (United Skin Specialists, September 2015); Pharos Capital Group (Dermatology and MedSpa, January 2016); Sterling Partners (Platinum Dermatology, May 2016); Frazier Healthcare Partners (United Derm Partners, December 2016); Goldman Sachs Capital Partners (California Skin Institute, January 2017); Sheridan Capital Partners (Dermatologists of Central States, May 2017); Susquehanna Private Capital (Skin Cancer Associates, April 2018); and Gryphon Investors (Water's Edge Dermatology, May 2018).

72. Eyesteve, "Return of Private Equity"; Kent, "Is a Private Equity Deal Right?"

73. Reider et al., "Past Lessons, Future Directions," 40–50.

74. Quoted in Kent, "Is a Private Equity Deal Right?"

75. Chen et al., "Private Equity in Ophthalmology and Optometry."

76. Minority investors included Bush O'Donnell Investment Advisors, Pine Street Capital Partners, Bay Capital Investment Partners, Eagle Private Capital, Bridgepoint Capital, and Plexus Capital.

77. Eli Global holds more than 132 companies that together yield $3 billion in annual revenues. Snyder, "Ophthalmology Investments Spread"; Yetter and Snyder, "Physicians First."

78. Koch, "As I See It," 56.

79. Yetter and Snyder, "Physicians First"; Reider et al., "Past Lessons, Future Directions."

80. Eyesteve, "Return of Private Equity."

81. Krause, "Why PE Firms Are Buying."

82. Fugazy, "Why Private Equity Firms"; Buckley et al., "Why Private Equity Has Eyes."

83. Mahdaui, "Private Equity," 38–40, 69.

84. Harbin and Markowitz, "Private Equity Buyouts."

85. Reider et al., "Past Lessons, Future Directions."

86. Quoted in Kent, "Is a Private Equity Deal Right?"

87. Michael W. Davis calls this "stealth branding" because the PE firms, in his opinion, purposely hide the fact that the practices are PE-owned. Davis interview.

88. Aprill, Herschman, and Patel, "Hot Physician Specialists."

89. Other energetic consolidators newly on the scene in 2017 included American Vision Partners, a platform formed by H. I. G. Capital with Barnet Dulaney Perkins Eye Center and Southwestern Eye Center. Acquiring eye care centers in Arizona and New Mexico, American Vision Partners via H. I. G. intends to spread throughout the Southwest. Sterling Partners, which bought Grand Rapids Ophthalmology and created Blue Sky Vision as its management services organization, aspires to grow the platform both organically and through acquisitions in Michigan and surrounding areas. Flexpoint Ford joined the PE acquisition of eye care platforms with its buyout of SouthEast Eye Specialists; it intends to be a main competitor in the US South. Riata Capital Group created Acuity Eyecare as a platform and as of January 2020 had purchased more than twelve optometry practices in ten states.

90. Gauge Capital aimed for Nevada and the surrounding states with its acquisition and recapitalization of Comprehensive EyeCare Partners. The platform, acquired in 2018, is the result of mergers among Nevada Eye Physicians, New Eyes of Southern Nevada, and Shepherd Eye Center. GMB Mezzanine Capital is a minority investor. Revelstoke Capital Partners has been more ambitious. The PE firm, which formed the platform CEI Vision Partners with Cincinnati Eye Institute, intended to start in Ohio, where it is based, extend CEI Vision throughout the Midwest, and then spread nationally. Similarly, in 2018, Quad-C Management, which purchased the management platform NJEye (formed by NJ Retina) also seeks to cover the United States, starting with acquisitions in the Northeast. LLR Partners created Eye Health America to consolidate eye care in the South, including Georgia, Florida, and South Carolina. Clemson Eye, the Eye Associates, and Piedmont Surgery Center, all purchased in March 2018, were the first practices owned by the platform. Pursuing practices in the West, ShoreView Industries formed its platform jointly with California Retina Associates.

91. Pringle, "FFL's Eyecare Partners." West Street Capital Partners is the PE division of Goldman Sachs. Pringle, "Goldman PE Arm."

92. Aprill, "Private Equity Investment in Orthopedics."

93. DJl Consulting, "Breaking Down PE's Push."

94. Aprill, "Private Equity Investment in Orthopedics."

95. In 2012, there were thirteen deals, there were twenty in 2014, twenty-six in 2015, thirty-seven in 2016, twenty-four in 2017, and thirty-nine in 2018. DJl Consulting, "Breaking Down PE's Push."

96. Murphy, "Rush Ortho Group."

97. Strode, "Orthopedics."

98. Quoted in Pringle, "Why Healthcare Sponsors."

99. DJl Consulting, "Breaking Down PE's Push."

100. The deal included several minority investors as well: C3 Capital, Eagle Private Capital, Harbert Credit Solutions, and Resolute Capital Partners. The company was first acquired in June 2011 by East Cooper Medical Center, a subsidiary of Tenet Healthcare.

101. Aprill, "Private Equity Investment in Orthopedics."

102. Jacofsky interview. Jacofsky cofounded the CORE Institute, based in Phoenix, Arizona, in 2005. It is the largest orthopedic facility in the state and has eight locations in Michigan as well.

103. "Value-based care" is a health care delivery model in which providers, including hospitals and physicians, are paid based on patient health outcomes.

104. Rocco in Meyer, "Physician Groups Crave Capital."

105. Pringle, "Varsity Orthopedics Care Partners."

106. OrthoBethesda was founded in 1965 and is based in Bethesda, Maryland. Dr. Edward Bieber is the managing partner.

107. Murphy, "Rush Ortho Group."

108. Pringle, "Varsity Orthopedics Care Partners."

109. Aprill, Herschman, and Patel, "Hot Physician Specialists." Gastro Health was cofounded by Dr. James Leavitt in Miami, Florida.

110. Oliver, "Is Private Equity Investment in GI?"

111. Kane, "Medscape Gastroenterologist Compensation Report."

112. Provident Healthcare Partners, "Private Equity Investment in Gastroenterology"; Suthrum, "It's Time to Talk."

113. Based in Fort Worth, Texas, and founded by Dr. James Weber, at the time it had 110 practices in Texas and a few in Louisiana. Waud Capital, "Waud Capital Forms Partnership."

114. Meyer, "Physician Groups Crave Capital."

115. Meyer, "Physician Groups Crave Capital."

116. The three practices were Regional GI, Main Line Gastroenterology Associates, and Digestive Disease Associates. Pringle, "Amulet Forms Pennsylvania Gastro Group."

117. According to Pringle, the founders of Peak, Drs. Buck Patel and Prashant Krishnan, will earn the same income as before the buyout and receive a significant financial share of the practice. At sale time, Peak owned twelve clinics and twenty-one ambulatory and hospital-based endoscopy centers. Pringle, "Colorado's Peak Gastroenterology."

118. Oliver, "Is Private Equity Investment in GI?"

119. Kane, "Medscape Gastroenterologist Compensation Report."

120. Aprill, Herschman, and Patel, "Hot Physician Specialists"; Weinzimmer, "Private Practice Consolidation Opportunity."

121. Initially founded by Dr. Sanford Siegel, CU is based in Owings Mills, Maryland. The company was formed through a merger of the earlier CU (consisting of fourteen physicians), Maryland Urology Associates (fifteen physicians), and a third group (seven physicians). United Urology is the management services organization. Chesapeake Urology, "United Urology Group Expands."

122. Founded in 2004, the Gahanna, Ohio, urology group also provides ancillary services, such as pharmacy, radiology, pathology, imaging, and diagnostics.

123. J. W. Childs Associates was soon rebranded as Prospect Hill Growth Partners after its cofounder John Childs was accused of participating in a prostitution ring.

124. Prior to that 2018 modification, the government paid higher rates for patients treated in hospital-owned ambulatory centers than in stand-alone surgery centers. Formed in 2006 by thirty-one physicians, by November 2018 IMP had fifty locations throughout the New York metropolitan area.

125. Lee Equity Partners bought a little more than 50 percent of the two groups, with the rest held by their 100 physician stakeholders. As a result of the consolidation, Solaris had 150 providers at sixty places in New York, Ohio, Kentucky, and Indiana. Pringle, "Lee Equity Unites."

126. Hilton, "Urologists Eye Private Equity."

127. Section 2991 of the Social Security Amendments provides an entitlement for all insured individuals with chronic renal failure to receive services. It is still not entirely clear why this catastrophic ailment was privileged, but the National Kidney Foundation did engage in intensive advocacy. For a comprehensive history of section 2991, see Retting, "Origins of the Medicare Kidney Disease Establishment."

128. Murphy, "Dialysis Centers."

129. Shinkman, "Big Business of Dialysis."

130. Dickson, "CMS Proposes $190 Million Raise."

131. Hiltzik, "Column."

132. Murphy, "Dialysis Centers."

133. One of the more successful enterprises in the initial days of dialysis consolidation, Renal Care Group, was established in 1995 by nephrologists of six companies who merged their practices and took the group public. They paid for the transaction with the $64 million they collected from the IPO. Once publicly traded, Renal Care Group proceeded to accumulate 425 dialysis centers until it merged in 2005 with Fresenius, which had 1,630 facilities of its own. The acquisition cost Fresenius $3.3 billion, an enormous sum at the time.

Liberty Dialysis Holdings was initially formed in 2002 by Mark Caputo and Robert Santelli with financing from Bain Capital; more borrowed capital came from Ignition Partners five years later and additional money from six investors during 2010: WP Global Partners, Bain, Ignition Partners, KRG Capital Partners, and InvestMichigan! Mezzanine Fund. Another company, Renal Advantage, was founded in 2005 also by Mark Caputo, this time with investment dollars from Welsh, Carson, Anderson & Stowe. Five years later the financiers gave themselves a $245 million dividend recap, seven months before unloading the company to Liberty Dialysis Holdings for $850 million. In early 2012 Liberty (including Renal Advantage) was acquired by Fresenius for $2.3 billion, with the associated PE firms all cashing in; the company had to divest fifty centers to satisfy Federal Trade Commission antitrust concerns.

Reliant Renal Care was established in 2007 by founder Barbara Bednar with $50 million in development capital from investors Ferrer Freeman & Company and DW Healthcare Partners. It, too, in 2017 was acquired by Fresenius Medical Care.

134. Hiltzik, "Column."

135. In 2016, U.S. Renal Care had merged with its nonprofit competitor DSI Renal for $640 million. Frazier Healthcare and NEA had formed DSI in 2011 after buying some centers from DaVita. Pringle, "U.S. Renal."

136. Pringle, "U.S. Renal"; Shinkman, "Big Business of Dialysis."

137. Abram, "Why Kidney Dialysis Patients Are Pushing"; Fields, "God Help You"; Kidney Buzz, "Intense Debate Sparked."

138. Fields, "God Help You."

139. Fields, "God Help You"; Shinkman, "Big Business of Dialysis."

140. Cited in Shinkman, "Big Business of Dialysis."

141. Quoted in Bort, "John Oliver Sees Ills." DaVita had to pay $253 million in damages for the deaths of three patients who were treated with GranuFlo, a product made by Fresenius that was recalled in 2011 by the US Food and Drug Administration. Fresenius settled a different wrongful death lawsuit for negligence in 2008. Fields, "God Help You."

142. Gander, Zhang, and Ross, "Association," cited in Carroll, "Patients at For-Profit Dialysis Centers."

143. Cooper, "Dialysis Centers on Every Corner."

144. Abelson and Thomas, "UnitedHealthcare Sues Dialysis Chain."

145. Associated Press, "Judge Blocks California Law."

146. Livingston, "Dialysis Companies."

147. Pringle, "Dialysis, Behavioral Health."

148. Hiltzik, "Column."

149. Hirsch, "Trump Administration"; Copley, "U.S. Seeks to Cut Dialysis Costs."

150. Cockrell and Mick, "Next Wave of Consolidation"; Cantrell, "This Venture Capital Fund"; Hicks, "Why Are Private Equity Investors."

151. One of the first PE investments in IVF treatment was IntegraMed Fertility, a publicly traded company since 1992; two private equity firms, Hercules Capital and Morgan Stanley Expansion Capital, held shares in the enterprise through an earlier PIPE. In 2012 it was taken private by Sagard Capital Partners for $169.5 million. By 2019, the practice management company had locations across thirty-two states.

152. Fertility issues have drawn venture capitalists into the business too. In 2017, more than $178 million flowed into startups developing fertility products, such as a test that promised a credit-score-style rating of a woman's fertility. Companies have launched expensive trials for finding genetically related causes of infertility and measuring hormone levels. One venture capital–supported enterprise, Modern Fertility, provides blood analysis that gauges how many eggs a woman has left in her ovaries and any hormonal imbalances. There are

also egg freezing services (e.g., Extend Fertility, financed through North Peak Capital). Robbins, "Investors See Big Money."

153. Quoted in Robbins, "Investors See Big Money."

154. Quoted in Robbins, "Investors See Big Money."

155. PR Newswire, "Ovation Fertility Announces."

156. Snyder interview.

157. Cantrell, "This Venture Capital Fund." These enterprises include Pacific Fertility Center (2017), Vivere Health (2017), Advanced Fertility Center of Chicago (2018), and Inception Fertility (2019). This was the second private equity LBO for Vivere, which had been created as a platform in 2010 by LLR Partners for $23 million; LLR had merged Piney Point Surgery Center and Houston Fertility Laboratory, both owned by Dr. Jimmy Gill and Dr. Gus Haddad. At Pacific Fertility Center, up to 2,000 frozen embryos were accidentally destroyed in a liquid nitrogen storage tank. Prelude has been facing a class action lawsuit since March 2018.

158. Sverica Capital Management must have been quite satisfied with this asset in the fertility niche because in 2019 it invested $31.5 million of development capital for the platform In Vitro Sciences, grabbing a minority stake; the company operates a network of fertility practices. Simultaneously, Sverica added Advanced Fertility Care, spun out of Women's Health USA, to In Vitro Sciences. In 2020, the business owned seventeen clinics and four in vitro labs and aimed to spread across the nation. Business Wire, "Sverica Capital Management Announces."

159. Schinfeld interview. The following quotes are also from this interview.

160. Somkuti interview.

161. Bruch et al., "Expansion of Private Equity Involvement."

162. Reddy, "Private Equity Investments."

163. Becker et al., "15 Private Equity in Healthcare."

164. DocWire News, "Economies of Urgent Care."

165. DocWire News, "Economies of Urgent Care."

166. Other PE investments in urgent care chains include NextCare Holdings (by Enhanced Healthcare Partners in 2010); WellStreet Urgent Care (by FFL Partners and Crane Street Capital in 2011); Fast Pace Urgent Care (by Shore Capital Partners in 2012 and then in an SBO by Revelstoke Capital Partners, WP Global Partners, and Yukon Partners in 2016); Physicians Immediate Care (by LLR Partners and Anthem in 2012); and Xpress Wellness Urgent Care (by Latticework Capital Management and BPEA Private Equity in 2018).

167. The business had been formed as Premier Urgent Care in 2010 by several emergency medicine physicians.

168. Becker et al., "15 Private Equity in Healthcare." It was a quick flip for Stat, which had been acquired from Spanos Barber Jesse & Co. only two years earlier.

169. Pringle, "Marriage of Summit Medical."

170. Evans, "Private-Equity Backed." Humana had acquired Concentra in 2010 for $790 million and sold it five years later for $1.05 billion. Headquartered in Addison, Texas, Concentra operates 520 urgent care facilities in forty-four states.

171. MedExpress had been acquired by Urgent Care MSO through an LBO sponsored by its owners, Sequoia Capital and General Atlantic, in 2012.

172. Gustafsson, Seervai, and Blumenthal, "Role of Private Equity."

173. Alternative, "Why Doesn't Private Equity."

174. Ojo, "Trends in Healthcare Staffing."

175. Headquartered in Nashville, Tennessee, Envision provides staffing across the nation for hospital emergency rooms and other departments; post-acute care; and ambulatory surgery. It also owns more than 260 outpatient surgery centers in thirty-five states. Ojo, "Trends in Healthcare Staffing."

176. Founded in 1972, EmCare was first acquired in 1997 by Laidlaw International for $335 million and then received growth capital from minority investor North Peak Capital prior to its sale to Envision Healthcare via Onex. Through its PE owners, EmCare merged and consolidated staffing enterprises, especially for emergency rooms, throughout the United States.

177. Sutherland, "It's the Greatest Health-Care Buyout"; Kincaid, "Envision Healthcare."

178. Comments by Conway, vice chair, CD&R, second morning fireside chat, Columbia Business School, Twenty-Fifth Conference.

179. Balance billing is when a provider bills a patient for the difference between its charge and the amount paid by the insurance company. This is not allowed when physicians, hospitals, or other health care providers participate in the patient's insurance network.

180. One in five patients in an ER is cared for by an outside company doctor who is not in their insurance network. Kincaid, "Envision Healthcare."

181. Kincaid, "Envision Healthcare."

182. Beecken Petty O'Keefe & Company also bought Medical Solutions, a nurse staffing company, from Tenex Capital Management and McCarthy Capital through a $40 million LBO in 2012 and sold it to PNC Erieview Capital and TPG Capital in 2017.

183. Between 2010 and 2016, TeamHealth bought fifty-one ER and physician specialist practices. Appelbaum and Batt, "Private Equity Tries to Protect."

184. Smith, "Private Equity: The Perps."

185. Appelbaum and Batt, "Private Equity Tries to Protect."

186. Some other staffing LBOs include American Physician Partners, formed in 2015 as a medical services organization through the buyout of Align MD and Elite Emergency Services. After being recapitalized in 2016 by Brown Brothers Harriman Capital Partners, receiving $244.5 million in debt financing in 2018 and acquisition funding from Carlyle Group in January 2019, the enterprise was put up for sale nine months later. Apparently, American Physician Partners provides in-network services and does not engage in balance billing; nonetheless, reflecting concern that the sale would be adversely affected by the controversy over surprise-billing practices, the company was removed from the market a few months later.

GrapeTree Medical Staffing, established in 2016, was recapitalized through a management LBO by New Mainstream Capital at the end of 2017. The enterprise provides medical staffing across the US Midwest. Integrated Care Physicians was formed by BelHealth Investment Partners in 2017 through the merger of Integrated Emergency Medicine Specialists and Integrated Care Physicians. It is continuing to expand in the Florida market. Emerald Health Services, founded in 2002, was acquired by Webster Equity Partners in March 2018.

Emergency Care Partners, a new platform, was formed by Varsity Healthcare Partners by merging Professional Emergency Management and Professional Emergency Physician Associates in September 2018. Five months later, Emergency Care Partners united with New Progressive Emergency Physicians, doubling its size, and added Regal Healthcare as a minority investor in February 2019. In September, it merged with another large staffing company, Illinois Emergency Medicine Specialists. As of January 2020, the combined entity had a labor force of 600 physicians and midlevel providers who treat roughly 900,000 ER patients annually in four states.

One of the largest takeovers in 2018, Sound Inpatient Physician Holdings (Sound Physicians) was carved out of Fresenius Medical Care, which had acquired the enterprise in 2014 for $600 million. Just four years later, Fresenius sold it through a $2.2 billion LBO to a consortium of five investors: Summit Partners, Silversmith Capital Partners, Revelstoke Capital Partners, Optum-Health, and Athyrium Capital Management. What a payday for Fresenius and its PE owners. Dorbian, "PE-Backed ECP"; Pringle, "PE-Backed American Physician Partners"; Phillips, "PE Firms Target"; Ojo, "Trends in Healthcare Staffing"; Pringle, "Varsity Healthcare Partners Recaps"; Pringle, "Varsity's Emergency Care Partners"; Appelbaum and Batt, "Private Equity Tries to Protect."

187. Appelbaum and Batt, "Private Equity and Surprise Medical Billing"; Markian Hawryluk, "Ever Heard of a Surgical Assistant? Meet a New Boost to Your Medical Bills," July 2020.

188. Appelbaum, "Private Equity Is a Driving Force."

189. Cited in Lewis, "Blackstone, KKR."

190. Appelbaum and Batt, "Private Equity Tries to Protect." California's 2016 legislation is one of the more stringent: it puts a cap on out-of-network charges, tying them to the median in-network rate of insurers or to 125 percent of the Medicare fee, whichever is higher.

191. Cited in Lewis, "Blackstone, KKR"; Luthi, "Surprise Medical Billing Legislation."

192. Appelbaum and Batt, "Private Equity Tries to Protect."

193. Appelbaum and Batt, "Private Equity Tries to Protect."

194. Appelbaum and Batt, "Private Equity Tries to Protect."

195. Cohrs, "How Congress' Surprise Billing."

196. The earlier Senate Health, Education, Labor and Pensions Committee proposal did not include an arbitration backstop, and the House Energy and Commerce legislation had set a narrow arbitration option, allowing providers to appeal charges of $1,250 or more. In the newly negotiated bill, the amount was set at $750.

197. GPs are exploring primary care, and in 2016 Pine Tree Equity Partners acquired InHealth MD Alliance. In January of the following year, Gauge Capital bought Miami Beach Medical Group. The arena may prove to be more valuable than the PE industry initially thought: only twelve months later Gauge helped itself to a $7.8 million dividend recap. Moreover, at least one primary care enterprise, Community Medical Group, is on its third flip. Community Medical Group was first bought by Pine Tree Equity Partners in 2013, tossed to six PE

firms (Alpine Partners, Ardian, Barings BDC, Mosaic Health Solutions, Nautic Partners, and ShumCapital) only two years later, and then landed at Centene in March 2018.

Chapter 5. Drilling for Gold

1. Molin, "Private Equity Dental Management."
2. Davis, "Private Equity Firms Target."
3. Davis, "GA Board Member Resigns."
4. Moriarty, "Unethical Private-Equity."
5. Freedberg, "Dental Abuse."
6. Freedberg, "Dental Abuse," 2.
7. Moriarty, "Unethical Private-Equity."
8. Joint Staff Report on the Corporate Practice of Medicine in the Medicaid Program, 2.
9. Freedberg, "Dental Abuse"; Ackerman, "Medicaid Dental Clinics."
10. Freedberg, "Dental Abuse."
11. Casamassimo interview.
12. Casamassimo interview.
13. Barker, "Private Equity Toolbox."
14. Tanzi interview. Michigan, Arizona, Maine, Minnesota, and Vermont have already enacted legislation allowing for dental therapists to perform certain procedures. The level of education and training depends on the state.
15. Davis interview. The following comments are all from this interview.
16. A few states, such as Missouri, have outlawed the fraudulent plans.
17. Tanzi interview. When my dentist decided to retire and sell his practice in 2006, he did not receive a single inquiry from private equity firms. Indeed, he told me that he had never heard of PE at the time. He did mention, however, that he lucked out in selling his practice to a dentist in the area since other retiring practitioners were having difficulty in doing so. Dobrowolski interview.
18. Casamassimo interview.
19. Davis interview.
20. Davis, "Doctors Selling Practices."
21. Davis interview.
22. Casamassimo interview. The following comments also are from this interview.
23. Molin, "Private Equity Dental Management."
24. Quoted in Davis, "Emerging Advocacy Groups."
25. Quoted in Davis, "Emerging Advocacy Groups."
26. Jackie Stanfield quoted in Davis, "Emerging Advocacy Groups."
27. Barrett, "Massive Dental Fraud Uncovered"; Moriarty, "Unethical Private-Equity."
28. The television investigations included WJLA-TV (Washington, DC, area) and ABC-TV's 20/20.
29. Barrett, "Massive Dental Fraud Uncovered"; Moriarty, "Unethical Private-Equity."
30. US Department of Health and Human Services, "OIG Excludes Pediatric Dental Management," 1.

31. Launched in Phoenix, Arizona, during 1997, ReachOut was known as Healthy Kids and Seniors Dental until 2004. In its early years, the company provided dental services to older people in nursing homes but divested that segment at the end of 2011. In addition to serving schoolchildren, the chain expanded to homeless shelters, foster programs, group homes, and mental health facilities. Freedberg, "Dental Abuse."

32. There were also two minority investors: Caymus Equity Partners and Audax Group.

33. Freedberg, "Dental Abuse"; McGuire Woods, "Dental Management Company Agrees."

34. Feldman,, "Ares Increases Stake in Dental Firm."

35. Moriarty, "Unethical Private-Equity."

36. Freedberg, "Dental Abuse"; McGuire Woods, "Dental Management Company Agrees."

37. University of Michigan, School of Dentistry, "Alumni Profile."

38. His company was formerly known as East Coast Dental Management.

39. Provident Healthcare Partners, "Private Equity Investment in Dental Care." Two minority growth investors—Gemini Investors and Seacoast Capital Partners—came on board in 2002, followed by Capital Resource Partners in 2004.

40. Rosenbaum and Heath, "Patients, Pressure and Profits."

41. In 2017, American Securities sold additional shares to minority investors Leonard Green & Partners and Ares Capital Corporation.

42. Private Equity Stakeholder Project, "Private Equity Health Care Acquisitions."

43. Business Wire, "Aspen Dental Management."

44. New York Attorney General, "A. G. Schneiderman Announces Settlement with Aspen."

45. New York Attorney General, "A. G. Schneiderman Announces Settlement with Aspen"; Feldman, "Ares Increases Stake in Dental Firm."

46. McGuire Woods, "Class Action Filed."

47. Rosenbaum and Health, "Patients, Pressure and Profits."

48. Rosenbaum and Health, "Patients, Pressure and Profits."

49. Davis interview.

50. Consumer Affairs, "Ratings for Aspen Dental."

51. See boycottaspendental.com.

52. The Effingham, Illinois–based Heartland had sold a minority stake in 2008 to CHS Capital, four years before the Ontario pension investors bought it.

53. Group Dentistry Now, "Taking a Deeper Look"; Cooper, "KKR to Acquire Majority Interest"; Mathis and Metcalf, "Private Equity Is Pouring Money."

54. Group Dentistry Now, "Taking a Deeper Look"; Cooper, "KKR to Acquire Majority Interest"; Mathis and Metcalf, "Private Equity Is Pouring Money."

55. Davis, "Private Equity Firms Target."

56. Cooper, "KKK to Acquire Majority Interest."

57. Davis interview.

58. All Smiles was founded by Richard Malouf. After the LBO by Valor Equity, the PE shop owned 72 percent of the company and Malouf owned 28 percent.

59. Dallas News Administrator, "All Smiles Dental Centers."

60. Freedberg, "Dental Abuse."

61. Premier Dental Holdings is the dental management organization for Western Dental.

62. Olmos, "Federal Agents Raid."

63. These included Kids Dental Kare (fourteen offices); Children's Dental Group (eight offices); Choice Family Dentistry Center in Perris, California (one office); and Smile Wide (fourteen offices). Phillips, "PE Firms Go in Big."

64. Coast Dental Services, founded in 1992 in Tampa, Florida, was taken private by its management team and merged with the newly formed Intelident Solutions in 2005. At the time, it had 106 dental centers in four states. In August 2011, Coast Dental bought Smilecare (founded in 1977 and acquired by Liberty Partners in 1997). In an SBO, Smilecare was bought by Western Dental via New Mountain Capital. The Guardian purchase added 63 offices in Texas, California, and Alabama, including 36 affiliated with South Texas Dental. The acquired DSO's other brands are Access Dental, Blue Hills Dental, and Vital Smiles. Western Dental's other affiliate is Brident Dental and Orthodontics.

65. Western Dental serves roughly 2.9 million people each year, mostly through Medicaid. It owns 312 affiliated offices in California, Texas, Arizona, Nevada, and Alabama. Business Wire, "Western Dental Completes."

66. Consumer Affairs, "Consumer Complaints, Western Dental Reviews."

67. See https://western-dental.pissedconsumers.com/review.html.

68. Located in Marietta, Georgia, Kool Smiles was founded by Drs. Tu Tran and Thien Pham in 2006.

69. Tailwind Capital also bought Lone Peak Dental Group, another DSO, in January 2017. At the end of 2018, Lone Peak was accused by the Washington State Department of Health of "dangerous and deceptive practices," including kickbacks for the use of general anesthesia; self-referral to affiliated oral surgery and orthodontia clinics, causing hardship for clients; and reusing disposable mouthpieces, against the manufacturer's instructions, to enhance earnings. Davis, "WSDA Files Complaint."

70. Latour, "To Remedy COVID-19 Impasse."

71. Davis, "Kool Smiles Dental—A Disturbing Peek."

72. US Department of Justice, "Dental Management Company Benevis."

73. Davis, "Kool Smiles Dental Quietly Changes."

74. In the middle of the investigation in 2016, Georgia governor Nathan Deal appointed Dr. Dale Mayfield (the long-time dental officer for Kool Smiles) to the Georgia Board of Dentistry. Michael Davis aptly remarks: "the fox guards the henhouse." After the conclusion of the investigation, Governor Deal had to ask Mayfield to resign. Davis, "Kool Smiles Dental—A Disturbing Peek."

75. The rebranded names are Sunnybrook Dentistry (Mississippi and Arkansas); Cortland Dental (Massachusetts); Pippin Dental (Indiana); Elstar Dental, Pinova Dental, and Jubilee Dental (Texas); Creston Dental and Braces (South Carolina); Pine Dental (Maryland and Virginia); Sutton Dental (Connecticut); Taylor Dental (Louisiana); Ruby Dental (Kentucky); and Dorsett Dental and Manzana Dental (Arizona). Davis, "Kool Smiles Dental Quietly Changes."

76. Davis, "Benevis Files for Chapter 11"; Latour, "To Remedy COVID-19 Impasse."

77. Founded in 1982 by Walter Knysz, GEDC is based in Bloomfield, Michigan.

78. Some of the acquisitions via Audax were Willow Creek Dental Care (July 2009); Dental Health Group (September 2008); Ramsey Salem DDS (March 2010); Nanston Dental Group (June 2010); Dr. John Dos Passos (November 2010); Family Smiles Dentistry (December 2010); Smilecare Dental Associates (December 2010); Wright Dental Care (July 2011); and Goodman Orthodontists (August 2011). Dental Health Group, formerly known as ConsoliDent, was subsequently sold separately to Cave Creek Management for $30 million in a tertiary LBO (October 2011). Provident Healthcare Partners, "Private Equity Investment in Dental Care."

79. "Dental Franchises Show Steady Growth."

80. Smilecare Dental Associates, which had been acquired by Great Expressions through Audax Group, was separately sold to Western Dental via New Mountain Capital and Court Square in June 2018.

81. See https://www.bbb.org/us/mi/southfield/profile/dentist/great-expres sions-dental-centers-0332-46000435/complaints.

82. Dorbian, "Riverside and Abry." North American Dental, founded in 2007 by Ken Cooper and Dr. Andrew Matta, was initially based in New Castle, Pennsylvania. Jacobs Holding is a Switzerland-based PE firm that keeps its portfolio companies for the long term. It also has no limited partners; the beneficiary is the Jacobs Foundation, a charitable organization that assists children and adolescents.

83. For instance, six months after Harvest purchased DCA, the company paid $330 million to acquire Northeast Dental Management. Formerly Garden State Dental Management, Northeast Dental had already been bumped to a number of PE firms: DFW Capital Partners and MCG Capital Corporation (2007), Sentinel Capital Partners (2012), and Harvest Partners (2016).

84. Metro Square Dental Associates, founded in 1992 by Jeffrey Cohen, was its first LBO.

85. Group Dentistry Now, "Why Private Equity Firms Like Dentists."

86. Steve Bilt and Brad Schmidt merged three dental companies to form Bright Now!

87. In 2018, Jefferson Dental Clinics had fifty-eight offices in Dallas–Fort Worth, Houston, and San Antonio, Texas.

88. For example, Dr. Dental Management, acquired by Abry Partners in January 2019, has developed into one of the largest DSOs in New England.

89. Pringle, "Healthcare Corner." Current PE investments include Frontier Dental Laboratories 02 Investment Partners), National Dentex (WCAS), Dental Services Group (Cressey & Company), and SmileDirectClub (CD&R).

90. Tanzi interview.

91. Phillips, "PE Firms Go in Big"; Fugazy, "Why Private Equity Firms."

92. PE owns Pacific Dental Services (My Kid's Dentist), Benevis (Kool Smiles), and Children's Choice Pediatric Dental Care (acquired as a platform by Amulet Capital Partners), among others.

93. Roub, "5 Dental Trends."

Chapter 6. Frail Elderly and Children

1. Mullaney, "Home Health Spending."
2. Spinger et al., "Private Equity Pursues Profits."
3. In the late 1980s, 90 percent of Medicaid long-term care dollars were for nursing homes and only 10 percent for HCBS; in 2018, nursing homes received only 43 percent of the total. Span, "In the Nursing Home."
4. Mullaney, "Home Health Spending."
5. The profit margin for inpatient rehabilitation is 13.9 percent, followed by skilled nursing homes (12.6 percent) and long-term acute care hospitals (4.6 percent). Livingston, "Reimbursement Limitations."
6. Cited in Abelson, "When a Health Insurer"; Flynn, "Home Health Care."
7. Kindred, Amedisys, and LHC Group are the largest companies, each accounting for 4–6 percent of the total. Holly, "Top 10 Largest"; McDermott and Palasota, "Visiting the Home Health Marketplace."
8. Holly, "Top 10 Largest"; McDermott and Palasota, "Visiting the Home Health Marketplace"; Shulas, "Private Equity Poised"; Holly, "Home Health"; Holly, "Skeptics Raise Concerns."
9. Holly, "With Medicare Advantage."
10. Cabin et al., "For-Profit Medicare Home Health."
11. Dickson, "CMS Preparing Rules."
12. Braff Group, "Home Health and Hospice."
13. Famakinwa, "Private Equity Likely."
14. McDermott and Palasota, "Visiting the Home Health Marketplace."
15. Famakinwa, "Calculating the Cost of PDGM."
16. Holly, "Encompass Health's April Anthony"; Goldberg, "Medicare Decides." On the other hand, the industry received a 2.1 percent net increase in overall payments ($400 million) for fiscal year 2019.
17. Famakinwa, "Calculating the Cost of PDGM."
18. Holly, "Encompass Health's April Anthony."
19. Goldberg, "Medicare Decides," 1.
20. Holly, "Skeptics Raise Concerns."
21. Cabin et al., "For-Profit Medicare Home Health." Profits are revenues minus total costs for the company. Nonprofit home health agencies can use any profits they earn to enhance quality of care and provide crucial but money-losing services to their clientele. They also tend to charge less than commercial enterprises and are far more willing to provide services to more costly, vulnerable individuals and those who are dependent on Medicaid.
22. Bernstein, "Father's Last Wish."
23. According to PHI, a New York–based national research, consulting, and direct care advocacy organization, one-sixth of homecare workers live in poverty, 90 percent are women, 62 percent are people of color, 31 percent are immigrants, and 53 percent depend on welfare. Famakinwa, "18% of Home Care Workers."
24. The average turnover rate in 2017 was 67 percent. Providers offering wages above the 90 percent median had the lowest turnover rate (38.1 percent) while those in the bottom 10 percent of pay had the greatest frequency (80.2 percent). Baxter, "Median Home Care Turnover."

25. The initial program, founded by Asian and Italian immigrant families in San Francisco, was called On Lok.

26. Participants are eligible for both programs. Prior to 2016, there were only 40,000 participants.

27. Varney, "Private Equity Pursues Profits," 1.

28. Spinger et al., "Private Equity Pursues Profits."

29. Thomas Scully, a general partner with WCAS since 2004, was previously the administrator of the Centers for Medicare and Medicaid Services from 2001 to 2004.

30. Abelson, "When a Health Insurer," 1.

31. In 2018, hospice utilization accounted for 3 percent of Medicare's budget ($17.5 billion).

32. Kacik, "Amedisys Aims to Acquire."

33. Hallman, "Hospice Inc."

34. US Department of Health and Human Services, "Vulnerabilities in the Medicare Hospice Program."

35. Hallman, "Hospice Inc."

36. US Department of Health and Human Services, "Vulnerabilities in the Medicare Hospice Program."

37. Hallman, "Hospice Inc."

38. Abelson, "When a Health Insurer."

39. US Department of Health and Human Services, "Vulnerabilities in the Medicare Hospice Program."

40. Hallman, "Hospice Inc."

41. US Department of Health and Human Services, "Vulnerabilities in the Medicare Hospice Program."

42. In 2017, the average amount was $191 per day for the first sixty-day period and $150 daily for any time after that. Payments vary by level of care: routine homecare; inpatient treatments for pain control and symptom management; short-term inpatient respite care; and homecare for intermittent emergencies. Since 2016, hospices have received higher amounts in the seven days before death if they provide skilled care to the patient. US Department of Health and Human Services, "Vulnerabilities in the Medicare Hospice Program."

43. Calma, "Top 10 Home and Hospice Providers."

44. Funding Universe, "Vencor, Inc. History."

45. Hilzenrath, "Vencor Faces $1 Billion Claim," E1.

46. Vencor was initially financed privately by Gene Smith; Michael Barr was the other cofounder.

47. Livingston, "Home Healthcare."

48. In 2017, Kindred sold the operations of fifty-four skilled nursing homes to BM Eagle Holdings, led by affiliates of Blue Mountain Capital Management, for $519 million, with the intention of shifting the rest of the eighty-nine facilities and seven assisted living places to them. It also bought some of the real estate that Ventas (its previous REIT) owned (thirty-six nursing home properties) for more than half a billion dollars and was given an option to purchase the rest. Kindred Healthcare, "Kindred Completes First Closing." At the end of 2017, Kindred's debt load was $3.3 billion.

49. Heller, "Kindred Healthcare to Pay."

50. Teichert, "Kindred Pays Feds."

51. Humana received 40 percent, and the rest was divided between TPG and WCAS. However, Humana retains the right to buy the remaining at-home division shares over time. The Kindred at-home division in 2018 was the nation's largest home health and second largest hospice business, as well as a significant provider of in-home personal care. It served patients in forty-one states.

52. At the time, Curo had 245 hospice locations in twenty-two states.

53. Hospice providers bought by Curo through GTCR include Hospice Plus (2010, Texas), Hospice Family Care (2012, Arizona), and Community Home Care and Hospice (2012, North Carolina).

54. Hospice providers bought by Curo through Thomas H. Lee and HealthView include SouthernCare (2014, North Carolina), which had experienced three prior LBOs, and New Century Hospice (2016 for $120 million, Georgia). In October 2020, Thomas H. Lee Partners returned to the hospice business when it purchased Care Hospice from Martis Capital (the PE firm had rebranded from Capricorn Healthcare in 2018). Founded in 2008 by J. Brad Hunter and acquired by Martis in 2017, Care Hospice had sixty locations in twelve states at the time of the leveraged buyout.

55. Wikipedia, "Gentiva Health Services."

56. This was an SBO for Girling, which was first acquired by TGF Management in 2005 for $100 million. Its services range from skilled nursing and rehabilitation to personal care. Auxi Health, a provider of home health care products and services in the US Midwest and Southeast, was founded by Monterey Capital Partners, which in 1999 cobbled together eight homecare agencies: Always Care Home Health Services, First Home Health, Hawkeye Health Services, Home MedCare, PharmaThera, Procare Home Health Services, Jackson Healthcare, and Missouri Home Care.

57. Willmer, "When Wall Street Took Over."

58. When Bain bought the company, Epic had seventy-seven locations in seventeen states. Or, "Webster Capital Explores Sale."

59. These acquisitions include PyraMed Health Services (bought by Epic in 2011); Americare Health Services (2012); Loving Care Agency* (2015); Medical Staffing Network Healthcare (2012); Sante Pediatric Services* (2012); CLARITY Service Group (2015); Option 1 Nutrition Solutions* (2015); Unifour Nursing (2015); Medco Medical Supply (2015); Liberty Healthcare Services (2016); Rehabilitation Associates (2016); Pediatric Special Care (2016); Spring View Home Healthcare (2016); Pediatria Healthcare (2016); and Firstaff Nursing Services (2016). The asterisk (*) indicates companies that had been flipped once before and had their own history of leveraged buyouts: Sante Pediatric Services (2009); Loving Care Agency (2007); and Option 1 Nutrition Solutions (2004 and again in 2007).

60. Or, "Webster Capital Explores Sale."

61. Willmer, "When Wall Street Took Over."

62. At the time of the IPO, PSA had 41 locations in twelve states, generating $46 million in annual revenues. From 1994 to 1998, PSA had acquired 38 pediatric care companies, had achieved $200 million in annual revenues, and operated 123 places

in twenty-five states. Funding Universe, "History of Pediatric Services of America, Inc."

63. US Department of Justice, "Pediatric Services of America."

64. These LBOs include Assure Home Health (private duty nursing for medically fragile children); Innovations Health Services (private duty nursing); Professional Pediatric Home* (home nursing services for children); Reach Pediatric Therapy* (pediatric homecare); Care Unlimited (homecare services for medically fragile children); and the Care Group (homecare services). The purchases marked with an asterisk (*) were secondary private equity LBOs.

65. The acquisition of PSA cost almost $300 million and that of Epic cost $950 million. Baxter, "Epic Merges with PSA."

66. Willmer, "When Wall Street Took Over."

67. Zepp interview. The following comments are also from this interview.

68. Funding Universe, "ResCare, Inc. History."

69. Private placement is the sale of stocks and bonds to preselected investors instead of on the open market through an IPO. ResCare received development capital from RFE Investment Partners, Nautic Partners, and North Peak Capital. Funding Universe, "ResCare, Inc. History."

70. Tully, "ResCare Whistleblowers."

71. "Possible ResCare Inc. Employee."

72. Tully, "ResCare Whistleblowers." The fine was later reduced to $15.5 million.

73. Sabella, "Teen's Death."

74. Sergent, "Workforce Board Terminates Contract."

75. Tully, "ResCare Whistleblowers."

76. Lawsuit Resource Center, "ResCare Overtime."

77. Nakamoto, "Major Problems."

78. Walgreens Boots Alliance was a minority investor. At this point ResCare owned entities that offered services in forty-four US states and Canada.

79. Globe News Wire, "Onex Completes Tale."

80. Gregory, "PharMerica Corporation Settles."

81. Gregory, "PharMerica Corporation Settles."

82. US Department of Justice, "Long-Term Care Pharmacy."

83. Advanced Homecare Management is based in Dallas, Texas. The company was purchased by Saunders Karp & Megrue, which merged with Apax in 2005.

84. In February 1984, HealthSouth had been incorporated by cofounders Richard M. Scrushy and Aaron Beam as AmCare, but the following year they changed its name to HealthSouth Rehabilitation Corporation. The hugely successful company experienced its first IPO in 1986, at which time it was publicly traded on the NASDAQ. In 1988 HealthSouth was moved to the New York Stock Exchange. By the early1990s, the company was one of the largest providers of outpatient and inpatient rehabilitative services in the United States. The now-multimillionaire owners and other executives engaged in an accounting fraud scheme beginning in 1996 in order to bolster HealthSouth's finances and enrich themselves. Among other methods of cooking the books, they misclassified expenses, overstated revenues, and understated the amount of cash on the balance sheet, including the net assets of their acquisitions. Until

they were caught in 2002, the annual gap between the actual figures and the ones they were reporting amounted to hundreds of millions of dollars. The perpetrators were convicted and jailed. In 2006, the company regained its financial footing, Scrushy's name was scrubbed out everywhere, and Health-South once more returned to the NYSE. McCann, "Two CFOs Tell."

85. Alacare operates twenty-three home health and twenty-three hospice locations in Alabama.

86. Mullaney, "Jordan, Great Lakes."

87. These include CIMA Hospice (2011), Farias Home Health Care (2012), SMC Home Health (2012), Tritrax Healthcare Services (2012), Visiting Nurses of Delaware (2012), Providence Homecare Services (2012), Healthcare Innovations Private Services (2013), Healing Touch Homecare Services (2014), Texas Gulf Coast Home Health and Home Care (2014), Primary Nurse Care (2014), PrimeCare Network (2014), Exceptional HomeCare (2015), Accord Home Care (2015), Rose of Texas Hospice (2015), Harris County Home Health Services (2015), Angelina Home Health Services (2015), Wise County Home Health (2016), Excel Home Health (2016), Cooper Home Health (2016), SimCor Home Care (2016), CareCycle Solutions (2016), HealthSense Cares (2017), Grapevine Mission Hospice (2017), Medistar Home Health (2017), Cypress Home Health (2017), Ross Health Care (2017), Kindred at Home (Oklahoma operations, 2017), Pyramid Home Health Services (2018), and Aspire Home Care (2018).

88. Based in Connecticut, NHHC has four subsidiary companies: Accredited Health Services, Allen Health Care Services, Medical Resources Home Health Corporation, and New England Home Care.

89. Mike McMaude, an operating partner at Frazier, became Abode's CEO in 2012.

90. Audax Group also came on board as a minority investor.

91. In seven short years, Abode Healthcare acquired home health and hospice agencies in twelve states.

92. Originally called CLP Healthcare Services (also known as Cloverleaf Partners), the company was renamed Compassus in 2009.

93. Two of these enterprises—Life Choice and Hospice Advantage—were well worn, each having experienced a prior LBO along with the usual buying sprees. By 2018, Compassus had 162 locations in more than thirty states.

94. Mokhiber, "Evercare Hospice to Pay."

95. Abelson, "When a Health Insurer."

96. In 2016, Optum paid $18 million in fines to settle the earlier False Claims Act violations.

97. Guardian had been picked over by Transition Capital Partners, Evolve Capital, and Progress Equity Partners in its initial management LBO in 2000, and later by Friedman Fleischer and Lowe after an SBO in 2005.

98. At that point, AccentCare owned forty-two health care companies in sixteen states. It also had thirty partnerships with insurance companies, physician groups, and major health systems. Bryant, "AccentCare to Be Acquired."

99. Bryant, "AccentCare to Be Acquired."

100. Caring Brands has more than 530 franchise locations in seven nations, including the United States, Australia, the United Kingdom, and Ireland. The

US division is based in Sunrise, Florida. See https://www.interimhealthcare.com.

101. Ross had earlier experienced the challenges of caring for his mother, who was out of state; Bonacuse had watched the trials of his mother as she cared for his grandmother. Ross interview. The information in the following paragraphs is from this interview.

102. The purchase included two minority investors, Glouston Capital Partners and Maven Hill Capital Partners. Home Helpers is based in Cincinnati, Ohio.

103. Care Advantage was founded in 1988 in Richmond, Virginia, by Deborah Johnston.

104. It has purchased Stay at Home Personal Care (2017), Care Solutions (2017), Ready Hands (2018), Paradise Homecare (2018), A Hopeful Home (2018), Direct Home Health (2018), Capital City Nurses (2019), and Allegiance Home Care (2019).

105. The business was established by Michael Newman in Roseville, California. Plenary Partners became a minority investor through the LBO.

106. Pringle, "Five Questions with NexPhase Capital."

107. Famakinwa, "PE-Backed Synergy HomeCare."

108. See https://healthcarecompare.com/home-health/ca-058076/.

109. Zang interview. The information in the following paragraphs is from this interview.

110. CarePatrol is a nationwide referral system for senior living facilities. In 2012, the Federal Trade Commission accused the conglomerate of false and deceptive advertising that asserted that it monitored and prescreened every place it recommended. CarePatrol was ordered to stop and desist from such claims, though some observers suggest that it continued doing so nonetheless. At any rate, the FTC order seemingly did give Riverside pause about acquiring the moneymaking company.

111. SC&H Capital, "How Private Equity Is Helping."

112. Famakinwa, "With New Franchise Sales on the Rise."

113. Pringle, "Varsity Healthcare Backs."

114. Calma, "Top 10 Home and Hospice Providers."

115. Kacik, "Amedisys Aims to Acquire"; Heller, "Kindred Healthcare to Pay."

116. From 2005 to 2019, LHC Group acquired nearly seventy agencies. Arguably, its most consequential purchase was Almost Family for $1 billion in 2019. Almost Family was established in 1976 and was placed on the NASDAQ eleven years later. A provider of home health and personal care, Almost Family was an avid devourer of businesses, acquiring more than twenty-six from 2002 through 2017. Among other purchases, in 2016 Almost Family acquired the assets of ResCare/BrightSpring Health Services. Another large acquisition was the Home Health Division of Community Health Systems for $128 million in 2017.

117. Pringle, "Post Capital, Ex-Addus Chief."

118. HCAP Partners became a minority investor at that time. Arosa+LivHome is the holding company of the entities.

119. Medoff interview and email. The information in the following paragraph is also from these sources.

120. Lebherz, "Lord of the Manor"; Funding Universe, "Manor Care, Inc. History."

121. Lebherz, "Lord of the Manor."

122. Blumenthal, "Barron's Insynt," C24.

123. Stevenson and Grabowski, "Private Equity Investment."

124. "Manor Care Plans Restructure."

125. HCP also bought a 9.9 percent stake in the nursing home operator for $95 million. Rubin, "Nursing Home Bankruptcies."

126. ManorCare also had to pay for property taxes, insurance, and upkeep at the homes. By 2012, the nursing homes could not afford their leases; net cash flows were insufficient to make the rent payments. Rubin, "Nursing Home Bankruptcies"; Rucinski, "A Bid to Save."

127. Whorisky and Keating, "Overdoses, Bedsores, Broken Bones."

128. Whorisky and Keating, "Overdoses, Bedsores, Broken Bones," 3.

129. Department of Justice quoted in Kosman, "Nursing Home CEO," 2.

130. The combined entity includes 13 acute care hospitals; 6 ambulatory surgery centers; and 300 assisted living, memory care, skilled nursing and rehabilitation, hospice, and home health facilities. Each of them merged its respective piece of the joint venture with its own ongoing operations. Rucinski, "A Bid to Save."

131. Mullaney and Spanko, "HCR ManorCare's Home Health"; Rucinski, "A Bid to Save"; Kacik, "Pro Medico Closes."

132. Pringle, "Grant Avenue Clinches First Deal."

133. Holly, "Immigration Reform."

134. Baida interview.

Chapter 7. Public Crisis, Private Gain

1. Brico, "Cost of Addiction Treatment"; Lopez, "Trump Just Signed."

2. The survey also showed that 2.5 percent of adolescents age twelve to seventeen (623,000 individuals) were afflicted with alcohol use disorder. National Institute on Alcohol Abuse and Alcoholism, "Alcohol Facts and Statistics."

3. For example, only 6.7 percent of adults with alcohol use disorder receive any treatment for their addiction. National Institute on Alcohol Abuse and Alcoholism, "Alcohol Facts and Statistics."

4. Corkery and Silver-Greenberg, "The Giant"; Johnson, "Quality Ratings Are Coming."

5. Oran, "Obamacare Helps Private Equity."

6. Quoted in Kodjak, "Investors Seek to Buy."

7. Swisher, "Methadone Treatment Raises Questions"; Freedberg, "Bain's For-Profit Methadone Clinics."

8. Lurie, "Mom, When They Look at Me"; Whalen and Cooper, "Private Equity Pours Cash."

9. By 2018, despite the availability of government penalties for insurance companies that do not comply with the law, there were still more problems in attaining full benefits for the treatment of mental health problems than for other disorders. These include the number of allowable visits, more circum-scribed definitions of medical necessity, fewer behavioral services within provider networks, and lower compensation for care. Moreover, an investiga-tion that year by ParityTrack, a group led by former congressman Patrick

Kennedy, discovered that only Illinois scored well in parity legislation; forty-three states had low marks. Johnson, "Mental Health Parity."

10. Brennan interview.

11. The US Food and Drug Administration first approved buprenorphine for treating addiction in 2002.

12. The Opioid Crisis Response Act is also called the SUPPORT for Patients and Communities Act.

13. Much of the state and local spending has come through relatively meager federal block grants.

14. Sforza et al., "How Some California Drug Rehab."

15. National Center on Addiction and Substance Abuse, "Addiction Medicine," ii.

16. National Center on Addiction and Substance Abuse, "Addiction Medicine," i.

17. Brennan interview. He also said that in 2016 addiction medicine was legitimized and codified: the American Board of Medical Specialties finally included a representative of the subspecialty on its board. Consequently, more physicians are treating substance abuse disorders, which means they can now address the rest of the ailments that affect addicted people, such as heart disease.

18. D'Aunno interview.

19. Kodjak, "Investors Seek to Buy."

20. Even though residential centers are licensed by states, the standards vary considerably and are minimal in most places.

21. Fletcher, Inside Rehab.

22. "Southern California Rehab Industry."

23. Fletcher, Inside Rehab.

24. Lanzone Morgan, "Problems with Drug Rehab Centers."

25. Fletcher, Inside Rehab.

26. Chopra, Letter to the House Energy and Commerce Committee, 2.

27. Cited in Sforza, "Lawmakers Resolve to Control."

28. Cited in Brico, "Cost of Addiction Treatment."

29. Some states, such as Florida, have prohibited kickbacks for referrals, but these are being circumvented. Chopra, Letter to the House Energy and Commerce Committee; Segal, "Doctor with a Phone."

30. Lurie, "Mom, When They Look at Me."

31. Brennan interview.

32. Oliver, "Rehab."

33. Lanzone Morgan, "Problems with Drug Rehab Centers."

34. Bain assumed CRC's previous debt in the deal.

35. At the time, Habit OPCO was the largest chain of methadone clinics in Massachusetts and also had sites elsewhere. The purchase price for the 22 clinics and 154 facilities (in five states) was $58 million. Healy, "Bain Capital Sees Opportunity"; McCambridge, "Bain Capital Buying Up"; Kodjak, "Investors Seek to Buy."

36. Healy, "Bain Capital Sees Opportunity"; Freedberg, "Bain's For-Profit Methadone Clinics."

37. Levine, "Dark Side of a Bain Success."

38. Freedberg, "Bain's For-Profit Methadone Clinics."

39. Healy, "Bain Capital Sees Opportunity."

40. Levine, "Dark Side of a Bain Success."

41. Levine, "Dark Side of a Bain Success."

42. Levine, "Dark Side of a Bain Success," 14.

43. Freedberg, "Bain's For-Profit Methadone Clinics."

44. Roche, "New Life Lodge Whistleblower."

45. Kodjak, "Investors Seek to Buy."

46. At that time, Acadia owned nearly 600 facilities in forty states, providing treatment for addictions, eating disorders, PTSD, and trauma injuries.

47. Trainer, "Not Buying Acadia Healthcare."

48. Little, "Acadia Healthcare."

49. Gluck, "Park Royal Hospital"; Carpenter, "Park Royal Hospital."

50. Little, "Acadia Healthcare."

51. Nisen, "Why Are Buyout Firms Ready?"

52. Swisher, "Methadone Treatment Raises Questions."

53. Swisher, "Methadone Treatment Raises Questions."

54. Shapiro Law Group, "Are Methadone Clinics Safe?"

55. Nilsen, "Methadone."

56. Swisher, "Methadone Treatment Raises Questions"; Schwartz, "Venture Capital and Methadone."

57. Beasley Allen Law, "Beasley Allen Files Suit."

58. Established in 1995, Foundations Recovery Network is based in Brentwood, Tennessee.

59. Founded in 1979 by Alan B. Miller, UHS owns acute care hospitals, outpatient facilities, and behavioral health facilities. In February 2018, it operated 350 inpatient facilities in thirty-seven states.

60. Service Employees International Union, "Universal Health Services."

61. McNeill, "New Report Reveals Major Problems."

62. Service Employees International Union, "Universal Health Services."

63. Adams, "What the Fuck Just Happened?"; Grohol, "Universal Health Services."

64. Pinnacle Treatment Centers is based in Mount Laurel, New Jersey.

65. At the same time, Golub Capital BDC and Prospect Partners bought a minority position in the company.

66. Founded in 1998 by Udi Barkai, Aegis Treatment Centers was yet another opioid treatment company that had piqued the interest of PE firms. In a January 2014 LBO, Housatonic Partners, Operand Group, and Mammoth Equity Partners each grabbed a minority share in the network of outpatient clinics. By 2019, Aegis had thirty-three centers, all in California and mostly publicly funded through Medi-Cal.

67. Rice interview. The information in the following paragraphs is from this interview.

68. Formerly known as Lakeview Health System, the company was co-founded by Patrick Healy in 2001 and is based in Jacksonville, Florida.

69. Other LBOs included Cottonwood Tucson (Arizona) and St. Gregory Retreat (Iowa), both in 2018.

70. Summit Behavioral Healthcare initially received venture capital in 2013 from an unknown source.

71. In 2014, Summit Behavioral Healthcare and cofounder Karen Prince had invested in Texas-based Great Oaks Recovery Center (also called Serenity at Summit); this center was not included in the merger.

72. For example, in July 2019 Delphi purchased Desert View Recovery in Palm Springs, California.

73. These PE firms were Petra Capital Partners, HealthInvest Equity Partners, NewSpring Capital, and SV Health Investors. LLR Partners joined in 2016. Page interview. The information in the following paragraphs is from this interview.

74. For seventy days of treatment, the charge is from $36,500 to $46,500. After thirty-five days, residents are moved to an outpatient apartment complex where they room with another recovering addict; they must purchase their own food.

75. Pringle, "Webster Shelves BayMark Auction."

76. Initially established in 2008 by Rupert McCormac and Steve Kester, Crossroads is based in Greenville, South Carolina.

77. Pringle, "Revelstroke's Crossroads Sales." Its buyouts were Starting Point of Florence (South Carolina), Center of Hope of Myrtle Beach (South Carolina), and EHC Medical Office (Tennessee).

78. Kolodner interview. The information in the following paragraphs is from this interview.

79. Liberation Way is based in Yardley, Pennsylvania; Life of Purpose Treatment (founded in 2013) is in Boca Raton, Florida; and City Line is in Fort Washington, Pennsylvania.

80. Turner, "How a Pa. Treatment Center."

81. Turner, "How a Pa. Treatment Center"; Levy, "Pennsylvania Treatment Firm Accused"; Ciavaglia, "After Charges Liberation Way to Close."

82. Turner, "Liberation Way Drug Treatment."

83. Levy, "Pennsylvania Treatment Firm Accused."

84. Bithoney, "Behavioral Health"; Or, "McCallum Pursues Sale."

85. Shepherd, "Are Wall Street's For-Profit Eating Disorder Clinics."

86. Or, "McCallum Pursues Sale"; Goode, "Centers to Treat Eating Disorders"; Attia et al., "Marketing Residential Treatment Programs." The first residential center for eating disorders was established in 1985.

87. Pollack, "Eating Disorders." The federal 2008 Mental Health Parity and Addiction Equity Act was the first step in mandating equal treatment of physical and mental diseases. But the act was relatively weak and depended on the states for interpretation, compliance, and enforcement.

88. Kantor told me that this was the Castlewood case. Kantor interview.

89. Kantor and Kantor is the only law firm in the United States that focuses on eating disorders treatment. https://www.kantorlaw.net/attorneys/lisa-s -kantor/.

90. Kantor interview. The information in the following paragraphs is from this interview.

91. Bithoney, "Behavior Health."

92. Balshem, "Private Equity Targeting."

93. Attia et al., "Marketing Residential Treatment Programs."

94. Attia et al., "Marketing Residential Treatment Programs"; Guarda, "Refeeding and Weight Restoration"; Goode, "Centers to Treat Eating Disorders."

95. Attia et al., "Marketing Residential Treatment Programs."

96. Goode, "Centers to Treat Eating Disorders," 1.

97. Attia interview. The information in the next paragraphs is also from this interview.

98. The Medicaid institutions for mental disease exclusion, a provision of the Social Security Act, prohibits using federal Medicaid money for services in mental health and substance use disorder residential treatment facilities larger than sixteen beds, even for medically necessary treatment, unless the beneficiary is over age sixty-five or under twenty-one.

99. Attia interview.

100. Anonymous, eating disorders specialist interview.

101. Shepherd, "Are Wall Street's For-Profit Eating Disorder Clinics."

102. Goode, "Centers to Treat Eating Disorders." The National Council for Behavioral Health reported in 2018 that thirty-two states received a failing grade in their parity laws and their enforcement. Pellitt, "Thirty-Two States."

103. News 4, "Castlewood Treatment Center."

104. Lerz interview. The information in the following paragraphs is from this interview.

105. At the time, Castlewood was only a ten-bed facility. It also owned a step-down outpatient clinic.

106. Bernhard, "Castlewood Eating Disorder Center."

107. Dunn, "A Dad's Journey."

108. See https://www.trinityhunt.com/portfolio/castlewood-treatment-center.

109. Anonymous, PE manager at unnamed PE firm interview.

110. Eating Recovery Center, based in Denver, Colorado, began as an inpatient psychiatric hospital and residential treatment center, mostly treating anorexia and bulimia.

111. To ensure that the rapidly growing chain had few empty beds, the two PE firms established a central call center and employed up to twenty "professional relations liaisons" who, like bottom feeders, contacted clinicians all over the United States. Goode, "Centers to Treat Eating Disorders."

112. Pringle, "CCMP to Buy."

113. For example, in December 2013, Monte Nido via its PE acquired and recapitalized Oliver-Pyatt Center, an eating disorder clinic in Miami, Florida. Kantor remarked that after this purchase the PE firm fired the entire executive team. Kantor interview. Monte Nido's first facility was located in Malibu, California.

114. Costin interview. The information in the following paragraphs is from this interview.

115. The cofounders are Stacie McEntyre, Chase Bannister, and Jeff Clark. Veritas Collaborative is based in Durham, North Carolina.

116. These consist of Timberline Knolls (based in Illinois, it was purchased for $90 million in 2010 from Dr. Kimberly Dennis); the Refuge (founded by Judy Crane in Florida, it was bought in 2013 for $14 million); McCallum Place Eating Disorder Centers (located in Missouri, it was founded by Dr. Patrick McCallum and bought in 2014 for $43.4 million); and Bellmont Behavioral Health (established in Pennsylvania, it was purchased by Acadia for $38.2 million in 2015).

117. Based in Los Alamitos, California, Center for Discovery was cofounded by Craig Brown.

118. Oliver, "Rehab." Cliffside Malibu boasts a lavish estate with magnificent views, comfortable single rooms, a pool, tennis and basketball courts, meditation areas, and gourmet food. It is mostly a cash-only facility, with some assistance for those with health care coverage. It was founded by Richard Taite.

119. The platform was created with founder and CEO Ward Keller, who left in 2009. In 2017, he and his wife, Carolyn Keller, opened KellerLife, a nondenominational faith-based eating disorder center in Chandler, Arizona.

120. Kohlberg had formed Alita Care as a parent holding company for its addiction treatment portfolio, including Sunspire Health; the Meadows became its subsidiary.

121. PR Newswire, "American Capital Receives $97 Million."

122. Knopper, "How Wickenburg, Arizona."

123. Kantor interview.

124. *Harlick v. Blue Shield of Cal.*, 686 F.3d 699, 53 Employee Benefits Cas. 2203, 12 Cal. Daily Op. Serv. 6075, 2012 Daily Journal D.A.R. 7340 (9th Cir. 2012).

Chapter 8. Capitalizing on Children with Autism Spectrum Disorders

1. Siegel, *Politics of Autism*.

2. See https://www.autismspeaks.org.

3. https://www.autismspeaks.org; Abramowitz and Bluce, "Why Are Investors Focused."

4. Pitney, *Politics of Autism*.

5. R&A Staff, "U.S. Autism Treatment Market."

6. Siegel, *Politics of Autism*.

7. This bill expanded on the Education for all Handicapped Children Act of 1975, which required states receiving federal special-education funds to provide a free, appropriate public education to handicapped children in the least restrictive setting. At the same time, the Developmental Disabilities Assistance and Bill of Rights Act provided limited state grants, along with a list of the rights of people with developmental disabilities. Pitney, *Politics of Autism*.

8. Siegel, *Politics of Autism*.

9. Siegel, *Politics of Autism*.

10. Pitney, *Politics of Autism*; Hammer, "Reining in Medicaid Spending"; Mosumeci and Foutz, "Medicaid's Role for Children."

11. Siegel, *Politics of Autism*.

12. Koegel interview. Koegel has authored *Positive Behavioral Support; Teaching Children with Autism; Pivotal Response Treatments for Autism; Overcoming Autism;* and *Growing Up on the Spectrum*.

13. Perkes, "As Demand for ABA Therapy Increases."

14. Furfaro, "Optimism Greets Investors' Sudden Interest."

15. R&A Staff, "U.S. Autism Treatment Market."

16. Provident Healthcare Partners, "Investment & Consolidation in Autism."

17. McEachin interview.

18. Frea interview.

19. Taylor interview. Located in New Jersey, the Alpine Learning Group was established in 1989.

20. Crittendon interview. The information in the following paragraphs is from this interview.

21. PE investors in autism therapy companies addressed in this chapter include Abry Partners, Altamont Capital, Altos Health Management, Arsenal Capital Partners, Baird Capital, Blackstone Group, DW Healthcare Partners, Five Arrows Capital Partners, General Atlantic, GI Partners, Golden Gate Capital Great Point Partners, Halifax Group, H. I. G. Growth Partners, Jefferson River Capital, KKR, LLR Partners, Martis Capital, MBF Healthcare Partners, Milestone Partners, NexPhase Capital, Petra Capital Partners, Pharos Capital, Post Capital Partners, Riverside Company, Shore Capital Partners, Thomas H. Lee Partners, TPG Capital, Trimaran Capital Partners, Vista Verde Group, Veronis Suhler Stevenson, Vista Capital Partners, Wellspring Capital Management, Wicks Group, and WindRose.

22. Frea interview.

23. Koegel interview.

24. Molko, *Autism Matters*, 11, 58.

25. McEachin interview. The Behavior Analyst Certification Board in 2014 added credentials for entry-level frontline workers treating individuals with mental health problems and developmental delays, including autism. McEachin et al., "Concerns about Registered Behavioral Technicians."

26. Koegel interview.

27. Molko, *Autism Matters*, 14, 63.

28. Koegel interview.

29. Frea interview.

30. Siegel, *Politics of Autism*.

31. McEachin interview.

32. Pitney, *Politics of Autism*.

33. Although PitchBook dates the PE firm investments in 2010, Heilveil said it was a year earlier. At the time, Autism Learning Partners had eleven offices in three states. Heilveil interview.

34. Heilveil interview.

35. Pringle, "Why Healthcare Investors."

36. Heilveil interview. The following information is also from this interview.

37. See https://www.gpp funds.com/portfolio.

38. Pringle, "Five Questions with FFL."

39. McClain interview. The information in the following paragraphs is from this interview.

40. For example, with backing from Post Capital, in 2016 Invo acquired Progressus Therapy, a company based in Tampa, Florida. Progressus was already a well-worn PE-owned therapy staffing provider, having had its first LBO in 2003 through Apollo Global Management. It was acquired next in 2006 by Sterling Partners; Post Capital was its third LBO in fourteen years.

41. McClain indicated that top staff received stock options when Invo was first sold to Post Capital Partners. Since selling her stake, she has become a

consultant, advising PE firms on how to choose an autism treatment company. The McClains signed a noncompete and nondisclosure document, which is no longer in effect. She and her husband also set up the Mary and Patrick McClain Foundation at the end of 2017 to assist people with developmental disabilities and chronic illnesses and those experiencing homelessness. She told me that they are funding the project themselves; at this point in their lives they want to give back to the community. McClain interview.

42. https://www.glassdoor.com/overview/work-at-autism-home-support -services.

43. MyTherapyCompany (Lafayette, Colorado) and Cumberland Therapy Services (founded in 1989 and divested from Orion Talent through a Centre Partners–led LBO in 2008) were both acquired by Shore Capital at the same time and combined under a holding company, Pediatric Therapy Services. McBurnie stayed on at his company for a year and remained as a director for another two years. He is currently a consultant. McBurnie interview.

44. AlphaVista Services, based in Sunnyvale, California, was founded by Pradeesh Thomas in 2007; Staffing Options Solutions, with headquarters in Indianapolis, Indiana, was founded by Sandy Burns in 1994.

45. McBurnie interview. The information in the following paragraph is also from this interview.

46. Pringle, "Why Healthcare Investors." Shore Capital Partners made investments in two other autism treatment establishments: Florida Autism Center (August 2015) and Behavioral Innovations (June 2017). Florida Autism Center, based in Lake Mary, Florida, was founded in 2005 by Chrystin Bullock. Behavioral Innovations, based in Irving, Texas, was cofounded by Lori Russo in 2000.

47. The Perfect Playground was founded in 2003 by Patrick DeMarco.

48. Established in 2001, Trellis Services is based in Sparks, Maryland. With headquarters in Burbank, California, Autism Spectrum Therapies was launched in 2001 by William Frea and Ronit M. Molko. A fast-growing company, it already had services in ten states at the time of the first PE purchase. Based in Los Angeles and set up in 2009 by Dan Campbell, Beach Cities Learning is a private school alternative for children with autism and other disabilities. It services children in grades 1–12.

49. Niager interview. The following information is also from this interview.

50. Behavioral Concepts was started in 2002 by Jeff Robinson, PhD. He is president and CEO of the company and will retire in 2021. I interviewed Robinson and asked about his experiences with private equity. However, like many other founders who have sold their businesses, he was reluctant to offer much information, most likely because of a nondisclosure agreement. Created by Katherine Johnson in 2002, Advances Learning Center is in Boston, Massachusetts. Melanie Kong-Shaw established Play Connections, a Beaverton, Oregon–based company. Founded in 2014 and centered in Elmhurst, Illinois, at the time of the buyout Total Spectrum had services in Illinois, Indiana, Michigan, and Wisconsin.

51. Frea interview. The information in the following paragraphs is from this interview.

52. Molko interview.

53. Molko, *Autism Matters*, 176.

54. Molko interview.

55. These include Spectrum Center Schools and Programs (2004), Ombudsman Educational Services (2005), Early Autism Project (2013), and Sage Care Therapy Services (2015).

56. Pringle, "ChanceLight."

57. Monk, "SC Woman Charged."

58. Kennedy, "The Boss."

59. Shulman, "Only a Fool." Claypool coauthored *We're in This Together* (2015) and authored *How Autism Is Reshaping Special Education* (2017).

60. Primack, "Trimaran Claws." Trimaran was created by Jay Bloom, Andrew Heyer, and Dean Kehler, who previously had been involved in Michael Milken's firm, Drexel Burnham Lambert.

61. ChanceLight has three main divisions: ChanceLight Education, ChanceLight Therapy, and ChanceLight Behavioral Health (autism and other disorders). As of April 2018, ChanceLight had 150 locations in twenty states. Pringle, "ChanceLight"; McNulty, "Halifax Acquires ChanceLight."

62. Business Wire, "H. I. G. Growth Partners Announces."

63. PR Newswire, "Jeffrey Newman Law Announces."

64. For example, Family Behavioral Resources expanded the company's ASD treatment to western Pennsylvania in 2012. Futures Behavioral Therapy, the sixth company acquired by CIS (2015), extended its reach of autism services in Massachusetts.

65. PR Newswire, "Jeffrey Newman Law Announces."

66. Private Equity Stakeholder Project, "H. I. G. Capital's Mental Health Company."

67. Fritts interview. Seven states had mandated commercial coverage for ABA services, and twenty-four states had pending legislation to do so.

68. The two enterprises were Quality Behavior Outcomes and the Behavioral Counseling and Research Center.

69. Fritts interview.

70. Business Wire, "Ned Carlson Appointed CEO."

71. Fritts interview.

72. Dorbian, "TPG Commits $300 Million."

73. Camelot System of Care, based in Austin, Texas, had been established as a platform by Charterhouse Group in 2006. It was sold again in 2011, independently from Camelot Education, to Sequel Youth and Family Services through an LBO financed by Levine Leichtman Capital Partners. Charterhouse Group increased the company's revenue by 300 percent during its five-year ownership, mostly through add-ons, de novo facilities, and increased capacity in existing places. Beltran, "Charterhouse Sells Camelot."

74. The Brown Schools owned boarding schools and wilderness camps for troubled children. Hensley-Clancy, "Hard Lessons."

75. Berardi et al., "Camelot under Siege."

76. Carr et al., "These For-Profit Schools."

77. Hensley-Clancy, "Hard Lessons."

78. Hensley-Clancy, "Hard Lessons."

79. Hensley-Clancy, "Hard Lessons"; Berardi et al., "Camelot under Siege"; Carr et al., "These For-Profit Schools."

80. Berardi et al., "Camelot under Siege."

81. Hensley-Clancy, "Hard Lessons."

82. Berardi et al., "After Allegations of Physical Abuse."

83. Rice, "How, Why MCSD Camelot."

84. Koffler was accused of using two schools, Sunshine Developmental School and K3 Learning, Inc., as a "personal ATM." Apparently, he and his family used the companies to pay for their credit card bills, maintenance on their boat, and a son-in-law's school tuition. They also set up a real estate company that charged Sunshine an exorbitant rent, which the family pocketed. The attorney general of New York, Eric Schneiderman, sternly warned: "We won't allow special education programs to be exploited for personal financial gain. These defendants used their programs as a way to defraud the government and cheat on their taxes—sticking law-abiding New Yorkers with the bill in the process." In 2016, the Koffler family agreed to pay $4.3 million to settle the charges. Taylor, "Education Company to Pay"; New York Attorney General, "A. G. Schneiderman, Acting Tax Commissioner Manion."

85. Aaron School serves children with learning disabilities in reading, writing, and math as well as attention, sensory, and social challenges. Rebecca School was first established in 2006, and Aaron School in 2003.

86. ParentAdvocates, "Schools for Children with Autism."

87. ParentAdvocates, "Schools for Children with Autism."

88. Sequel Youth and Family Services, bought by Altamont from Alaris Royalty, a Canadian private equity firm, in September 2017, provides an array of programs for youngsters with behavioral, emotional, and physical challenges across twenty-one states. Just prior to the lucrative sale, Alaris grabbed a debt-funded dividend recap for itself. Children under the care of Sequel-owned facilities have not fared well. There were fifty-six substantiated violations between 2018 and 2020 alone, and a Black teenager died at Lakeside for Children in Kalamazoo, Michigan. Unsafe, squalid living conditions and "dangerous restraint and verbal abuse heaped on children by staff" were found in Sequel's Courtland facility by an Alabama Disabilities Advocacy Program investigation in early 2020. Before closing down Red Rock Canyon School in 2019, Utah had threatened to revoke its license because at least nine staff members were charged with child abuse, and the school overall was dangerously understaffed. In 2020, Sequel Pomegranate's license was also at risk by the Ohio Department of Mental Health and Addiction Services after rampant sexual abuse, violence, and unwarranted use of restraints on youngsters. Unsafe conditions were documented at Sequel's Kingston Academy (Tennessee) and Clarinda Academy (Iowa). O'Grady, "Understaffed, Unlicensed, and Untrained."

89. Quinn, "New Jersey Halts Admissions."

90. Bernstein, "Deletion of Word"; Vogell, "What Happened to Adam"; Steele, "AdvoServ."

91. Vogell, "What Happened to Adam"; Vogell, "Unrestrained."

92. Mulford and Washburn, "Bellwether Group Homes."

93. Steele, "AdvoServ."

94. Hudak, "Plagued by Abuse Claims and Deaths."

95. Miller and Madan, "Beset by Rapes."

96. Fallstrom, "Carlton Palms Facility."

97. Hudak, "Plagued by Abuse Claims and Deaths."

98. Quinn, "New Jersey Halts Admissions," 4.

99. Hudak, "Plagued by Abuse Claims and Deaths"; Quinn, "New Jersey Halts Admissions."

100. Mulford and Washburn, "Bellwether Group Homes."

101. Centria offers rehabilitation, private duty nursing, and supportive care for dementia patients as well. However, in 2010, probably because of greater amounts of funding, it began to focus on autism. The Novi, Michigan–based company was founded in 2009 by Scott Barry.

102. Anderson, "Abuse Caught on Video."

103. Anderson, "Abuse Caught on Video"; Wisely and Anderson, "How Michigan's Largest Autism Therapy Provider Lost"; Rochester, Wisely, and Anderson, "Centria Healthcare Accused of Fraud."

104. Anderson, "Abuse Caught on Video"; Wisely and Anderson, "How Michigan's Largest Autism Therapy Provider Lost"; Rochester, Wisely, and Anderson, "Centria Healthcare Accused of Fraud."

105. Anderson, "Abuse Caught on Video."

106. Pringle, "Thomas H. Lee Partners."

107. DeLombaerde, "Pharos Buys Adolescent Treatment Center." Cofounded in 2000 by Larry Carter and Jeff Smith, Logan River Academy is based in Utah.

108. See https://wwwshutdownloganriver.com/testimonials.

109. The business was established in New Britain, Connecticut, and Gwen Killheffer continued as Solterra's principal after its purchase.

110. Plano-based ABA of North Texas was founded by Susan Krejci in 2012.

111. Pringle, "Blackstone Walks Away."

112. KKR closed this $1.45 billion inaugural health care growth fund in November 2017. The PE firm intends to invest in health care businesses such as diagnostics, medical devices, and care providers.

113. See https://www.linkedin.com/in/keithjones.

114. Pringle, "KKR's BlueSprig."

115. Headquartered in Salt Lake City, Alternative Behavior Strategies was created by Jeff Skibitsky in 2011.

116. Perkes, "As Demand for ABA Therapy Increases." In 2005, Hopebridge was cofounded by Amy Ellis in Indianapolis, Indiana. By 2019, it had thirty-eight clinics in Georgia, Indiana, Kentucky, and Ohio. Pringle, "Arsenal's Deal."

117. The initial LBOs were Autism Centers of Michigan (founded in 2012) and WeBehave of Coral Gables (founded in 2011).

118. Centered in Van Nuys, California, 360 Behavioral Health was founded by Leili Zarbakhsh in 2003.

119. Established in 2012 by Gregg and Sandy Maggioli, Lighthouse's head-quarters is in Mishawaka, Indiana.

120. The Texas-based business was founded in 2016 by Ryan and Holly Lambert. Pringle, "NexPhase's Action Behavioral Centers."

121. Business Wire, "ACES and General Atlantic."

Chapter 9. Hijacking an Industry

1. Levine and Graybow, "Special Report."

2. According to Levine and Graybow, "Special Report," the for-profit ambulance industry is an outgrowth of the funeral home business, which carried sick or injured people in hearses.

3. Fire departments were 49 percent of providers; the government, 14.5 percent; hospitals, 7 percent; and other, 11.5 percent. Calams, "Private vs. Public Ambulance Services."

4. McCallion, "Ambulance Companies Change Hands."

5. Ivory, Protess, and Bennett, "When You Dial 911," A1.

6. Hsia is a professor of emergency medicine at the University of California, San Francisco. The study was published in JAMA Network Open and is cited by Steven Ross Johnson, who notes that this is the first national investigation addressing disparities in ambulance arrival times. Johnson, "Poor Communities Wait Longer."

7. Pell et al. "Effect of Reducing Ambulance Response," quoted in Johnson, "Poor Communities Wait Longer."

8. Air medical transportation, including helicopters and fixed-wing planes, is equipped with life support and other equipment for emergency situations, such as accidents, heart attacks, and strokes, and also carries organs, medical supplies, health providers, and patients from one hospital to another.

9. Tozzi, "Air Ambulances Are Flying More"; Perritt, "Arm and a Leg."

10. Williams, "Air Methods Sold."

11. Perritt, "Arm and a Leg." Susannah Luthi reports that 80 percent of air transports are used for interfacility transfers rather than for accidents. Luthi, "Congress Angles."

12. Certificate-of-need laws are regulatory mechanisms for establishing or expanding health care facilities and services in a given area. When certificates of need are required, a state health planning agency must approve major capital expenditures for certain health care facilities.

13. Luthi, "Congress Angles."

14. Galli, Zimmerman, and Ross, "Sky Rage."

15. Rowland, "Why the Flight."

16. Luthi, "Congress Angles."

17. Perry, "Up in the Air." Taxpayers, too, pay a price. Researchers at Johns Hopkins University found that the national median charge to Medicare for an air ambulance in 2016 was 4.1 to 9.5 times higher than what it had paid for the same services in 2012. The expenditures mounted from $24,000 to $39,000. Meyer, "Air Ambulance Charges."

18. Appelbaum and Batt, "Private Equity Tries to Protect."

19. Luthi, "Congress Angles"; Tozzi, "Air Ambulances Are Flying More."

20. Luthi, "Air Ambulances May Be Banned."

21. Lobbyists for air ambulances include the Association of Air Medical Services and Save Our Air Medical Resources, representing Air Methods, PHI Air Medical, and Air Medical Group Holdings. Both lobbying organizations advocate increased Medicare reimbursement rates for the industry as well. On

the other hand, the Association of Critical Care Transport, representing eighty air and ground medical transport operators, is in favor of curtailing balance billing. Head, "FAA Reauthorization Act."

22. Perritt, "Arm and a Leg," 334.

23. Perritt, "Arm and a Leg."

24. Perritt, "Arm and a Leg," 340.

25. Veillette, "How to Develop."

26. AP News, "Physician Questions."

27. AP News, "Physician Questions"; Perritt, "Arm and a Leg."

28. US Government Accountability Office, "Air Ambulance."

29. Luthi, "Congress Angles."

30. Quoted in Tribble, "Air Ambulances."

31. Funding Universe, "American Medical Response, Inc. History."

32. Funding Universe, "American Medical Response, Inc. History."

33. McCallion, "Ambulance Companies Change Hands."

34. Pringle, "KKR, on a Healthcare Tear"; Meikle, "Envision Health."

35. Conway, second morning fireside chat, Columbia Business School, Twenty-Fifth Conference.

36. AMR did not escape lawsuits over its billing practices. It faced a US Justice Department investigation of allegedly fraudulent claims in New York, and in 2010 settled a long-running class action suit against it brought by Spokane, Washington, residents who said they were overcharged for ambulance rides. Levine and Graybow, "Special Report."

37. Other acquisitions include Abbot Ambulance, along with its affiliates Mission Care of Illinois, Health Solutions Center, and Access2Care, serving Illinois and Missouri (bought in 2007); Community Emergency Medical Services, formerly Marlboro-Hudson Ambulance Service, founded in 1965 and serving central Massachusetts; Lifeguard Transportation Services, serving Atlanta, Georgia, and Dallas, Texas (bought in 2007); River Medical, serving western Arizona (bought in 2008); Skyservice Air Ambulance, founded in 1989 and serving Los Angeles (bought in 2009 via Gibralt Capital); Blythe Ambulance Service, founded in 1979 and serving Blythe, California (bought in 2011); Doctor's Ambulance Service, founded in 1974 and serving Laguna Hills, California (bought in 2011); MedStat EMS, founded in 2007 and serving central and northern Mississippi (bought in 2014); Life Line Ambulance, founded in 1956 and serving Prescott, Arizona (bought in 2014); Vital Emergency Medical Service, founded in 2006 and serving Worcester, Massachusetts (bought in 2015); ComTrans, founded in 1995 and serving Phoenix, Arizona (bought in 2016); and Kurtz EMS, founded in 1977 and serving New Lenox, Illinois (bought in 2017).

38. Berlin, "LPCI Air Medical." There were two other investors, Koch Equity Development and Ardian.

39. Funding Universe, "Rural/Metro Corporation History."

40. Funding Universe, "Rural/Metro Corporation History."

41. McCallion, "What's Next for Rural/Metro."

42. Levine and Graybow, "Special Report."

43. McCallion, "What's Next for Rural/Metro."

44. Ivory, Protess, and Bennett, "When You Dial 911."

45. Air Evac, founded in 1985 in West Plains, Missouri, by Bill Chritton, had multiple bases in nine states in 2004. Meier, "Air Ambulances." By 2017, despite its questionable practices, Air Evac emerged as the foremost provider of air medical services. Pringle, "Air Medical Resources Group."

46. Meier, "Air Ambulances," A1.

47. Other LBOs via Brockway and MVP include TJ Holding Company, which held Medtrans Corporation and Executive Air Taxi (bought in 2006); Southwest Heliservices (bought in 2006); and EagleMed (bought in 2009, formerly known as Kansas Air Life).

48. Beltran, "Bain Takes $200M Dividend."

49. Some of the REACH purchases via Bain were Cal-Ore Life Flight (bought in 2011), Reno Flight Services (bought in 2014), EAL Leasing (bought in 2014), and Expedition Helicopter (also known as Summit Air Ambulance, bought in 2015).

50. Ardian also participated in the deal. Pringle, "Air Medical Resources Group."

51. These included Guardian EMS, Aircare, Hawaii LifeFlight, Gallup Medflight, Medstar, Valley Med Flight, Alaska Regional Life Flight, Mountain Star, and AeroCare Medical Transport.

52. As of April 2021, Guardian was involved in a lawsuit against North Dakota, claiming that the state's 2017 law imposing caps on out-of-network charges violates the Airline Deregulation Act of 1978. It won an earlier lawsuit in opposition to the state's 2015 legislation that had created a main air ambulance carrier list; to join, the business had to agree to become an in-network provider with Blue Cross Blue Shield of North Dakota. Springer, "ND Defends Lawsuit."

53. Pringle, "KKR, on a Healthcare Tear."

54. In April 2019 AMGH acquired SenBar Aviation, a supplier of air transportation in New Mexico, Texas, Maine, Massachusetts, Virginia, and North Carolina. The company owns nine jet and turboprop airplanes and six helicopters.

55. Brickley, "Turnaround Executive Lynn Tilton."

56. Tilton was also accused of defrauding all the PE's investors by hiding the real value of loans in Patriarch's overall portfolio. After Tilton resigned from the Zohar funds, executives there claimed that she had been "looting cash and assets from the businesses they managed." Brickley and Corrigan, "Lynn Tilton's Firm"; Noto, "Private Ambulance Service."

57. Ivory, Protess, and Daniel, "What Can Go Wrong," 1.

58. Brickley and Corrigan, "Lynn Tilton's Firm"; Dwyer, "Bankruptcy of TransCare"; Brickley, "Turnaround Executive Lynn Tilton."

59. By 2017 Air Methods had 300 bases across forty-eight states. It operates under different brands, depending on the state. It also provides aircraft tourism in Las Vegas, the Grand Canyon, and Hawaii. Perry, "Up in the Air"; Funding Universe, "Air Methods Corporation History."

60. Funding Universe, "Air Methods Corporation History."

61. The following are a few of Air Methods's other PE buyouts: CJ Systems Aviation (formerly Corporate Jets, bought in 2007), United Rotorcraft Solutions (bought in 2011), OF Air Holdings (bought in 2011), Sundance

Helicopters (bought in 2012), American Jets (bought in 2013), Helicopter Consultants of Maui (also known as Blue Hawaiian Helicopters, bought in 2013), Baptist LifeFlight (bought in 2014), Texas AirLife (bought in 2015), and TriState CareFlight (bought in 2016).

62. Funding Universe, "Air Methods Corporation History."

63. By 2016 Rocky Mountain Helicopters was the largest HEMS operator in the United States, accounting for one-fifth of all Medicare-funded trips; its three subsidiaries were among the companies that charged the highest fees. Meyer, "Air Ambulance Charges."

64. Galli, Zimmerman, and Ross, "Sky Rage"; Perry, "Up in the Air"; Head, "FAA Reauthorization Act."

65. In 2011, Voce Capital Management had acquired a 4.9 percent stake in the company through a PIPE. Huber, "Air Methods CEO."

66. See https://www.linkedin.com/jobs/view/hedge-fund-research-analyst-at-voce-capital-management-llc-753149353/.

67. Williams, "Air Methods Sold"; also see https://www.american-securities.com.

68. Air Methods's profits increased sevenfold from 2004 to 2014. Appelbaum and Barr, "Private Equity Tries to Protect."

69. Stanberry interview.

70. Tribble, "Air Ambulances."

71. Stanberry interview. The information in the following paragraph is also from this interview.

72. Ivory, Protess, and Bennett," When You Dial 911."

Conclusion. Infiltrating Our Health Care System

1. American Medical Association, "Report 11," 6.

2. Tozzi, "Prognosis."

3. Satz, *Why Some Things*.

4. Lieberthal, health private equity panel, Columbia Business School, Twenty-Sixth Conference.

5. Mitchell, "CalPers CIO Unveils"; Fernyhough and Carmean, "US PE Breakdown"; Cox, Fernyhough, and Carmean, "Private Fund Strategies Report." CalPERS's chief investment officer, Yu "Ben" Meng, proposed a steady increase in the percentage of the fund's PE investments over ten years, a plan that elicited negative responses from a few board members and fund beneficiaries because of the added risk. Mitchell, "CalPers CIO Unveils." Meng abruptly resigned in August 2020 seemingly because of conflict of interest disclosures. As reported in *Naked Capitalism*, he had personal investments in PE firms, including Blackstone and Carlyle. Under his leadership, CalPERS in 2020 allocated money to both shops; Blackstone obtained $1 billion. Smith, "CalPERS Chief Investment Officer."

6. Lewis, "Private Equity Fundraising Totals"; Lykken, "Following a Decade-Long Uptick"; Cox, Wiek, Fernyhough, and Carmean, "Private Fund Strategies Report." Some PE firms, such as Apollo Global Management and Oaktree Capital, have been raising private debt vehicles for decades.

7. Canderle, "Modern Private Equity."

8. Lewis, "Private Equity Fundraising Totals"; Mclean, "Too Big to Fail."

9. Cox, Fernyhough, and Carmean, "COVID-19's Influence," 2.

10. Borrowing at the fund level, which adds debt on the older vehicle's pool of assets over and above existing leverage on the portfolio companies per se, requires fund term amendments from the PE shop's LPs. Witkowsky, "GPs Ask LPs."

11. Breaking with tradition, a few PE firms decided to take at least some responsibility for workers at their portfolio companies and first responders in the communities in which they do business. MiddleGround Capital, established in 2018, said it would subsidize testing and days lost for any of the 3,000 employees afflicted with the coronavirus at the five enterprises it owns. Leonard Green & Partners, KKR, and Bain Capital created accounts of $10 million, $50 million, and $40 million, respectively, for emergency relief. Advent International pledged $25 million; Blackstone Group, $15 million; Thoma Bravo, $2 million; BlackRock, $50 million; and Apollo Global Management's founder (Leon Black), $20 million. Witkowsky, "KKR Pledges." These amounts are negligible, of course, relative to their capacity. KKR, for example, had fully $218 billion under its management at the end of 2019.

12. Cox, Fernyhough, and Carmean, "COVID-19's Influence"; McElhaney, "Private Equity Investments." Some firms, however, retained their ambitious fundraising endeavors. Bain Capital, for example, sought $9 billion or more by the end of 2020 for its latest buyout fund. Likewise, BDT Capital Partners, Sterling Partners, and One Rock Capital Partners sought $9.1 billion, $1.75 billion, and $1.5 billion, respectively. McElhaney, "Private Equity Investments."

13. Gottfried, "Private-Equity Firms Scramble," 3.

14. Canderle, "Modern Private Equity."

15. The survey of more than 400 practices was conducted by the Massachusetts Health Policy Commission and the Massachusetts chapter of the American College of Physicians from the end of May 2020 through the beginning of June. Kacik, "Massachusetts Physician Practices."

16. For example, the more than hundred-year-old Easton Hospital in Lehigh Valley, Pennsylvania (my hometown) by the spring of 2020 was on the verge of collapse. The facility was acquired in 2001 by Community Health Systems Inc. and in 2017 by Cerberus Capital Management, which merged the facility with its Steward Hospital chain. As part of its deal, Cerberus sold the hospital's properties to Medical Properties Trust, a real estate investment trust, collecting $304 million. Already burdened by substantial debt and now forced to pay rent, the Easton facility exploited the pandemic by demanding and receiving $8 million in emergency funds from Governor Tom Wolf in exchange for keeping the hospital open through April 2020. It was acquired by St. Luke's University Health Network at the end of June. A number of employees lost their jobs, but if Easton had shut down, the entire staff (694 people) would have become unemployed. Batt and Appelbaum, "Hospital Bailouts Begin"; Harris, "Easton Hospital Notifies State."

17. Levy, opening keynote speaker, Columbia Business School, Twenty-Sixth Conference.

18. Pringle, "Bracing for the Long Haul."

19. Falconer, "Brookfield Sees COVID-19." Brookfield is the majority owner of Oaktree Capital, which sought $15 billion for its latest credit fund.

20. Over the years, certain private equity firms have amassed billions for special funds that provide rescue capital, debt investments, or PIPE deals. At the beginning of the pandemic they had $64 billion immediately available for deployment. Taking advantage of the coronavirus-induced downturn, Bain Capital upped the cap on its latest distressed debt and special situations fund to $3.5 billion. Ares Capital also lifted the ceiling on its special opportunities fund from $2 billion to $3.5 billion. In two months, KKR raised $4 billion for its newly created credit fund, KKR Dislocation Opportunities Fund. Oaktree Capital solicited LPs for a newly established distressed fund, aiming to accrue $15 billion. In addition, Apollo Global Management recast a traditional buyout fund ($24.6 billion) to concentrate on distressed-for-control credit transactions. Other PE firms that participated in such investing previously include Cerberus Capital Management, Leonard Green & Partners, and Centerbridge Partners. Davis, "Ask PitchBook"; Falconer, "Bain Capital's Latest"; Haverstock, "Apollo Loses 2.3B."

21. Sherman and Hirsch, "Private Equity Eyes Industries"; Lykken, "Flush with Cash"; Cox, Fernyhough, and Carmean, "COVID-19's Influence."

22. Tse and Baker, "Private Equity Firms Fight." Roark Capital, for example, in April 2020 entered into a PIPE deal with the Cheesecake Factory for $200 million in convertible preferred stock; the PE firm's dividend is 9.5 percent, and when the stock hits a certain price the securities will convert to common shares. Likewise, Apollo Global Management teamed up with Silver Lake to purchase $2 billion in preferred stock from Expedia; they, too, will receive a 9.5 percent dividend and potentially a replacement with common shares.

23. Holly, "No 'Strings Attached.'"

24. Lewis, "Fed's Stimulus."

25. During the first quarter of 2020 the AIC spent $640,000; the National Venture Capital Association disbursed another $569,000 to protect its interests. Lewis and Thorne, "Ask PitchBook."

26. To be eligible, companies had to have 500 or fewer employees, $15 million or less in net worth, and $5 million or less in net income, after federal taxes, for the last two years before the date of application.

27. Thorne, "Over 8,000 Privately Backed Companies."

28. Perlberg, "Rescue Cash Too Hot."

29. Perlberg, "Private Equity's Backdoor Path."

30. Schwellenbach and Szakonyi, "Inside the Pandemic Cash Bonanza."

31. Mclean, "Too Big to Fail."

32. Mclean, "Too Big to Fail."

33. According to a survey by *Pensions and Investments*, the 200 largest US defined-benefit plans already have an average of 8.7 percent of their assets invested in PE. Cited in Witkowsky, "U.S. Government Offers Guidance."

34. Witkowsky, "U.S. Government Offers Guidance"; Appelbaum, "CEPR Statement"; Bain, "Private Equity Gets a Big Win."

35. Gara, "Vanguard Pushes into Private Equity."

36. Kacik, "Healthcare Spending to Consume."

37. PE executives could still use the capital gains rate for money that they invest themselves. This was the second time Pascrell proposed the Carried Interest Fairness Act; in 2019, the legislation remained stuck in committee.

38. Lewis, "Elizabeth Warren Proposes Legislation"; Editorial, "Private Equity Must Be Less Private."

39. Research by Ludovic Phalippou, a professor of finance at the University of Oxford's Saïd Business School, found that PE funds did not produce greater returns relative to public companies for at least fourteen years, especially if one allows for their hefty fees. At an SEC online meeting, he told participants that in 2019, investors paid 6–7 percent overall in PE charges, as compared to 0.74 percent for managed equity mutual funds. Flood, "Buyout Groups Blasted." Other researchers have echoed the concern over what they view as overstated returns. A report by Harvard economist Josh Lerner indicates that after the deduction of fees, over a ten-year period PE and S&P 500 returns were roughly equivalent. Similarly, in a study of 330 pension funds and other institutional investors worldwide, the consultancy company CEM reported that between 1996 and 2018 PE firms—again, after the deduction of fees—underperformed a mix of small-cap indexes. Cited in Haverstock, "PE Has Failed to Outperform Stocks"; Hurley, "Alternatives a 'Loser's Game' "; Wiggins, "US Stock Market Beats"; Flood, "Cheap Tracker Funds." Richard Ennis, an eminent consultant in the field, has suggested that the alternative investment industry has been bringing in "consistent negative returns for more than a decade and will probably keep doing so for the years ahead." In a study of forty-six public pension funds (including CalPERS) and educational endowments from mid-2008 to mid-2018, Ennis determined that they underperformed passive index funds measurably. Ennis interviewed in Hurley, "Alternatives a 'Loser's Game.' " In addition, these investigators argue that PE firms are using suspect criteria and benchmarks. Phalippou writes that they can misrepresent yields through the use of internal rates of return; the metric is often inaccurate and can be manipulated by the PE firms. He insists that the SEC should ban the use of IRR altogether. Phalippou, *Private Equity Laid Bare*. PE titans, of course, crusade against such conclusions.

Books

Alexander, Brian. *Glass House: The 1% Economy and the Shattering of the All-American Town* (New York: St. Martin's, 2017).

Anders, George. *Merchants of Debt: KKR and the Mortgaging of American Business* (New York: Basic, 1992).

Appelbaum, Eileen, and Rosemary Batt. *Private Equity at Work: When Wall Street Manages Main Street* (New York: Russell Sage, 2014).

Brown, Wendy. *Undoing the Demos: Neoliberalism's Stealth Revolution* (New York: Zone, 2015).

Bruck, Connie. *The Predators' Ball* (New York: Penguin, 1989).

Burrough, Bryan, and John Helyar. *Barbarians at the Gate: The Fall of RJR Nabisco* (New York: HarperCollins, 2009).

Canderle, Sebastien. *The Debt Trap: How Leverage Impacts Private-Equity Performance* (Hampshire, England: Harriman House, 2016).

———. *Private Equity's Public Distress: The Rise and Fall of Candover and the Buyout Industry Crash* (N.p.: Sebastien Canderle, 2011).

Carey, David, and John Morris. *King of Capital: The Remarkable Rise, Fall, and Rise Again of Steve Schwarzman and Blackstone* (New York: Crown, 2012).

Fletcher, Anne M. *Inside Rehab* (New York: Penguin, 2013).

Foroohar, Rana. *Makers and Takers: The Rise of Finance and the Fall of American Business* (New York: Crown, 2016).

Granpeesheh, Doreen. *Evidence-Based Treatment for Children with Autism: The CARD Model* (Waltham, MA: Academic, 2014).

Harvey, David. *A Brief History of Liberalism* (New York: Oxford University Press, 2005).

Kelly, Jason. *The New Tycoons: Inside the Trillion Dollar Private Equity Industry that Owns Everything* (Hoboken, NJ: Wiley, 2012).

Kosman, Josh. *The Buyout of America: How Private Equity Is Destroying Jobs and Killing the American Economy* (New York: Penguin, 2009).

Molko, Ronit. *Autism Matters: Empowering Investors, Providers, and the Autism Community to Advance Autism Services* (Charleston, SC: ForbesBooks, 2018).

Phalippou, Ludovic. *Private Equity Laid Bare* (Scotts Valley, CA: Createspace Independent Publishing, 2017).

Pitney, John J., Jr. *The Politics of Autism: Navigating the Contested Spectrum* (Boulder, CO: Rowman & Littlefield, 2015).

Recovered: Journeys through the Autism Spectrum and Back. Directed by Michele Jaquis, 2008.

Satz, Debra. *Why Some Things Should Not Be for Sale: The Moral Limits of Markets* (New York: Oxford University Press, 2010).

Siegel, Bryna. *The Politics of Autism* (New York: Oxford University Press, 2018).

Yu, Jonathan Stanford. *From Zero to Sixty on Hedge Funds and Private Equity* (Columbia, SC: CreateSpace Independent Publishing Platform, Mar. 2018).

Zeisberger, Claudia Michael Prahl, and Bowen White. *Mastering Private Equity: Transformation via Venture Capital, Minority Investments and Buyouts* (New York: Wiley, 2017).

Private Databases, Research, and Intelligence Services

Associated Press. "Judge Blocks California Law on Dialysis Clinics," *Modern Healthcare*, Dec. 31, 2019. https://www.modernhealthcare.com/legal/judge -blocks-california-law-dialysis-clinics.

Beltran, Luisa. "Bain Takes $200M Dividend on Air Medical," *PE Hub*, June 3, 2013. https://www.pehub.com/buyouts/bain-takes-$200m-dividend-on-air -medical.

———. "Charterhouse Sells Camelot System of Care," *PE Hub*, Mar. 7, 2011. https://www.pehub.com/charterhouse-sells-camelot-system-of-care/.

———. "Investcorp's Maniscalco: Minority GP Stakes Produce Higher Cash-on-Cash Yields," *PE Hub*, Apr. 1, 2019. https://www.pehub.com/buyouts/investcorps -maniscalco-minority-GP-stakes-produce-high-cash-on-cash-yields.

———. "Leonard Green Gets Its Money Back with Mister Car Wash's Second Dividend," *PE Hub*, May 2, 2019. https://www.pehub.com/leonard-green-gets -its-money-back-with-mister-car-washs-second-dividend/.

Bluth, Rachel. "GoFundMe CEO: 'Gigantic Gaps' in Health System Showing Up in Crowdfunding," *Kaiser Health News*, Jan. 16, 2019. https://www.khn.org/news /gofundme-ceo-gigantic-gaps-in-health-system-showing-up-in-crowdfunding/.

Christ, Ginger. "Physician Shortage Could Top 100,000 by 2033, AAMC Predicts," *Modern Healthcare*, June 26, 2020. https://www.modernhealthcare.com /physicians/physician-shortage-could-top-100,000-by-2033-aamc-predicts.

Cohrs, Rachel. "How Congress' Surprise Billing Compromise Fell Short," *Modern Healthcare*, Dec. 23, 2019. https://www.modernhealthcare.com /politics/policy/how-congress-surprise-billing-compromise-fell-short.

Cordeiro, Nico. "US PE Breakdown: 2017 Annual," Merrill Corporation, 2018. https://www.theleadleft.com/wp-content-uploads/2018/01/PitchBook_2017 _Annual_US_PE_Breakdown.pdf.

Cox, Dylan, Wylie Fernyhough, and Zane Carmean. "COVID-19's Influence on the US PE Market," *PitchBook Data, Inc.*, Mar. 30, 2020. www.pitchbook.com /news/reports/q1-2020-pitchbook-analysts-note-covid-19s-influence-on-the -us-market.

———. "Private Fund Strategies Report, 2019 Annual," *PitchBook Data, Inc.*, Feb. 19, 2020. www.pitchbook.com/news/reports/2019-annual-private-fund -strategies-report.

Cox, Dylan N., and Darren Klees. "Measuring SBOs Effect on Fund Performance," *PitchBook Data, Inc.*, Oct. 15, 2018. www.pitchbook.com/news /reports/4q-2018-pitchbook-analyst-note-measuring-sbos-effect-on-fund -performance.

Davis, Alexander. "Ask PitchBook: What's Up with Distressed-Debt Investing?," *PitchBook Data, Inc.*, Apr. 27, 2020. www.pitchbook.com/news/articles/ask -pitchbook-whats-up-with-distressed-debt-investing.

Devine, Murray. "USPE Breakdown: 2Q," *PitchBook Data, Inc.*, July 11, 2018. www.pitchbook.com/news/reports/2q-2018-us-pe-breakdown.

Dickson, Virgil. "CMS Preparing Rules for Nursing Home Staff Fines, Home Personal Care Oversight Transformation Hub," *Modern Healthcare*, Oct. 8, 2018. https://www.modernhealthcare.com/article/20181008/transforma tion-hub.

———. "CMS Proposes $190 Million Raise for Dialysis Centers," *Modern Health-care*, July 11, 2018. https://www.modernhealthcare.com/article/20180711 /news/cms-proposes-$190-million-raise-for-dialysis-centers.

DJl Consulting. "Breaking Down PE's Push into Orthopedics," *PitchBook Data, Inc.*, Nov. 26, 2019. www.pitchbook.com/news/articles/dji-consulting -breaking-down-pes-push-into-orthopedics.

———. "The Dynamics Driving Dealmaking in US Healthcare Services: Interview with Dana Jacoby," *PitchBook Data, Inc.*, July 8, 2019. https://www .pitchbook.com/news/articles/djl-consulting-the-dynamics-driving-deal making in-us-healthcare-services.

Dorbian, Iris. "PE-Backed ECP Completes Merger with IEMS," *PE Hub*, Sept. 16, 2019. https://www.pehub.com/pe-backed-ecp-completes-merger-with-iems/.

———. "Riverside and Abry Exits NADG," *PE Hub*, Oct. 2, 2019. https://www .pehub.com/riverside-and-abry-exits-nadg/.

———. "TPG Commits $300 Million to New Autism Services Company Kadiant," *PE Hub*, Feb. 1, 2019. https://www.pehub.com/tpg-commits-$300-million-to -new-autism-services-company-kadiant.

Dowd, Kevin. "Carlyle Closes New Mega-Fund on 18.5 B," *PitchBook Data, Inc.*, July 30, 2018. https://pitchbook.com/news/articles/carlyle-closes-new-mega -fund-on-185b.

———. "11 Big Things: Brick-and-Mortar Goes Bust," *PitchBook Data, Inc.*, May 10, 2020. https://pitchbook.com/news/articles/11-big-things-brick-and -mortar-goes-bust.

———. "This Day in Buyout History: KKR, Bain Capital Complete the Biggest LBO Ever," *PitchBook Data, Inc.*, Nov. 17, 2017. https://pitchbook.com/news /articles/this-day-in-buyout-history-kkr-bain-capital-complete-the-biggest -lbo-ever.

Evans, Melanie. "Private-Equity Backed Urgent-Care Developer Taps Dignity Health for California Expansion," *Modern Healthcare*, Feb. 9, 2016. https:// www.modernhealthcare.com/article/20160209/NEWS/160209862/private -equity-backed-urgent-care-developer-taps-dignity-health-for-california -expansion.

Fernyhough, Wylie, and Jordan Beck. "US PE Breakdown: 2018 Annual," *PitchBook Data, Inc.*, Jan. 10, 2019. https://pitchbook.com/news/reports/2018 -annual-us-pe-breakdown.

Fernyhough, Wylie, and Zane Carmean. "US PE Breakdown: 2019 Annual," *PitchBook Data, Inc.*, Jan. 19, 2020. https://files.pitchbook.com/website/files /pdf/2019_Annual_US_PE_Breakdown.pdf

Fernyhough, Wylie, Stephen George Davis, and Darren Klees. "US PE Middle Market Report, 1Q 2019," *PitchBook Data, Inc.*, 2019. https://www.readkong.com/page/us-pe-middle-market-report-8734809.

Fernyhough, Wylie, and Darren Klees. "IRS & IRRs: How Tax Reform Will Impact PE," *PitchBook Data, Inc.*, June 29, 2018. https://pitchbook.com/newsletter/irs-irrs-how-tax-reform-will-impact-pe/.

Gamble, Harry. "Is Private Equity Helping or Hurting Healthcare," *Modern Healthcare*, July 10, 2018. https://www.modernhealthcare.com/article/20180710/news/is-private-equity-helping-or-hurting-healthcare.

Gelfer, James, Bryan Hanson, and Darren Klees. "Addictive Dealmaking: Part 1," *PitchBook Data, Inc.*, Apr. 16, 2018. https://pitchbook.com/news/reports/2q-2018-pitchbook-analyst-note-addictive-dealmaking.

Gelfer, James, and Darren Klees. "Echo Buyouts," *PitchBook Data, Inc.*, June 7, 2018. https://pitchbook.com/news/reports/2q-2018-pitchbook-analyst-note-echo-buyouts.

Goldberg, Stephanie. "Medicare Decides a Cost-Saving Strategy Costs Too Much," *Modern Healthcare*, Aug. 19, 2019. https://www.modernhealthcare.com/home-health/medicare-decides-cost-saving-strategy-costs-too-much.

Grant, Teddy. "LPs Grow Uneasy about Attacks on Private Equity by Politicians: Survey," *PE Hub*, Oct. 23, 2019. https://pehub.com/buyouts/lps-grow-uneasy-about-attacks-on-private-equity-by-politicians-survey.

Haverstock, Eliza. "Apollo Loses 2.3B, but Credit Unit Provides Hope," *PitchBook Data, Inc.*, May 1, 2020. https://pitchbook.com/news/articles/apollo-loses-23b-but-credits-unit-provides-hope.

———. "PE Has Failed to Outperform Stocks, Research Says, but LPs Aren't Turning Away," *PitchBook Data, Inc.*, June 25, 2020. https://pitchbook.com/news/articles/pe-stocks-lps-arent-turning-away.

Hawryluk, Markian. "Ever Heard of a Surgical Assistant? Meet a New Boost to Your Medical Bills," *Kaiser Health News*, July 22, 2020. https://khn.org/news/ever-heard-of-a-surgical-assistant-meet-a-new-boost-to-your-medical-bills/.

Hirsch, Marla Durben. "Trump Administration to Overhaul Kidney Disease Care, Reimbursement," *Modern Healthcare*, July 10, 2019. https://www.modernhealthcare.com/politics-policy-trump-administration-to-overhaul-kidney-disease-care.

Johnson, Steven Ross. "Mental Health Parity Remains a Challenge 10 Years after Landmark Law," *Modern Healthcare*, Oct. 5, 2018. https://www.modernhealthcare.com/article/20181005/NEWS/181009925/mental-health-parity-remains-a-challenge-10-years-after-landmark-law.

———. "Poor Communities Wait Longer for Ambulances, Causing Health Disparities," *Modern Healthcare*, Nov. 30, 2018. https://www.modernhealthcare.com/article/20181130/NEWS/181139991/poor-communities-wait-longer-for-ambulances-causing-health-disparities.

———. "Quality Ratings Are Coming to Addiction Treatment Provider Space," *Modern Healthcare*, Dec. 18, 2018. https://www.modernhealthcare.com/article/20181218/NEWS/181219904/quality-ratings-are-coming-to-addiction-treatment-provider-space.

Kacik, Alex. "Advanced Practice and Nurse Practitioners Bring More Profit, Productivity to Medical Practices," *Modern Healthcare*, July 20, 2018. https://www.modernhealthcare.com/article/20180720/NEWS/180729986/advanced-practice-and-nurse-practitioners-bring-more-profit-productivity-to-medical-practices.

———. "Amedisys Aims to Acquire Compassionate Care Hospice for $340 Million," Oct. 10, 2018. https://www.modernhealthcare.com/article/20181010/NEWS/181019988/amedisys-aims-to-acquire-compassionate-care-hospice-for-340-million.

———. "For the First Time Ever, Less than Half of Physicians Are Independent," *Modern Healthcare*, May 31, 2017. https://www.modernhealthcare.com/article/20170531/NEWS/170539971/for-the-first-time-ever-less-than-half-of-physicians-are-independent.

———. "Healthcare Credit Ratings Dip amid M&A Binge," *Modern Healthcare*, Oct. 29, 2018. https://www.modernhealthcare.com/article/20181029/NEWS/181029897/healthcare-credit-ratings-dip-amid-m-a-binge.

———. "Healthcare Spending to Consume 20% of GDP by 2028," *Modern Healthcare*, Mar. 24, 2020. https://www.modernhealthcare.com/healthcare-economics/healthcare-spending-consume-20-gdp-2028#:~:text=U.S.%20healthcare%20spending%20is%20expected,according%20to%20a%20new%20report.

———. "Health Systems Driving Prices Higher with Physician Group Purchases," *Modern Healthcare*, Sept. 4, 2018. https://www.modernhealthcare.com/article/20180904/NEWS/180909986/health-systems-driving-prices-higher-with-physician-group-purchases.

———. "How US Tax Reform Will Impact PE," *PitchBook Data, Inc.*, July 6, 2018. https://pitchbook.com/news/articles/how-us-tax-reform-will-impact-pe.

———. "Massachusetts Physician Practices Considering Closure, Consolidation," *Modern Healthcare*, June 10, 2020. https://www.modernhealthcare.com/operations/massachusetts-physician-practices-considering-closure-consolidation.

———. "Monopolized Healthcare Market Reduces Quality, Increases Cost," *Modern Healthcare*, Apr. 13, 2017. https://www.modernhealthcare.com/article/20170413/NEWS/170419935/monopolized-healthcare-market-reducesquality-increases-cost.

———. "Pro Medico Closes HCR ManorCare Acquisition," *Modern Healthcare*, July 27, 2018. https://wwwmodernhealthcare.com/article/20180727/news.

Knauth, Dietrick. "CalPers Committed $1 Bln to PE in Final Months of 2018," *PE Hub*, Feb. 13, 2019. https://pehub.com/buyous/calpers-committed-$1-bln-to-pe-in-final-months-of-2018/.

———. "Oregon Defends Paying PE Fees, Commits to Genstar," *PE Hub*, Mar. 14, 2019. https://www.pehub.com/buyouts/oregon-defends-paying-high-PE-fees-commits-to-genstar/.

———. "PE Fundraising Remains Resilient Going into 2019," *PE Hub*, Dec. 24, 2018. https://www.pehub.com/buyouts/pe-fundraising-remeains-resilient-going-into-2019/.

Kolakowski, Mark. "World's Top Ten Private Equity Firms," *Investopedia*, Feb. 21, 2021. https://www.investopedia.com/articles/markets/011116 /world's-top-10-private-equity-firms-apo-asp.

Krause, Patrick. "Why PE Firms Are Buying Orthopedic and Ophthalmology Practices," *PE Hub*, Aug. 3, 2017. https://www.pehub.com/2017/08/why-pe -firms-are-buying-orthopedic-and-ophthalmology-practices.

LaMantia, Jonathan. "Physician Practices Increasingly Turn to Private Equity for Capital," *Modern Healthcare*, Apr. 26, 2019. https://www.modernhealth care.com/finance/physician-practices-increasingly-turn-to-private-equity -for-capital.

Lewis, Adam. "Bain Capital, KKR to Back Hardship Fund for Toys R US Work- ers," *PitchBook Data, Inc.*, Sept. 28, 2018. https://pitchbook.com/news /articles/bain-capital-kkr-to-back-hardship-fund-for-toys-r-us-workers.

———. "Blackstone, KKR Draw Ire from Congress over Surprise Medical Bills," *PitchBook Data, Inc.*, Sept. 17, 2019. https://pitchbook.com/news/articles /blackstone-kkr-draw-ire-from-congress-over-surprise-medical-bills.

———. "Congress Confronts Bain Capital, KKR over Toys R US Liquidation," *PitchBook Data, Inc.*, July 6, 2018. https://pitchbook.com/news/articles /congress-questions-bain-capital-kkr-over-toys-r-us-liquidation.

———. "Elizabeth Warren Proposes Legislation to Rein in Private Equity 'Vampires,'" *PitchBook Data, Inc.*, July 18, 2019. https://pitchbook.com/news /articles/elizabeth-warren-proposes-legislation-to-rein-in-private-equity -vampires.

———. "Fed's Stimulus Offers Relief to Private Equity Despite Critics' Objections," *PitchBook Data, Inc.*, Apr. 16, 2020. https://pitchbook.com/news/article/fed -stimulus-offers-relief-to-private-equity-despite-critics-objections.

———. "5 PE-Backed Retail Deals That Didn't End in a Disaster," *PitchBook Data, Inc.*, Dec. 7, 2018. https://pitchbook.com/news/articles/five-pe-backed-retail -deals-that-didnt-end-in-disaster.

———. "John Oliver Takes on PE over Mobile Home Investments," *PitchBook Data, Inc.*, Apr. 8, 2019. https://pitchbook.com/news/article/john-oliver -takes-on-pe-over-mobile-home-investments.

———. "PE-Backed Distressed Exits in Freefall," *PitchBook Data, Inc.*, Feb. 23, 2018. https://pitchbook.com/news/articles/pe-backed-distressed-exits-in -freefall/.

———. "PE Firms Keep Deploying Dividend Recaps Despite the Risks," *PitchBook Data, Inc.*, Aug. 15, 2019. https://pitchbook.com/news/articles/pe-firms-keep -deploying-dividend-recaps-despite-the-risks.

———. "Private Equity Deprives World of Cute Valentine's Day Candies (for Now)," *PitchBook Data, Inc.*, Feb. 13, 2019. https://pitchbook.com/new/articles /private-equity-deprives-world-of-cute-valentine's-day-candies-for-now/.

———. "Private Equity Fundraising Totals Sure to Tumble due to the Coronavi- rus," *PitchBook Data, Inc.*, Mar. 31, 2020. https://pitchbook.com/news/articles /private-equity-fundraising-totals-sure-to-tumble-thanks-to-the-corona virus.

———. "Q&A: How PE Firms Are Dealing with Fallout from the Latest Tax Changes," *PitchBook Data, Inc.*, July 10, 2018. https://pitchbook.com/news

/articles/qa-heres-how-pe-firms-are-dealing-with-fallout-from-the-latest-tax
-changes/.

———. "Retail Roundup: Gymboree, Shopko File for Bankruptcy, Sears Gets
Saved," *PitchBook Data, Inc.*, Jan. 17, 2019. https:/pitchbook.com/news
/articles/retail-roundup-gymboree-shopko-file-for-bankruptcy-sears-gets
-saved/.

———. "Sycamore Set to Take $1B out of Staples," *PitchBook Data, Inc.*, Mar. 25,
2019. https://pitchbook.com/news/articles/sycamore-set-to-take-$1-billion
-out-of-staples/.

———. "The US PE Middle Market in 9 Charts," *PitchBook Data, Inc.*, Aug. 22, 2018.
https://pitchbook.com/news/articles/the-us-middle-market-in-9-charts.

Lewis, Adam, and James Thorne. "Ask PitchBook: Has Private Investor Lobbying for Pandemic Loans Been Successful?," *PitchBook Data, Inc.*, May 21, 2020.
https://pitchbook.com/news/articles/Ask-pitchbook-has-private-investor
-lobbying-for-pandemic-loans-been-successful.

———. "Private Equity's Campaign Funding Spree Points to 2020's High Stakes,"
PitchBook Data, Inc., Nov. 3, 2020. https://pitchbook.com/news/articles
/private-equity-election-spending-2020-high-stakes.

Lightbrown, Sean. "SBOs and Beyond: PE Playing Pass the Parcel," *PitchBook
Data, Inc.*, Nov. 27, 2018. https://pitchbook.com/news/articles/SBOs-and
-beyond-PE-playing-pass-the-parcel/.

Livingston, Shelby. "Dialysis Companies to Feel Squeeze from California's
Reimbursement Bill," *Modern Healthcare*, Oct. 14, 2019. https://www
.modernhealthcare.com/politics-policy/dialysis-companies-feel-squeeze
-calif-reimbursement-bill.

———. "Reimbursement Limitations on Home Healthcare Are Being Loosened,"
Modern Healthcare, Oct. 27, 2018. https://www.modernhealthcare.com
/article/20181027/NEWS/181029949/reimbursement-limitations-on-home
-healthcare-are-being-loosened.

Loughead, Katherine. "How Well-Funded Are Pension Plans in Your State?," *Tax
Foundation*, May 17, 2018. https://taxfoundation.org/state-pensions-funding
-2018/.

Luthi, Susannah. "Air Ambulances May Be Banned from Balance Billing,"
Modern Healthcare, June 22, 2019. https://www.modernhealthcare.com
/government/air-ambulances-may-be-banned-from-balance-billing.

———. "Congress Angles for Air Ambulance Cost Transparency," *Modern
Healthcare*, Oct. 8, 2018, 8–9.

———. "Surprise Medical Billing Legislation Threatened by Provider Lobbying," *Modern Healthcare*, Aug. 26, 2019. https://www.modernhealthcare.com
/government/surprise-medical-billing-legislation-threatened-provider
-lobbying#:~:text=Surprise%20medical%20billing%20legislation%20
threatened%20by%20provider%20lobbying,Susannah%20Luthi&text
=Physician%20groups'%20public%20relations%2C%20advertising,the%20
entire%20effort%20will%20collapse.

Lykken, Alex. "The Consequences of PEs Fundraising Arms Race," *PitchBook
Data, Inc.*, Jan. 18, 2019. https://pitchbook.com/news/articles/the-conseque
nces-of-pes-fundraising-arms-race.

———. "Flush with Cash, PE Firms Confront Their New Reality," *PitchBook Data, Inc.*, Mar. 23, 2020. https://pitchbook.com/news/article/flush-with -cash-pe-firms-confront-their-new-reality.

———. "Following a Decade-Long Uptick, Direct Lending Continues to Rise," *PitchBook Data, Inc.*, Feb. 11, 2020. https://pitchbook.com/news/articles /following-a-decade-long-uptick-direct-lending-continues-to-rise.

———. "How US Tax Reform Will Impact PE," *PitchBook Data., Inc.*, July 6, 2018. https://pitchbook.com/news/articles/how-us-tax-reform-will-impact-PE.

———. "Inside PE's Record-Breaking Push into Healthcare," *PitchBook Data, Inc.*, May 25, 2018. https://pitchbook.com/news/articles/inside-pes-record -breaking-push-into-healthcare.

———. "Making a Case for SBO," *PitchBook Data, Inc.*, June 8, 2018. https:// pitchbook.com/news/articles/making-a-case-for-the-sbo.

———. "The Next Financial Crisis Could Crush PE's Middle Market," *PitchBook Data, Inc.*, nNov. 2, 2018. https://pitchbook.com/news/articles/the-next -financial-crisis-could-crush-pes-middle-market.

———. "PE Firms Aren't Keeping Portfolio Companies as Long as They Used To," *PitchBook, Data, Inc.*, Jan. 24, 2020. https://pitchbook.com/news/articles/pe -firms-arent-keeping-portfolio-companies-as-long-as-they-used-to.

———. "PE Firms Look to VC-Backed Companies with Increasing Interest," *PitchBook Data, Inc.*, July 13, 2018. https://pitchbook.com/news/articles/pe -firms-look-to-vc-backed-companies-with-increasing-interest.

Marham, Isabel. "LP Perspectives Survey 2020: Seven LP Opinions That Matter," *PE Hub*, Dec. 10, 2019. https://buyouts.com/lp-perspectives-survey -2020-seven-lp-opinions-that-matter/.

Meikle, Brad. "Envision Health Sets $100M Offering," *PE Hub*, July 1, 2013. https://www.pehub.com/buyouts/envision-health-sets-$100m-offering.

Meyer, Harris. "Air Ambulance Charges Study Could Boost Senate Surprise Bill Legislation," *Modern Healthcare*, July 1, 2019. https://www.modernhealthcare .com/payment/air-ambulance-charges-study-could-boost-senate-surprise -bill-legislation.

———. "Concerns Grow as Private Equity Buys Up Dermatology Practices," *Modern Healthcare*, July 24, 2019. https://www.modernhealthcare.com /finance/concerns-grow-as-private-equity-buys-up-dermatology.

———. "Healthcare Lawyers Tout Surge in Care Transactions as Transforma- tional," *Modern Healthcare*, July 7, 2018. https://www.modernhealthcare .com/article/20180707/TRANSFORMATION03/180709939/healthcare -lawyers-tout-surge-in-care-transactions-as-transformational.

———. "Medical Group Deals Force Growing Antitrust Scrutiny as Price Worries Rise," *Modern Healthcare*, July 6, 2019. https://www.modernhealthcare.com/legal /medical-group-deals-force-growing-anitrust-scutiny-as-price-worries-rise.

———. "Physician Groups Crave Capital but Worry about Future Sale," *Modern Healthcare*, Aug. 31, 2019. https://www.modernhealthcare.com/physicians /physician-groups-crave-capital-but-worry-about-future-sale.

———. "Specialty Physician Groups Attracting Private Equity Investment," *Modern Healthcare*, Aug. 31, 2019. https://www.modernhealthcare.com /physicians/specialty-physician-groups-attracting-private-equity-investment.

Mitchell, Justin. "CalPers CIO Unveils Major New Leverage-Backed Push into Private Equity and Private Credit," *Buyouts Insider*, June 16, 2020. https://www.buyoutsinsider.com/calpers-cio-unveils-major-new-leverage-backed-push-into-private-equity-and-private-credit.

———. "LPs Would Like More Vigorous Defense of PE Industry: Coller," *Buyouts Insider*, Dec. 2, 2019. https://www.buyoutsinsider.com/lps-would-like-more-vigorous-defense-of-PE-industry-coller.

Morris, Shawn. "Comment: Guest Expert," *Modern Healthcare*, June 3, 2019, 29.

Murphy, H. Lee. "Dialysis Centers Are the Health Industry's Growth Story," *Modern Healthcare*, July 11, 2018. https://www.modernhealthcare.com/article/20180711/NEWS/180719976/dialysis-centers-are-the-health-industry-s-growth-story.

O'Grady, Eileen, "Understaffed, Unlicensed, and Untrained: Behavioral Health under Private Equity," Private Equity Stakeholder Project, Oct. 6, 2020. https://pestakeholder.org/understaffed-unlicensed-and-untrained-behavioral-health-under-private-equity/.

Pringle, Sarah. "Air Medical Resources Group Attracts PE Interest as It Nears Sale," *PE Hub*, Feb. 28, 2017. https://www.pehub.com/air-medical-resource-group-said-to-near-sale/.

———. "Amulet Forms Pennsylvania Gastro Group via $130 Mln Deal," *PE Hub*, May 29, 2019. https://www.pehub.com/amulet-forms-pennsylvania-gastro-group-via-130-mln-deal/.

———. "Arsenal's Deal for Hopebridge Valued at $255 Mln," *PE Hub*, May 7, 2019. https://www.pehub.com/arsenals-deal-for-hopebridge-valued-at-255-mln/.

———. "Blackstone Walks Away with the Win for Autism-Treatment Company CARD," *PE Hub*, Apr. 13, 2018. https://www.pehub.com/buyouts/blackstone-walks-away-with-the-win-for-autism-treatment-company-card.

———. "Bracing for the Long Haul," *Buyouts Insider*, May 5, 2020. https://www.buyoutsinsider.com/bracing-for-the-long-haul/.

———. "CCMP to Buy Eating Recovery Center," *PE Hub*, Aug. 30, 2017. https://www.pehub.com/ccmp-to-buy-eating-recovery-center/.

———. "ChanceLight, Trimaran Portfolio Company, Weighs Sale," *PE Hub*, Jan. 24, 2018. https://www.pehub.cpm/buyouts/chancelight-trimaran-portfolio-company-weighs-sale.

———. "Colorado's Peak Gastroenterology Goes to Varsity Healthcare," *PE Hub*, Dec. 6, 2019. https://www.pehub.com/colorados-peak-gastroenterology-goes-to-varsity-healthcare.

———. "Dialysis, Behavioral Health Light Up December Deal Flow," *PE Hub*, Dec. 20, 2018. https://www.pehub.com/page/5/?s=dialysis%2c+behavioral+health+lights+up+december+deals&sort&date-range-min=19-12-2018&date-range-max=21-12-2018.

———. "FFL's Eyecare Partners Hits the Auction Block," *PE Hub*, Oct. 28, 2019. https://www.pehub.com/buyouts/ffls-eyecare-partners-hits-the-auction-block.

———. "Five Questions with FFL's Aaron Money on PE Investment In Autism Treatment," *PE Hub*, Nov. 7, 2018. https://www.pehub.com/buyouts/five-questions-with-ffl's-aaron-money-on-pe-investment-in-autism-treatment.

———. "Five Questions with NexPhase Capital's Andy Kieffer," PE Hub, Apr. 27, 2018. https://www.pehub.com/buyouts/five-questions-with-nexphase -capital's-andy-kieffer.

———. "Goldman PE Arm Buys MyEyeDr in $2.7B Deal, Producing 3.5x Return for Atlas Partners," PE Hub, June 3, 2019. https://www.pehub.com/buyouts /goldman-pe-arm-buys-myeyedr-in-2.7b-deal-producing-3.5x-return-for -atlas-partners.

———. "Grant Avenue Clinches First Deal, Carving Out HCR ManorCare Units," PE Hub, Feb. 4, 2020. https://www.pehub.com/grant-avenue-clinches-first -deal-carving-out-hcr-manorcare-units.

———. "Healthcare Corner: 'Selfie Generation' Makes Waves in the Dental Market," PE Hub, July 22, 2019. https://www.pehub/buyouts/healthcare -corner-selfie-generation-makes-waves-in-the-dental-market.

———. "KKR, on a Healthcare Tear, Builds Medical-Transport Giant," PE Hub, Aug. 14, 2017. https://www.pehub.com/buyouts/kkr-on-a-healthcare-tear -builds-medical-transport-giant.

———. "KKR's BlueSprig Snags Shore Capital's Florida Autism Center in $120M Deal," PE Hub, Mar. 6, 2020. https://pehub.com/kkrs-bluesprig-snags-shore -capitals-florida-autism-center-in-120m-deal.

———. "Lee Equity Unites Two Urology Groups to Create Solaris," PE Hub, June 16, 2020. https://www.pehub.com/lee-equity-unites-two-urology -groups-to-create-solaris.

———. "Marriage of Summit Medical and Warburg's CityMD Is First of Its Kind," PE Hub, June 27, 2019. https://www.pehub.com/buyouts/marriage-of -summit-medical-and-warburgs-citymd-is-first-of-its-kind.

———. "NexPhase's Action Behavioral Centers Returns to Auction Block," PE Hub, Sept. 16, 2019. https://www.pehub.com/buyouts/nexphases-action -behavioral-center-returns-to-auction-block.

———. "PE-Backed American Physician Partners Fields First Round Bids," PE Hub, Sept. 25, 2019. https://www.pehub.com/buyouts/pe-backed-american -physician-partners-fields-first-round-bids.

———. "Post Capital, Ex-Addus Chief Join in New Home-Care Platform," PE Hub, Feb. 6, 2019. https://www.pehub.com/buyouts/post-capital-ex-addus-chief -join-in-new-home-care-platform.

———. "Revelstroke's Crossroads Sales Process Heads to First Round," PE Hub, Apr. 12, 2019. https://www.pehub.com/buyouts/revelstokes-crossroads-sales -process-heads-to-first-round.

———. "Thomas H. Lee Partners Buys Centria in $400Mln-Plus Deal," PE Hub, Dec. 6, 2019. https://www.pehub/Thomas-h-lee-partners-buys-centria-in -$400-mln-plus-deal.

———. "21st Century Oncology, Owned by Debt Holders, Launches Auction amid Comeback," PE Hub, Oct. 18, 2019. https://www.buyoutsinsider.com/21st -century-oncology-owned-by-debt-holders-launches-auction-amid-comeback/.

———. "U.S. Renal, Backed by Leonard Green, Frazier Healthcare, Explore Sale," PE Hub, Dec. 18, 2018. https://www.pehub.com/u-s-renal-backed-by -leonard-green-frazier-healthcare-explores-sale/.

———. "Varsity Healthcare Backs Pediatric Home-Health Provider Angels of Care," *PE Hub*, Apr. 25, 2019. https://pehub.com/buyouts/varsity-healthcare -backs-pediatric-home-health-provider-angels-of-care.

———. "Varsity Healthcare Partners Recaps Newly Created Emergency Care Partners," *PE Hub*, Sept. 13, 2018. https://www.pehub.com/varsity-healthcare -partners-recaps-newly-created-emergency-care-partners/.

———. "Varsity Orthopedics Care Partners Adds the Steadman Clinic," *PE Hub*, Nov. 14, 2019. https://www.pehub.com/buyouts/Varsity-orthopedics-care -partners-adds-the-steadman-clinic.

———. "Varsity's Emergency Care Partners Merges with Northeastern Peer, Adds Regal Healthcare to Investor Base," *PE Hub*, Feb. 11, 2019. https://www .pehub.com/varsitys-emergency-care-partners-merges-with-northeastern -peer-adds-regal-healthcare-to-investor-base/.

———. "WCAS, Linden, Cressey Drive Healthcare Fundraising Momentum in 2018," *PE Hub*, Dec. 27, 2018. https://www.pehub.com/buyouts/wcas-linden -cressney-drive-healthcare-fundraising-momentum-in-2018.

———. "Webster Shelves BayMark Auction, Eyes Further Growth," *PE Hub*, Jan. 3, 2020. https://www.pehub.com/webster-shelves-baymark-auction -eyes-further-growth.

———. "Why Healthcare Investors Are Flocking to Opportunities in Autism," *PE Hub*, Feb. 5, 2018. https://www.pehub.com/buyouts/why-healthcare-investors -are-flocking-to-opportunities-in-autism.

———. "Why Healthcare Sponsors Are Pivoting to Orthopedics," *PE Hub*, Jan. 29, 2019. https://www.pehub.com/buyouts/why-healthcare-sponsors -are-pivoting-to-orthopedics.

Teichert, Erica. "Kindred Pays Feds Largest Penalty Ever Recorded for Integrity Agreement Violations," *Modern Healthcare*, Sept. 20, 2016. https://www .modernhealthcare.com/article/20160920/NEWS/160929995/kindred-pays -feds-largest-penalty-ever-recorded-for-integrity-agreement-violations#: ~:text=Kindred%20Healthcare%20will%20pay%20a,such%20penalty%20 issued%20to%20date.

Thorne, James. "Over 8,000 Privately Backed Companies Got Billions in PPP Loans, SBA Data Shows," *PitchBook Data, Inc.*, July 8, 2020. https://pitchbook .com/news/articles/privately-backed-companies-got-billions-in-ppp-loans.

"Venture Capital, Private Equity and M&A Glossary." *PitchBook Data, Inc.*, July 10, 2017. https://pitchbook.com/blog/private-equity-and-venture -capital-glossary.

Weitemeyer, Joseph. "Ninety-Nine PE-Backed Companies Receive Distressed Credit Ratings," *PE Hub*, Oct. 21, 2019. https://www.pehub.com/buyouts /ninety-nine-PE-backed-companies-receive-distressed-credit-ratings/.

———. "Retail Leads Long List of 2018 Distressed Companies," *PE Hub*, Jan. 7, 2019. https://pehub/buyouts/retail-leads-long-list-of-2018-distressed -companies/.

Witkowsky, Chris. "Deal of the Year Awards Intro 2019," *Buyouts Insider*, Mar. 18, 2019. https://www.buyoutsinsider.com/deal-of-the-year-awards -intro-2019/.

———. "Editor's Letter: PE's 'Silent Middle' on Display at Congressional Hearing," *Buyouts Insider*, Dec. 2, 2019. https://www.buyoutsinsider/pres -silent-middle-on-display-at-congressional-hearing/.

———. "GPs Ask LPs for More Ability to Use Fund-Level Leverage to Prop Up Older Investments," *Buyouts Insider*, June 10, 2020. https://www.buyoutsinsider .com/gps-ask-lps-for-more-ability-to-use-fund-level-leverage-to-prop-older -investments.

———. "Holding PE Partners Liable in Bankruptcies Gets Public Paddling," *Buyouts Insider*, Nov. 20, 2019. https://www.buyoutsinsider.com/holding-PE -partners-liable-in-bankruptcies-gets-public-paddling.

———. "KKR Pledges $50M Fund for Pandemic Relief Efforts," *Buyouts Insider*, Apr. 7, 2020. https://www.buyoutsinsider.com/kkr-pledges-50m-fund-for -pandemic-relief-effforts.

———. "Larger Funds, Specialization, Big Fundraising Trends for 2019," *PE Hub*, Dec. 3, 2018. https://www.buyoutsinsider.com/larger-funds-specialization -big-fundraising-trends-for-2019/.

———. "U.S. Government Offers Guidance That Opens Access to Private Equity in 401(k)s," *Buyouts Insider*, June 5, 2020. https://www.buyoutsinsider.com/u-s -government-offers-guidance-that-opens-access-to-private-equity-in-401ks.

Journal Articles, Reports, and Other Nongovernmental Sources

Abramowitz, Adam, and Jonathan Bluce. "Why Are Investors Focused on Autism Services," *Intrepid Investment Bankers*, 2018. https://intrepidib.com /why-are-investors-focused-on-autism-services/.

Alternative, Peter. "Why Doesn't Private Equity Like Staffing," *Mirus Capital Advisors*, 2013. https://merger.com/private-equity-staffing/.

American Medical Association. "Report 11 of the Council on Medical Service (A-19), Corporate Investors (Reference Committee G)," July 2019. https://ama -assn.org/system/files/2019-07/a19-cms-report-11.pdf.

Aprill, Robert. "Private Equity Investment in Orthopedics: Provident Perspective," *Provident Healthcare Partners*, 2018. https://www.providenthp.com /provident-perspective-private-equity-investment-in-orthopedics/.

Aprill, Robert, Gary W. Herschman, and Anjana D. Patel. "Hot Physician Specialists for Private Equity Investment," *Becker's Spine*, June 13, 2017. https://www.beckersasc.com/asc-transactions-and-valuation-issues/hot -physician-specialties-for-private-equity-investment-2.html.

Attia, Evelyn, et al. "Marketing Residential Treatment Programs for Eating Disorders: A Call for Transparency," *Psychiatric Services*, Mar. 14, 2016. https://ps.psychiatryonline.org/doi/full/10.1176/appi.ps.201500338.

Balshem, Deborah. "Private Equity Targeting Emerging Eating Disorder Treatment Space," *Merger Market*, Apr. 6, 2015. https://www.providenthp.com /wp-content/uploads/2015/04/MM_PE-Eating-Disorder-Space_04.08.15.pdf.

Barker, Nicholas H. "The Private Equity Toolbox for Dental Practices and Dental Businesses: More than Just a Checkbook," *Dentistry IQ*, July 11, 2017. https:// www.dentistryiq.com/articles/apex360/2017/07/the-private-equity-toolbox -for-dental-practices-and dental-businesses-more-than-just-a-checkbook.

Barrett, Stephen. "Massive Dental Fraud Uncovered," *Dental Watch*, Aug. 23, 2011. https://www.dentalwatch.org/news/forba.html.

Baxter, Amy. "Epic Merges with PSA to Create Pediatric Home Health Power-house," *Home Health Care News*, Jan. 17, 2017. https://homehealthcarenews.com/2017/01/epic-merges-with-psa-to-create-pediatric-home-health-powerhouse.

———. "Median Home Care Turnover Hit 66.7% in 2017," *Home Care News*, Apr. 19, 2018. https://homehealthcarenews.com/2018/04/median-home-care-turnover-hit-66-7-in-2017/.

BDO. "Healthcare's Consolidation Funnel, Told through Private Equity," BDO, Dec. 2019. https://www.bdo.com/insights/industries/healthcare/bdo-pitchbook-healthcare-s-consolidation-funnel,-t.

———. "Tenth Annual Private Equity Perspective Survey," Feb. 2019. htpp://www.bdo.com/insights/industries/private-equity/bdo-5-tenth-annual-private-equity-perspective-survey/.

Beasley Allen Law. "Beasley Allen Files Suit against Fraudulent Drug Treatment Centers," *Beasley Allen Law*, May 18, 2010. https://www.beasleyallen.com/news/beasley-allen-files-suit-against-fraudulent-drug-treatment-centers.

Becker, Scott, et al. "15 Private Equity in Healthcare—An Updated Review of Selected Niche Investment Areas," *McGuire Woods*, Mar. 29, 2018. https://www.mcguirewoods.com/client-resources/Alerts/2018/3/15-Private-Equity-Healthcare-Review-Selected-Investment-Areas.

Bernstein, Carl. Keynote speech, Fortieth Annual Rocco Tressolini Lectureship in Law, Lehigh University, Bethlehem, PA, Sept. 24, 2019.

Bithoney, Bill. "Behavioral Health: A Market Ripe for Growth and Consolidation," BDO, Mar. 2015. https://www.bdo.com/insights/industries/healthcare/behavioral-health-a-market-ripe-for-growth.

Braff Group. "Home Health and Hospice," 2018. https://thebraffgroup.com/market-sectors/home-health-and-hospice.

Brico, Elizabeth. "The Cost of Addiction Treatment Keeps Poor People Addicted," *Talk Poverty*, Nov. 1, 2017. https://talkpoverty.org/2017/11/01/cost-addiction-treatment-keeps-poor-people-addicted.

Bruch, Joseph D., et al. "Expansion of Private Equity Involvement in Women's Health Care," *JAMA Internal Medicine* 180, no. 11, Nov. 2020: 1542–1545.

Bryant, Baily. "AccentCare to Be Acquired by PE Giant Advent International: Updated," *Home Health Care News*, May 16, 2019. https://homehealthcarenews.com/2019/05/accentcare-to-be-acquired-by-PE-giant-advent-international.

———. "New Amedisys—ClearCare Personal Care Network Spreading Like Wildfire," *Home Health Care News*, Aug. 5, 2019. https://homehealthcarenews.com/2019/08/new-amadisys-clearcare-personal-care-network-spreading-like-wildfire.

Buckley, Holly, et al. "Why Private Equity Has Eyes on Vision Care," *McGuire Woods*, Nov. 27, 2018. https://www.thehealthcareinvestor.com/2018/11/articles/healthcare-services-investing/why-private-equity-has-eyes-on-vision-care.

Bundy, Clint. "The Dermatology Market: A Tidal Wave of Private Equity," *Practical Dermatology*, Sept. 2018. https://www.practical dermatology.com /2018/09/the-dermatology-market-a-tidal-wave-of-private-equity.

Butler-Young, Sheena. "Private Equity Pumped Billions into Dozens of Shoe Brands—Then They All Went Bankrupt," *Footwear News*, June 18, 2018. https://footwearnews.com/2018/business/retail/private-equity-bankruptcy -retail-fashion-shoe-brands-nine-west-payless-1202575710/.

Cabin, William, et al. "For-Profit Medicare Home Health Agencies' Costs Appear Higher and Quality Appears Lower Compared to Nonprofit Agencies," *Health Affairs* 33, no. 8, Aug. 2014: 1460–1465.

Calams, Sarah. "Private vs. Public Ambulance Services: What's the Differ-ences?," EMS1, Oct. 23, 2017. https://www.ems1.com/private-public-dispute /articles/private-vs-public-ambulance-services-whats-the-difference -WTgJNJgR4KlljlV9/.

Calma, Carlo. "Top 10 Home and Hospice Providers," *Home Health Care News*, Nov. 16, 2017. https://homehealthcarenews.com/2017/11/top-10-home-and -hospice-providers/.

Chen, Evan M., et al. "Private Equity in Ophthalmology and Optometry," *American Academy of Ophthalmology* 127, no. 4, Apr. 2020: 445–455.

Chesapeake Urology. "United Urology Group Expands National Presence with Colorado Affiliations," Dec. 5, 2018. https://www.coloradouro.com/news /united-urology-group-expands-national-presence-with-colorado -affiliations/.

Cockrell, Geoff, and Sarah Mick. "The Next Wave of Consolidation in PPM Models: Podiatry, Allergy and Fertility," *McGuire Woods*, Mar. 6, 2018. https://www.thehealthcareinvestor.com/2018/03/articles/health-care-the -next-wave-of-consolidation-in-ppm-models-podiatry-allergy-and-fertility.

Coker Capital Advisors. "Autism Services Sector," *Coker Capital's Newsletter*, Nov. 2017. https://www.cokercapital.com.

Columbia Business School. Twenty-Fifth Annual Private Equity Conference, Marriott Marquis, New York, Feb. 8, 2019.

———. Twenty-Sixth Annual Private Equity Conference, Athletic Club, New York, Feb. 7, 2020.

Davis, Michael. "Benevis Files for Chapter 11 Bankruptcy," *Dentistry Today*, Aug. 13, 2020. https://www.dentistrytoday.com/news/today's-dental-news /item/6793-benevis-files-for-chapter-11-banktuptcy.

———. "Doctors Selling Practices to Corporate Dentistry; or Dancing with the Devil," *Dentist the Menace*, Jan. 2, 2017. https://blog.dentistthemenace.com /2017/01/doctors-selling-practices-to-coporporate-dentistry-or-dancing-with -the-devil.

———. "Emerging Advocacy Groups Support Small Businesses," *Dentistry Today*, Apr. 20, 2018. https://www.dentistrytoday.com/news/todays-dental -news/item/3191-emerging-advocacy-groups-support-small-business -dentistry.

———. "GA Board Member Resigns after Kool Smile Dental Settlements," *Today's Dental News*, Jan. 31, 2018. https://www.dentistrytoday.com/news/todays -dental-news/item/2878-ga-board-member-resigns-after-kool-smiles-dental

-settlement#:~:text=Dale%20G.,request%20of%20Governor%20Nathan%20
Deal.&text=This%20action%20came%20in%20the,Department%20of%20
Justice%20.

———. "Kool Smiles Dental—A Disturbing Peek behind the Curtain," *Concerned Dentists of Texas*, Aug. 12, 2017.

———. "Kool Smiles Dental Quietly Changes the Names of Its Clinics," *Dentistry Today*, May 6, 2019. https://www.dentistry today.com/news/todays-dental -news/item4763.

———. "Private Equity Firms Target DSOs through Leveraged Buying," *Today's Dental News*, July 13, 2018.

———. "WSDA Files Complaint against Lone Peak Management," *Dentistry Today*, Nov. 19, 2018. https://dentistrytoday.com/news/todays-dental-news /item/4076/wsda-files-complaint against-lone-peak-management.

DocWire News. "The Economies of Urgent Care Centers," *DocWire News*, May 14, 2019. https://www.docwirenews.com/docwire-pick/the-economics-of -urgent-care-centers/.

Editorial. "Private Equity Must Be Less Private," *Pensions and Investments*, Aug. 19, 2019. https://www.pionline.com/editorial/private-quity-must-be -less-private.

Epprecht, Liz. "Corporate Practice of Medicine Laws," *MDRanger*, Nov. 9, 2018. https://www.mdranger.com/blogs/corporate-practice-of-medicine-laws.

Falconer, Kirk. "Bain Capital's Latest Distressed, Special Situations Fund Passes $2Bn Mark," *Buyouts Insider*, Apr. 24, 2020. https://www.buyoutsinsider.com /bain-capitals-latest-distressed-special-situations-fund-passes-2bn-mark/.

———. "Brookfield Sees COVID-19 Creating 'One of the Greatest Environments' for Distressed Debt," *Buyouts Insider*, May 14, 2020. https://www.buyouts insider.com/brookfield-sees-covid-19-creating-one-of-the-great-environm ents-for-distressed-debt/.

Famakinwa, Joyce. "Calculating the Cost of PDGM: A Case Study with Phoenix Home Care," *Home Health Care News*, Jan. 28, 2020. https://homehealth carenews.com/2020/01/calculating-the-cost-of-pdgm-a-case-study-with -phoenix-home-care/.

———. "18% of Home Care Workers Live below the Federal Poverty Line," *Home Health Care News*, Sept. 4, 2019. https://homehealthcarenews.com/2019/09/13 -of-home-care-workers-live-below-the-federal-poverty-line/.

———. "PE-Backed Synergy HomeCare Sees Medicare Advantage as 'Huge Opportunity,'" *Home Health Care News*, Sept. 2019. https:// homehealthcarenews.com/2019/09/pe-backed-synergy-homecare-sees -medicare-advantge-as-huge-opportunity.

———. "Private Equity Likely to Deploy $1.5 Trillion War Chest in Home-Based Care Market," *Home Health Care News*, Feb. 18, 2020. https://homehealth carenews.com/2020/private-equity-likely-to-deploy-$1.5-trillion-war-chest -in-home-based-care-market.

———. "With New Franchise Sales on the Rise, ComForCare Revamps Recruit-ment Process," *Home Health Care News*, Sept. 3, 2020. https://homehealth carenews.com/2020/09/with-new-franchise-sales-on-the-rise-comforcare -revamps-recruitment-process/.

Feldman, Marcos. "Ares Increases Stake in Dental Firm Fined $1.7 Million by State Attorneys General for Deceptive Practices," *UNITE HERE*, Sept. 2017. https://www.pecloserlook.org/wp-content/uploads/AspenDentalReport-1 .pdf.

Flood, Chris. "Buyout Groups Blasted at SEC Meeting for 'Misleading Numbers,'" *Financial Times*, Sept. 20, 2020. https://www.ft.com/content/4ae144cb -9056-41c2-a80a-36348de5296a.

———. "Cheap Tracker Funds Trounce Private Equity," *Financial Times*, Dec. 12, 2020. https://www.ft.com/content/0640d664-083e-4439-8fe4-faa06eee6e17.

Flynn, Maggie. "Home Health Care among Top Industries for Return on Equity," *Home Health Care News*, Nov. 6, 2017. https://homehealthcarenews.com/2017 /11/home-health-care-among-top-industries-for-return-on-equity.

Fred, Herbert L., and Mark S. Scheid. "Physician Burnout: Causes, Consequences and (?) Cures," *Texas Heart Institute Journal* 45, no. 4, Aug. 2018: 198–202.

Funding Universe. "Air Methods Corporation History." https://www.fundinguniv erse.com/company-histories/air-methods-corporation-history/.

———. "American Medical Response, Inc. History." https://www.fundinguniverse .com/company-histories-air-methods-corporation-history/.

———. "History of Pediatric Services of America, Inc." https://www.fundinguni verse.com/company/-histories/pediatric-services-of-america-inc.

———. "Manor Care, Inc. History." https://fundinguniverse.com/company -histories/manor-care-inc-history/.

———. "ResCare, Inc. History." https://fundinguniverse.com/company-histories .res-care-inc-history/.

———. "Rural/Metro Corporation History." https://www.fundinguniverse.com /company-histories/rural-metro-corporation-history.

———. "Vencor, Inc. History." https://www.fundinguniverse.com/company -histories/vencor-inc-history/.

Furfaro, Hannah. "Optimism Greets Investors' Sudden Interest in Autism Therapy," *Spectrum*, July 9, 2018. https://www.spectrumnews.org/news /optimism-greets-investors-sudden-interest-in-autism-therapy.

Gander, Jennifer C., Xingyu Zhang, and Katherine Ross, "Association between Dialysis Facility Ownership and Access to Kidney Transplants," *JAMA* 322, no. 10, Sept. 10, 2019: 957–973.

Gondi, Suhas, and Zirui Song. "Potential Implications of Private Equity Investments in Health Care Delivery," *JAMA* 321, no. 11, Feb. 28, 2019: 1047–1048.

Gregory, Golden Arnall. "PharMerica Corporation Settles Anti-Kickback Allegations by Paying over $9 Million to Government," *JD Supra*, Oct. 21, 2015. https://www.jdsupra.com/legalnews/pharmerica-corporation-settles -anti-kickback-allegations-by-paying-over-$9-million.

Grohol, John M. "Universal Health Services (UHS) Skewered (Again) by New Report," *Psych Central*, July 8, 2018. https://psychcentral.com/blog /universal-health-services-skewered-again-by-new-report.

Guarda, Angela. "Refeeding and Weight Restoration in Anorexia Nervosa," *Eating Disorder Catalogue*, Jan. 4, 2016. https://www.edcatalogue.com /refeeding-and-weight-restoration-in-anorexia-nervosa.

Gustafsson, Lovisa, Shanoor Seervai, and David Blumenthal. "The Role of Private Equity in Driving Up Health Care Prices," *Harvard Business Review*, Oct. 29, 2019. https://hbr.org/2019/10/the-role-of-private-equity-in-driving -up-health-care-prices.

Haas, Robert, and Roberto Pagani. "How PE Operation Teams Create Wealth," *A.T. Kearney*, 2014. https://www.atkearney.com/private-equity/article/?/a /how-PE-operations-teams-create-value/.

Hammer, Mark. "Reining in Medicaid Spending," *American Interest*, Sept. 5, 2018. https://www.the-american-interest.com/2018/09/05/reining-in -medicaid-spending.

Harbin, Thomas S. "Private Equity Buyouts of Ophthalmology Practices," *990 .org*, June 7, 2017. https://990.org/senior-orphthalmologists/scope/article /private-equity-buyouts-of-ophthalmology-practices.

Harbin, Thomas S., and Gary Markowitz. "Private Equity Buyouts of Ophthalmology Practice—Update 2018," *American Academy of Ophthalmologists*, July 26, 2018. https://www.aao.org/senior-ophthamologists/scope/article /private-equity-buyouts-of-ophthalmology-practices-update-2018.

Hicks, Fleur. "Why Are Private Equity Investors Turning to Fertility?," *Onefourzero Group*, May 31, 2019. https://onefourzerogroup.com/why-are -private-equity-investors-turning-to-fertility.

Hilton, Lisette. "Urologists Eye Private Equity Partners," *Urology Times*, Mar. 8, 2019. https://www.urologytimes.com/business-urology/urologists-eye -private-equity-partners.

Holly, Robert. "Encompass Health's April Anthony: Knee-Jerk Therapy Reactions May Prove Costly," *Home Health Care News*, Jan. 26, 2020. https:// www.homehealthcarenews.com/2020/01/encompass-health's-april-anthony -knee-jerk-therapy-reactions-may-prove-costly.

———. "Home Health, Hospice Experiencing Unprecedented M&A Action," *Home Health Care News*, Sept. 24, 2018. https://homehealthcarenews.com /2018/09/home-health-hospice-experiencing-unprecedented-m-&-a-actrion.

———. "Immigration Reform, Minimum Wage Increase Top of Mind for Bayada," *Home Health Care News*, Feb. 11, 2019. https://homehealthcarenews.com/2019 /02/immigration-reform-minimum-wage-increase-top-of-mind-for-bayada.

———. "In Dynamic Industry, At-Home Care Providers See Scale as a Leg Up," *Home Health Care News*, Apr. 2019. https://homehealthcarenews.com/2019/04 /in-dynamic-industry-at-home-care-providers-see-scale-as-a-leg-up.

———. "No 'Strings Attached': CMS Sending $30 Billion to Home Health Agencies, Other Medicare Providers," *Home Health Care News*, Apr. 9, 2020. https://homehealthcarenews.com/2020/04/no-strings-attached-cms -sending-$30-billion-to-home-health-agencies-other-medicare-providers.

———. "Skeptics Raise Concerns as Private Equity Investment in Home Health Industry Rises," *Home Health Care News*, June 15, 2018. https://homehealth carenews.com/2018/06/skeptics-raise-concerns-as-private-equity-investment -in-home-health-industry-rises.

———. "The Top 10 Largest Home Health Providers in 2019," *Home Health Care News*, Nov. 14, 2019. https://homehealthcarenews.com/2019/11/the-top-10 -largest-home-health-providers-in-2019.

———. "With Medicare Advantage in Mind, Newly Merged Home Care Company Seeks National Growth," *Home Health Care News*, Nov. 8, 2018. https://home healthcarenews.com/2018/11/with-medicare-advantage-in-mind-newly -merged-home-care-company-seeks-national-growth/.

Hsia, Renee Y., Delphine Huang, and N. Clay Mann. "A US National Study of the Association between Income and Ambulance Response Time in Cardiac Arrest," *JAMA Network Open*, Nov. 30, 2018. https://jamanetwork.com /journals/jamanetworkopen/fullarticle/2716993.

Hurley, Ben. "Alternatives a 'Loser's Game': Ennis Knupp Founder," *Investment Magazine*, July 6, 2020. https://www.investmentmagazine.com.au/2020/07 /alternatives-a-losers-game-ennis-knupp-founder/.

Kane, Leslie. "Medscape Gastroenterologist Compensation Report: 2019," Apr. 24, 2019. https://www.medscape.com/slideshow/2019-compensation -gastroenterologist-6011330.

Kaufman, Hall, and Associates. "Industry Flash Report—Physicians, Skokie, Illinois," *Kaufman, Hall*, Mar. 2018. https://www.kaufmanhall.com/sites /default/files/physician-groups-flash-report-march_2018.pdf.

Kennedy, Eleanor. "The Boss: Mark Claypool, ChanceLight Behavioral Health, Therapy and Education," *ChanceLight*, Feb. 13, 2017. https://chancelight .com/news/boss-mark-claypool-chancelight-behavioral-health-therapy -education.

Kent, Christopher. "Is a Private Equity Deal Right for You? Part 1," *Review of Ophthalmology*, Apr. 10, 2018. https://www.reviewofophthalmology.com /article/is-a-private-equity-deal-right-for-you.

Kidney Buzz. "Intense Debate Sparked regarding Poor Dialysis Patient Care and Infections," Jan. 9, 2018. https://www.kidneybuzz.com/intense-debate -sparked-regarding-poor-dialysis-patient-care-and-infections.

Kindred Healthcare. "Kindred Completes First Closing for Its Skilled Nursing Facility Business Divestiture," Aug. 31, 2017. https://www.kindredhealthcare .com/news/2017/08/31/kindred-completes-first-closing-for-its-skilled -nursing-facility-business-divestiture.

Koch, Paul S. "As I See It: You May Want to Think Twice about Private Equity," *Ophthalmology Management* 22, Mar. 2018: 16, 56.

Konda, Sailesh, and Joseph Francis. "Corporatization and the Rise of Private Equity in Dermatology: The Landscape of Private Equity in Dermatology and Concerns about Private Equity-Backed Models: Part 1," *Next Steps in Derm*, Nov. 14, 2018. https://www.nextstepsinderm.com/navigating-your-career /the-landscape-of-private-equity-in-dermatology-and-concerns-about-pe -backed-models.

———. "Corporatization and the Rise of Private Equity in Dermatology: Private Equity-Backed Concerns and How to Prevent Private Equity-Backed Consolidation: Part 2," *Next Steps in Derm*, Nov. 21, 2018. https://www.nextstepsind erm.com/navigating-your-career-private-equity-backed-model-concerns-and -how-to-prevent-private-equity-backed-consolidation/.

Konda, Sailesh, et al. "Future Considerations for Clinical Dermatology in the Setting of 21st Century American Policy Reform: Corporatization and the Rise of Private Equity in Dermatology," *Journal of the American Academy of*

Dermatology, Oct. 5, 2018. https://www.jaad.org/article/S0190-9622(18)32667-7
/fulltext.

Kraft, Stephen. "Physician Practice Management Companies: A Failed Concept," *Physician Executive*, Mar. 2002: 54–57.

Kronemyer, Bob. "6 Concerns about Practice Consolidation," *Dermatology Times*, Jan. 11, 2018. https://www.dermatologytimes.com/dermatology/6
-concerns-about-practice-consolidation.

Lanzone Morgan. "Problems with Drug Rehab Centers," *Lanzone Morgan*, Sept. 25, 2017. https://www.lanzonemorgan.com/drug-rehab-center-abuse-cases
/problems-with-drug-rehab-centers.

Latour, Abby. "To Remedy COVID-19 Impasse, Private Equity Owner Hands Benevis to Private Lender," *S&P Global Market Intelligence*, Oct. 20, 2020. https://www.spglobal.com/marketintelligence/en/news-insights/latest
-news-headlines/to-remedy-covid-19-impasse-private-equity-owner-hands
-benevis-to-private-lender-60805464.

Lawsuit Resource Center. "ResCare Overtime Class Action Lawsuit," *Overtime Pay Laws*, Sept. 2015. https://www.overtimepaylaws.org/rescare-overtime
-class-action-lawsuit.

Lebow, David. "Trumpism and the Dialectics of Neoliberal Reason," *Perspectives on Politics* 17, no. 2, June 2019: 380–395.

Levy, Marc. "Pennsylvania Treatment Firm Accused of Exploiting Addicts, Insurer," *Insurance Journal*, Mar. 27, 2019. https://www.insurancejournal
.com/news/east/2019/03/27/521935.htm.

Little, Penn. "Acadia Healthcare: Very Scary Findings from a 14-Month Investigation," *Seeking Alpha*, Nov. 16, 2018. https://seekingalpha.com/article/4222788
-acadia-healthcare-very-scary-findings-from-a-14-month-investigation.

Mahdaui, Shareef. "Private Equity: What You Need to Know," *Ophthalmology Management* 21, Sept. 1, 2017: 38–69.

Margosian, Emily. "Pulling Back the Curtain on Private Equity," *Dermatology World*, Jan. 10, 2018: 32–41.

———. "Skin in the Game," *Dermatology World*, July 2015: 40–44.

McCallion, Teresa. "Ambulance Companies Change Hands: Is the Move to Private Equity Firms a Bad Thing for U.S. Ambulance Companies," *Journal of Emergency Medical Services*, May 18, 2011. https://www.jems.com/articles
/2011/05/ambulance-companies-change-hands-is-the-move-to-private
-equity-firms-a-bad-thing-for-us-ambulance-companies.html.

———. "What's Next for Rural/Metro after Recent Bankruptcy Filing," *Journal of Emergency Medical Services*, Aug. 31, 2013. https://www.jems.com/operations
/what-s-next-ruralmetro-after-recent-bank/.

McCambridge, Ruth. "Bain Capital Buying Up Methadone Clinics," *Nonprofit Quarterly*, Mar. 26, 2014. https://nonprofitquarterly.org/bain-capital-buying
-up-methadone-clinics/.

McCue, Michael, and Jon Thompson. "The Impact of HCA's Leveraged Buyout on Hospital Performance," *Journal of Healthcare Management* 57, no. 5, 2012: 342–356.

McEachin, John, et al. "Concerns about Registered Behavioral Technicians in Relation to Effective Autism Intervention," *Behavioral Analysis Practice* 10, no. 2, Sept. 27, 2016: 154–163.

McGuire Woods. "Class Action Filed against Aspen Dental," *McGuire Woods*, Nov. 2012. https://www.mcguirewoods.com/client-resources/alerts/2012/11 /class-action-filed-against-aspen-dental.

———. "Dental Management Company Agrees to Be Excluded from Medicare and Medicaid," *McGuire Woods*, Apr. 8, 2014. https://www.mcguirewoods .com/client-resources/alerts/2014/4/dental-management-company-agrees-to -be-excluded-from-medicare-and-medicaid.

McNulty, John. "Halifax Acquires ChanceLight," *Private Equity Professional*, May 16, 2018. https://peprofessional.com/2018/05/halifax-acquires -chancelight.

Molin, Jim Du. "Private Equity Dental Management Companies Come under Fire," *Wealthy Dentist*, Dec. 22, 2018. https://www.thewealthydentist.com /blog/3219/private-equity-dental-management-companies-come-under-fire.

Moriarty, Jim. "Unethical Private-Equity Owned Dental Clinics Receive Well Deserved Attention," *Moriarty.com*, July 2012. https://www.moriarty.com /abusivedentalclinics/content/White_Paper_PDFs/7-26-12-1Unethical -private-equity-owned-dental-clinics-edits.pdf.

Mosumeci, MaryBeth, and Julia Foutz. "Medicaid's Role for Children with Special Health Needs: A Look at Eligibility, Services and Spending," *Henry J. Kaiser Family Foundation*, Feb. 22, 2018. https://www.kff.org/medicaid/issue -brief/medicaids-role-for-children-with-special-needs-a-look-at-eligibility -services-spending.

Mulford, Kim, and Lindy Washburn. "Bellwether Group Homes Ask for State Funds to Avoid 'Health Emergency' for Their Residents," *New Jersey Record*, June 14, 2019.

Mullaney, Tim. "Home Health Spending Projected to Outpace All Other Types of Care," *Home Health Care News*, Feb. 14, 2018. https://homehealthcarenews.com /2018/02/home-health-spending-projected-to-outpace-all-other-types-of-care/.

———. "Jordan, Great Lakes, National Home Health Rebrand as Elara Caring," *Home Health Care News*, July 17, 2018. https://homehealthcarenews.com/2018 /07/jordan-great-lakes-national-home-health-rebrand-as-elara-caring/.

Mullaney, Tim, and Alex Spanko. "HCR ManorCare's Home Health and Hospice Businesses to Get New Owner," *Home Health Care News*, Mar. 4, 2018. https://homehealthcarenews.com/2018/03/hcr-manorcares-home-health -and-hospice-business-to-get-new-owner/.

Murphy, Kara, and Nirad Jain. "Global Healthcare, Private Equity, and Corporate M&A Report," *Bain Report*, Apr. 18, 2018. https://bain.com/insights /global-healthcare-private-equity-and-corporate-ma-report-2018/.

National Center on Addiction and Substance Abuse at Columbia University. "Addiction Medicine: Closing the Gap between Science and Practice," June 2012. https://www.datafiles.samhsa.gov/study-publication/addiction -medicine-closing-gap-between-science-and-practice-nid13893.

Nisen, Max. "Why Are Buyout Firms Ready to Risk It on Acadia?," *National Real Estate Investor*, Oct. 22, 2018. https://www.nreionline.com/alternative -properties/why-are-buyout-firms-ready-to-risk-it-on-acadia.

Noto, Anthony. "Private Ambulance Service Backed by 'Wonder Woman of Wall Street' Files Bankruptcy," *New York Business Journal*, Feb. 25, 2016. https://

www.bizjournal.com/newyork/news/2016/02/25/private-ambulance-service
-backed-by-wonder-woman-of-wall-street-files-bankruptcy.

Ojo, Otegbolo. "Trends in Healthcare Staffing," *Provident*, 2018. https://www
.providenthp.com/expertise/trends-in-healthcare-staffing/.

Oliver, Eric. "Is Private Equity Investment in GI the Next Tech Boom? 6 Insights," *Gastroenterology & Endoscopy News*, Dec. 12, 2017. https://www
.beckersasc.com/gastroenterology-and-endoscopy/is-private-equity
-investment-in-gi-the-next-tech-boom-6-insights.

Pazanowski, Mary Anne. "Private Equity Investment in Health Care Stays
Strong (Corrected)," *Bloomberg Law*, Sept. 21, 2018. https://wwwbna.com
/private-equity-investment-in-health-care-stays-stron-corrected.

Pell, Jill P., et al. "Effect of Reducing Ambulance Response Times on Deaths from
Out of Hospital Cardiac Arrest: Cohort Study," *British Medical Journal* 322,
no. 7299, June 9, 2001: 1385–1388. https://www.ncbi.nlm.nih.gov/pmc/articles
/PMC32251/.

Pellitt, Stephanie. "Thirty-Two States Get a Failing Grade on Parity," *National
Council for Behavioral Health*, Oct. 4, 2018. https://www.thenationalcouncil
.org/capitol-connector/2018/10/32-states-get-a-failing-grade-on-parity
/#:~:text=The%20report%20assigns%20failing%20grades,and%20sub
stance%20use%20disorder%20treatment.

Perritt, Henry H. "An Arm and a Leg: Paying for Helicopter Air Ambulances,"
Journal of Law, Technology and Policy 1, no. 2, 2016: 317–404.

Perry, Angela Elizabeth. "Up in the Air: Inadequate Regulation for Emergency
Air Ambulance Transportation," *Consumers Union*, Mar. 2017. https://
advocacy.consumerreports.org/research/up-in-the-air-inadequate
-regulation-for-emergency-air-ambulance-transportation/#:~:text=Up%20
In%20The%20Air%3A%20Inadequate%20Regulation%20for%20Emer
gency%20Air%20Ambulance%20Transportation,-April%206%2C%20
2017&text=Patients%20are%20at%20a%20disadvantage,provider%20
should%20pick%20them%20up.

Phillips, Lisa. "PE Firms Go in Big for Dental Deals," *Levin Associates*, July 20,
2018. https://healthcare.levinassociates.com/2018/07/20/pe-firms-go-in-big
-for-dental-deals/.

———. "PE Firms Target Healthcare Staffing Services," *Levin Associates*,
Nov. 19, 2018. https://healthcare.levinassociates.com/2018/11/19/pe-firms
-target-healthcare-staffing-services/.

"Possible ResCare Inc. Employee Travel Time Class Action." May 8, 2007, *Big
Class Action*. https://www.bigclassaction.com/lawsuit/rescare-employees
.php.

Provident Healthcare Partners. "Investment & Consolidation in Autism,"
Provident Perspective, Jan.–Mar. 2018. https://www.providenthp.com
/investment-consolidation-in-autism/.

———. "Private Equity Investment in Dental Care," *Provident Perspective*,
Oct. 2017. https://www.providenthp.com/private-equity-investment-in
-dental-care.

———. "Private Equity Investment in Gastroenterology," *Insight*, 2018. https://
www.providenthp.com/private-equity-investment-in-gastroenterology.

R&A Staff. "The U.S. Autism Treatment Market Expected to Reach $2.23 Billion by 2022," *BusinessWire*, May 1, 2018. https://www.businesswire.com/news /home/20180501005785/us-autism-treatment-market-expected-to-reach-$2 .23-billion-by-2022.

Reddy, Rajesh. "Private Equity Investments in Women's Health and Obstetrics and Gynecology Practices," *Obstetrics and Gynecology* 136, no. 6, Dec. 2020: 1217–1220.

Reider, Alan, et al. "Past Lessons, Future Directions: A Roundtable Discussion of Private Equity in Ophthalmology and Current Consolidation Efforts," *CRS Today*, Oct. 2017. https://crstoday.com/articles/2017-aug/past-lessons-future -directions/.

Resnick, Jack S., Jr. "Dermatology Practice Consolidation Fueled by Private Equity Investment. Potential Consequences for the Specialty and Patient," *JAMA Dermatology* 154, no. 1, 2018: 13–14.

Retting, Richard A. "Origins of the Medicare Kidney Disease Establishment: The Social Security Amendments of 1972," in Carl W. Gottschalk, ed., *Biomedical Politics* (Washington, DC: National Academies Press, 1991), 1–51.

Roub, Michael. "5 Dental Trends (DSO) for the Next 5 Years," *Inflection 360*, Apr. 5, 2018. https://inflection360.com/five-dental-trends-dso-for-the-next-5-years.

Schwartz, Jason. "Venture Capital and Methadone," *Addiction & Recovery News*, Apr. 4, 2013. https://recoveryreview.blog/2013/04/02/10077/.

Schwellenbach, Nick, and David Szakonyi. "Inside the Pandemic Cash Bonanza for Private Equity-Backed Firms," *Daily Beast*, POGO, and Anti-Corruption Data Collective, July 15, 2020. https://www.pogo.org/investigation/2020/07 /inside-the-pandemic-cash-bonanza-for-private-equity-backed-firms.

Service Employees International Union. "Universal Health Services: Behind Closed Doors," Mar. 17, 2015. https://closed1293.rssing.com/chan-56427609 /all_p1.html.

Shapiro Law Group. "Are Methadone Clinics Safe?," *Shapiro Law Group*, Nov. 21, 2014. https://www.shapirolawgroup.com/are-methadone-clinics-safe.

Shinkman, Ron. "The Big Business of Dialysis Care," *New England Journal of Medicine Catalyst*, June 9, 2016. https://catalyst-nejm.org/the-big-business-of -dialysis care.

Stevenson, David G., and David C. Grabowski. "Private Equity Investment and Nursing Home Care: Is It a Big Deal?," *Health Affairs* 27, no. 5, Sept.–Oct. 2008: 1399–1408.

Strode, Roger D. "Orthopedics: The New Darling of Private Equity," *Health Care Law Today*, June 1, 2018. https://journals.lww.com/jbjsjournal/subjects/Ethics /Abstract/2020/06030/The_Corporate_Practice_of_Medicine_Ethical.17.aspx.

Suthrum, Praveen. "It's Time to Talk about Private Equity in Gastroenterol-ogy," *KevinMD*, Nov. 14, 2018. https://www.kevinmd.com/blog/2018/11/its -time-to-talk-about-private-equity-in-gastroenterology.

Tan, Sally, et al. "Trends in Private Equity Acquisition of Dermatology Practices in the United States," *JAMA Dermatology* 155, no. 9, July 24, 2019: 1013–1021.

University of Michigan, School of Dentistry. "Alumni Profile: Marcy Borofsky, DDS, 1984," *Dentistry News*, Oct. 30, 2018. https://news.dent.umich.edu/2018 /10/30/alumni-profile-marcy-borofsky-dds-1984.

Vaughan, James S., Catherine J. Robbins, and Todd Rudsenske. "Private Equity Investment in Health Care Services," *Health Affairs*, Sept. 2008. https://healthaffairs.org/doi/full/10.1377/hlthaff.27.51389.

Waud Capital. "Waud Capital Forms Partnership with TDDC to Create the GI Alliance," *Waud Capital*, Nov. 7, 2018. https://www.waudcapital.com/news/waud-capital-forms-partnership-with-tddc-to-create-the-gi-alliance.

Weinzimmer, Bernard. "Private Practice Consolidation Opportunity in the Fragmented Urology Specialty," *Provident Perspective*, Aug. 2019. https://www.providenthp.com/private-practice-consolidation-opportunity-in-the-fragmented-urology-specialty.

Weissman, Cale Guthrie. "Toys 'R' US, Private Equity, and Stagnant Salaries," *Fastcompany*, Sept. 4, 2018. https://www.fastcompany.com/90227917/toys-r-us-private-equity-and-stagnant-salaries.

Wharton School. Twenty-Fifth Private Equity and Venture Capital Conference, "Finding the Silver Lining," New York Athletic Club, New York, Mar. 22, 2019.

Wiggins, Kaye. "US Stock Market Beats Private Equity's Returns for First Time," *Financial Times*, Feb. 24, 2020. https://www.ft.com/content/e73396be-54a4-11ea-8841-482eed0038b1.

Yetter, Eric J., and J. Andrew Snyder. "Physicians First: The Physician Seller's Guide to Private Equity Firms Investing in Ophthalmology," *Physicians First*, Nov. 2018.

Newspapers, Magazines, Blogs, and Other Mass Media

Abelson, Reed. "When a Health Insurer Also Wants to Be a Hospice Company," *New York Times*, June 22, 2018.

Abelson, Reed, and Katie Thomas. "UnitedHealthcare Sues Dialysis Chain over Billing," *New York Times*, July 1, 2016.

Abram, Susan. "Why Kidney Dialysis Patients Are Pushing to Improve Dialysis Center," *Health Line*, June 4, 2018. https://www.healthline.com/health-news-/why-kidney-dialysis-patients-are-pushing-to-improve-dialysis-centers.

Ackerman, Todd. "Medicaid Dental Clinics Targeted, Accused of Mistreatment," *Houston Chronicle*, Apr. 30, 2016.

Adams, Rosalind. "What the Fuck Just Happened?," *BuzzFeed News*, Dec. 7, 2016. https://www.buzzfeednews.com/article/rosalindadams/intake#.jomko%20jkm.

Anderson, Elisha. "Abuse Caught on Video at Michigan's Biggest Autism Therapy Provider," *Detroit Free Press*, Oct. 5, 2018. https://www.freep.com/story/news/investigations/2018/10/05/.

AP News. "Physician Questions Single-Engine Helicopters after Crash," *AP News*, May 26, 2018. https://apnews.com/article/cf11161e0b3c46cc9f1bc7e375ec3fcd.

Appelbaum, Eileen. "CEPR Statement on New Labor Guidance Allowing Risky Private Equity Investments in Workers' 401(k) Accounts," *Center for Economic and Policy Research*, June 5, 2020. https://cepr.net/cepr-statement-on-new-labor-department-guidance-allowing-risky-private-equity-investments-in-workers-401k-accounts/.

———. "How Private Equity Makes You Sicker," *American Prospect*, Oct. 7, 2019. https://prospect.org/health/how-private-equity-makes-you-sicker.

———. "Private Equity Is a Driving Force behind Devious Surprise Billing," Hill, May 16, 2019. https://thehill.com/opinion/healthcare/444011-private-equity-is-a-driving-force-behind-devious-surprise-billing.

Appelbaum, Eileen, and Rosemary Batt. "Private Equity and Surprise Medical Billing," *Institute for New Economic Thinking*, Sept. 4, 2019. https://www.ineteconomics.org/perspectives/blog/private-equity-and-surprise-medical-billing.

———. "Private Equity Tries to Protect Another Profit Center," *American Prospect*, Sept. 9, 2019. https://prospect.org/articles/private-equity-tries-to-protect-another-profit-center.

Aschoff, Nicole M. "Ban Private Equity," *Jacobin Magazine*, June 16, 2019. http://www.jacobinmag.com/2019/06/private-equity-blackstone-workers-inequality/.

Asmail, M. Asif. "Investing in War," *Center for Public Integrity*, May 19, 2014. https://publicintegrity.org/national-security-investing-in-war.

Bain, Benjamin. "Private Equity Gets a Big Win with U.S. Nod to Tap 401(k) Plans," *Bloomberg News*, June 3, 2020. https://www.bloomberg.com/news/articles/2020-06-03/private-equity-gets-a-big-win-with-u-s-nod-to-tap-401k-plans.

Barr, Alistair. "Baker to Retire from Carlyle Group," *MarketWatch*, Mar. 7, 2005. https://www.marketwatch.com/story/james-baker-to-retire-from-carlyle-group/.

Batt, Rosemary, and Eileen Appelbaum. "Hospital Bailouts Begin—For Those Owned by Private Equity Firms," *American Prospect*, Apr. 2, 2020. https://prospect.org/economy/hospital-bailouts-begin-for-those-owned-by-private-equity-firms/.

Berardi, Francesca, et al. "After Allegations of Physical Abuse against Students, Several Cities Are Questioning Camelot Education," *Slate*, Mar. 2017. https://slate.com/news-and-politics/2017/03/camelot-education-under-scrutiny-in-philadelphia-houston-and-columbus-georgia.html.

———. "Camelot under Siege," *Slate*, Mar. 2017. https://www.propublica.org/article/camelot-under-siege.

Berfield, Susan, et al. "Tears 'R' Us: The World's Biggest Toy Store Didn't Have to Die," *Bloomberg Businessweek*, June 6, 2018. https://www.bloomberg.com/businessweek/tears-r-us-the-world's-biggest-toy-store-didnt-have-to-die.

Berlin, Andrew. "LPCI Air Medical Lands US $2.2 Billion of Debt for AMR Purchase," *Reuters*, Aug. 11, 2017. https://www.reuters.com/article/air-medical-acquisition/lpc-air-medical-lands-us2-2bn-of-debt-for-amr-purchase-idUSL1N1KX0T7.

Bernhard, Blyth. "Castlewood Eating Disorder Center Changes Name following Malpractice Lawsuits," *St. Louis Today*, July 24, 2018. https://www.stltoday.com/news/local/metro/castlewood-eating-disorder-center-changes-name-following-malpractice-lawsuits.

Bernstein, Nina. "Deletion of Word in Welfare Bill Opens Foster Care to Big Businesses," *New York Times*, May 4, 1997.

———. "A Father's Last Wish, and a Daughter's Anguish," *New York Times*, Sept. 26, 2014.

Blumenthal, Robin Goldwyn. "Barron's Insynt—Manor Care's Approach: Short-Term Rehabilitation," *Wall Street Journal*, Mar. 2000, C24.

Bort, Ryan. "John Oliver Sees Ills in For-Profit Dialysis Centers," *Newsweek*, May 15, 2017. https://www.newsweek.com/jphn-oliver-sees-ills-in-for-profit-dialysis-centers.

Brentwood Capital Advisors. "Overall Market Update and Economic Review: 3Q 2018," Dec. 2018. http://www.brentwoodcap.com/wp-content/uploads/2018/12/BCA-Quarterly_3Q2018-HC-Services-1.pdf.

Brickley, Peg. "Turnaround Executive Lynn Tilton to Testify about Failed Ambulance Company," *Fox Business*, June 8, 2017. https://www.foxbusiness.com/features/turnaround-executive-lynn-tilton-to-testify-about-failed-ambulance-company.

Brickley, Peg, and Tom Corrigan. "Lynn Tilton's Firm Took Millions from Failing Ambulance Operator," *Wall Street Journal*, Feb. 14, 2017.

Business Wire. "ACES and General Atlantic Announce Strategic Partnership," *Yahoo!*, Jan. 15, 2020. https://finance.yahoo.com/news/aces-general-atlantic-announce-strategic-partnership.

———. "Aspen Dental Management to Acquire ClearChoice Management Services," Nov. 16, 2020. https://www.businesswire.com/news/home/20201116005367/en/aspen-dental-management-to-acquire-clearchoice-management-services.

———. "H. I. G. Growth Partners Announces the Formation of Community Intervention Services and Completes the Acquisition of South Bay Mental Health," *Business Wire*, Apr. 17, 2012. https://www.businesswire.com/home/20120417005989/en/H.I.G.-growth-partners-announes-the-formation-of-community-intervention-services-and-completes-the-acquisition-of-south-bay-mental-health.

———. "Ned Carlson Appointed CEO of Trumpet Behavioral Health," *Business Wire*, Aug. 21, 2017. https://www.businesswire.com/news/home/20170821005130/en/ned-carlson-appointed-ceo-of-trumpet-behavioral-health.

———. "Sverica Capital Management Announces Investment in In Vitro Sciences," *Sverica*, Oct. 22, 2019. https://sverica.com/news-article/sverica-capital-management-announces investment-in-in-vitro-sciences.

———. "Western Dental Completes Transformational Acquisitions of a DSO Supporting 63 Dental Offices in California, Texas, and Alabama," *Business Wire*, Dec. 5, 2018. https://www.businesswire.com/news/home/20181205005227/en/Western-Dental-Enters-Definitive-Agreement-Acquire-DSO.

Canderle, Sebastien. "Modern Private Equity and the End of Creative Destruction," *CFA Institute*, May 13, 2020. https://blogs.cfainstitute.org/investor/2020/05/13/modern-private-equity-and-the-end-of-creative-destruction/.

Cantrell, Amanda. "This Venture Capital Fund Wants to Get You Pregnant," *Institutional Investor*, May 15, 2019. https://www.institutionalinvestor.com/article/b1ff3x6hcl5wbb/This-Venture-Capital-Fund-Wants-to-Get-You-Pregnant.

Carpenter, Jacob. "Park Royal Hospital Faces More Trouble with Lawsuit over Suicide of Psychiatric Patient Theodore Ousback Jr.," *Naples Daily News* (FL), Jan. 9, 2016. https://www.naplesnews.com/news/health/park-royal-hospital -faces-more-trouble-with-lawsuit-over-suicide-of-psychiatric-patient -theodore-ousback-jr.

Carr, Sarah, et al. "These For-Profit Schools Are 'Like a Prison,'" *Slate* and *Phillyvoice*, Mar. 9, 2017. https://www.phillyvoice.com/these-for-profit -schools-are-like-a-prison.

Carroll, Linda. "Patients at For-Profit Dialysis Centers Less Likely to Get Kidney Transplants," *Reuters*, Sept. 10, 2019. https://www.reuters.com/article/us -health-dialysis/patients-at-for-profit-dialysis-centers-less-likely-to-get -kidney-transplants.

Ciavaglia, Jo. "After Charges Liberation Way to Close Its Doors," *Intelligencer*, Apr. 13, 2019. https://www.theintell.com/news/20190412/after-charges -liberation-way-to-close-its-doors.

Confessore, Nicholas. " 'Too Rich for Conflicts': Trump Appointee May Have Many, Seen and Unseen," *New York Times*, Nov. 10, 2017.

Consumer Affairs. "Consumer Complaints, Western Dental Reviews," *Consumer Affairs*, 2018. www.consumeraffairs.com/dentists/dds_western_dental.html ?page=2.

———. "Ratings for Aspen Dental," *Consumer Affairs*, Dec. 26, 2018. https://www .consumeraffairs.com/dentists/dds_oh_aspen_dental.html.

Cooper, Katie. " 'Dialysis Centers on Every Corner' in Southern California," *KCET*, Oct. 30, 2018. https://www.kcet.org/shows/socal-connected/dialysis -centers-on-every-corner-in-southern-california-the-business-of-kidney -disease-is-booming.

Cooper, Laura. "KKR to Acquire Majority Interest in Heartland Dental," *Wall Street Journal*, Mar. 7, 2018.

Copley, Caroline. "U.S. Seeks to Cut Dialysis Costs with More Home Care versus Clinics," *Reuters*, Mar. 3, 2019. https://www.reuters.com/article/us-usa -healthcare-dialysis/u-s-seeks-to-cut-dialysis-costs-with-more-home-care -versus-clinics.

Corkery, Michael, and Ben Protess. "How the Twinkie Made the Superrich Even Richer," *New York Times*, Dec. 10, 2016.

Corkery, Michael, and Jessica Silver-Greenberg. "The Giant, under Attack," *New York Times*, Dec. 27, 2017.

Court, Emma. "Doctor's Offices Are a Hot Investment—What Does That Mean for Profit vs. Patient Care," *Market Watch*, June 13, 2018. https://www .marketwatch.com/story/doctors-are-being-bought-up-by-private-equity -and-its-your-health-on-the-line-2018-06-08.

Covert, Bryce. "You Buy It, You Break It," *Atlantic*, July–Aug. 2018. https://www .magzter.com/stories/News/The-Atlantic/You-Buy-It-You-Break-It.

Creswell, Julie, and Reed Abelson. "A Giant Hospital Chain Is Blazing a Profit Trail," *New York Times*, Aug. 14, 2012.

Dallas News Administrator. "All Smiles Dental Centers Turning Away Young Medicaid Patients, Closing Clinics," *Dallas News*, July 26, 2012. https://www .dallasnews.com/news/news/2012/07/26/all-smiles-dental-centers-turning -away-young-medicaid-patients-closing-clinics.

Dayen, David. "Toys 'R' US Workers Take on Private-Equity Barons: 'You Ought to Be Ashamed,'" *Nation*, June 5, 2018. https://www.thenation.com /article/toys-r-us-workers-take-on-private-equity-barons-you-ought-to-be -ashamed.

———. "Will the Tax Act Set Back Private Equity?," *American Prospect*, July 2, 2018. https://prospect.org/power/will-tax-act-set-back-private-equity/.

DeLombaerde, Geert. "Pharos Buys Adolescent Treatment Center," *Nashville Post*, Oct. 24, 2016. https://www.nashvillepost.com/business/health-care /behavioral/article/20838228/pharos-buys-adolescent-treatment-center.

"Dental Franchises Show Steady Growth," *USA Today*, Apr. 7, 2013. https://www .usatoday.com/story/money/business/2013/04/07/dental-franchises-show -steady-growth.

DePillis, Lydia. "Rich Investors May Have Let a Hospital Go Bankrupt. Now, They Could Profit from the Land," *CNN Business*, July 29, 2019. https://www .cnn.com/2019/07/29/economy/hahneman-hospital-closing-philadelphia /index/html.

Donmoyer, Ryan J. "Baucus Drops Higher Private-Equity Levy from Tax Bill," *Bloomberg News*, Dec. 3, 2010. https://www.bloomberg.com/news/articles /2010-12-03/tax-boost-for-hedge-fund-executives-dropped-from-bill/.

Dunn, Steven R. "A Dad's Journey with an Eating Disorder: Castlewood/ Alsana," *Castlewood Victims Unite*, Oct. 1, 2018. https://www.castlewood victimsunite.org/single-post/2018/10/01/a-dads-journey-with-an-eating -disorder-castlewood-alsana.

Dwyer, Jim. "Bankruptcy of TransCare Strains New York's Emergency Services," *New York Times*, Apr. 14, 2016.

Espinoza, Javier. "Private Equity Plays Risky Game of Musical Chairs," *Financial Times*, Sept. 24, 2018.

Eyesteve. "The Return of Private Equity to Ophthalmology," *Eyesteve*, Nov. 15, 2017. https://eyesteve.com/private-equity-ophthalmology.

Fallstrom, Jerry. "Carlton Palms Facility for Severely Disabled to Close after State Moves to Yank License," *Orlando Sentinel*, Oct. 29, 2018. https://www .orlandosentinel.com/news/lake/os-carlton-palms-for-disabled-to-close -20180510-story.html.

Faludi, Susan C. "Safeway LBO Yields Vast Profits but Exacts a Heavy Toll," *Wall Street Journal*, May 16, 1990, 3.

Fields, Robin. "God Help You, You're on Dialysis," *Atlantic*, Dec. 10, 2010. https://www.theatlantic.com/magazine/archive/2010/12/-god-help-you -youre-on-dialysis/308308/.

Foltin, Craig, et al. "Public Pension Underfunding," *SF Strategic Finance*, Sept. 1, 2018. https://sfmagazine.com/post-entry/september-2018-public-pension -underfunding/.

Frakt, Austin. "Medical Mystery: Something Happened to U.S. Health Spending after 1980," *New York Times*, May 14, 2018.

Freedberg, Sydney P. "Bain's For-Profit Methadone Clinics: Drug Users Turn Death Dealers as Methadone from Bain Hits the Street," *Bloomberg News*, Feb. 7, 2013. https://www.pnhp.org/news/2013/Feb./bains-for-profit -methadone-clinics-drug-users-turn-death-dealers-as-methadone-from -bain-hits-the-street.

———. "Dental Abuse Seen Driven by Private Equity Investments," *Bloomberg News*, May 16, 2012. https://www.bloomberg.com/news/articles/2012-05-17/dental-abuse-seen-driven-by-private-equity-investments.

Fugazy, Danielle. "Why Private Equity Firms like Veterinarians, Ophthalmologists and Dentists," *Middle Market*, Apr. 19, 2018. https://www.themiddlemarket.com/news/private-equity-firms-are-investing-in-veterinatians-ophthalmologists-and-dentists.

Galli, Cindy, Stephanie Zimmerman, and Brian Ross. "Sky Rage: Bills, Debt, Lawsuits Follow Helicopter Medevac Trips," *ABC News*, Mar. 16, 2016. https://abcnews.go.com/US/sky-rage-bills-debt-lawsuits-follow-helicopter-medevac/story?id=37669153.

Galston, William A. "The Perils of Corporate Concentration," *Wall Street Journal*, June 20, 2018.

Gara, Antoine. "Vanguard Pushes into Private Equity by Accessing Dealmaking like Stephen Schwarzman, Robert Smith, and Orlando Bravo," *Forbes*, Feb. 5, 2020. https://www.forbes.com/sites/antoinegara/2020/02/05/vanguard-pushes-into-private-equity-by-accessing-dealmakers-like-stephen-schwarzman-robert-smith-and-orlando-bravo.

Gelles, David, and David Yaffe-Bellany. "Shareholder Value Is No Longer Everything, Top CEOs Say," *New York Times*, Aug. 19, 2019.

George, John. "City Councilwoman Introduces Bill to Prevent the Next Hahnemann," *Philadelphia Business Journal*, Oct. 10, 2019. https://www.bizjournals.com/philadelphia/news/2019/10/10/city-councilwoman-introduces-bill-to-prevent-the.html.

Globe News Wire. "Onex Completes Sale of BrightSpring Health Services," *Globe News Wire*, Mar. 5, 2019. http://www.globenewswire.com/en/news-release/2019/03/05/1748473/0/en/Onex-Completes-Sale-of-BrightSpring-Health-Services.html.

Gluck, Frank. "Park Royal Hospital Patient Care Deficiencies Highlighted in Federal Inspection Reports," *USA Today*, Nov. 16, 2017.

Goode, Erica. "Centers to Treat Eating Disorders Are Growing, and Raising Concerns," *New York Times*, Mar. 14, 2016.

Gottfried, Miriam. "Private-Equity Firms Scramble to Shore Up Coronavirus-Hit Holdings," *Wall Street Journal*, Apr. 13, 2020.

Gottfried, Miriam, and Rachel Louise Ensign. "The New Business Banker: A Private-Equity Firm," *Wall Street Journal*, Aug. 12, 2018.

Gottfried, Miriam, and Ryan Tracy. "Risky Deals Return to Leveraged-Buyout Market," *Wall Street Journal*, Oct. 24, 2018.

Group Dentistry Now. "Taking a Deeper Look at KKR's Investment in Heartland Dental, the Largest DSO in Country," *Group Dentistry Now*, Mar. 13, 2018. https://groupdentistrynow.com/taking-a-deeper-look-at-kkr-investment-in-heartland-dental.

———. "Why Private Equity Firms Like Dentists, Veterinarians, and Ophthalmologists," *Group Dentistry Now*, May 1, 2018. https://groupdentistrynow.com/why-private-equity-firms-like-dentists-veterinarians-and-ophthalmologists.

Gustafson, Krystina. "Payless ShoeSource Files for Chapter 11 Bankruptcy," *CNBC News*, Apr. 4, 2017. https://www.cnbc.com/2017/04/payless-shoesource -files-for-chapter-11-bankruptcy.html.

Hafner, Katie. "Why Private Equity Is Furious over a Paper in a Dermatology Journal," *New York Times*, Oct. 26, 2018.

Hafner, Katie, and Griffin Palmer. "Skin Cancers Rise, Along with Questionable Treatments," *New York Times*, Nov. 20, 2017.

Hallman, Ben. "Hospice Inc.: How Dying Became a Multibillion Dollar Industry," *Huffington Post*, June 19, 2014. https://projects.huffingtonpost.com/hospice-inc.

Harris, Jon. "Easton Hospital Notifies State of 694 Layoffs, Possible Closure by End of June if Sale Collapses," *Morning Call* (PA), May 5, 2020.

Head, Elan. "FAA Reauthorization Act Could Mean Changes for Air Ambulance Industry," *Vertical Magazine*, May 24, 2018. https://www.verticalmag.com /news/faa-reauthorization-act-could-mean-changes-for-air-ambulance -industry.

Healy, Beth. "Bain Capital Sees Opportunity in Methadone Clinics," *Boston Globe*, Apr. 13, 2014. https://preservedstories.com/2014/04/13/bain-capital -sees-opportunity-in-methadone-clinics-boston-globe-april-13-2014/.

Heller, Matthew. "Kindred Healthcare to Pay $125M over Medicare Fraud," CFO, Jan. 12, 2016. https://www.cfo.com/fraud/2016/01/kindred-healthcare-pay -125m-medicare-fraud/#:~:text=Matthew%20Heller&text=Kindred%20 Healthcare%2C%20the%20largest%20U.S.,patients%20to%20inflate%20 Medicare%20billings.

Hensley-Clancy, Molly. "Hard Lessons," *BuzzFeed News*, Mar. 22, 2017. https:// www.buzzfeednews.com/article/mollyhensleyclancy/hard-lessons.

Hiltzik, Michael. "Column: Dialysis Firms' Profits Are Obscene, What Will Happen if California Tries to Cap Them?," *Los Angeles Times*, July 20, 2018.

Hilzenrath, David S. "Vencor Faces $1 Billion Claim: U.S. Seeking Medicare Repayments," *Washington Post*, Mar. 14, 2000, E1.

Hirsch, Lauren, and Lauren Thomas. "Life after Liquidation: Toys R US Stores Will Be Back This Holiday Season, This Time with a Tech Partner," CNBC, July 18, 2019. https://www.cnbc.com/2019/07/18/toys-r-us-plots-comeback -this-holiday-season-this-time-with-a-tech-partner/.

Hoffman, Liz. "How Four Private-Equity Firms Cleaned Up on Multiplans," *Wall Street Journal*, May 6, 2016.

Huber, Mark. "Air Methods CEO: Air EMS Market Oversaturated," *AIN Online: Business Aviation*, Oct. 6, 2015. https://www.ainonline.com/aviation-news /business-aviation/2015-10-06/air-methods-ceo-air-ems-market-over saturated.

Hudak, Stephen. "Plagued by Abuse Claims and Deaths, Carlton Palms Finally Closes Doors to Florida's Disabled," *Orlando Sentinel*, Oct. 25, 2018. https:// www.orlandosentinel.com/news/lake/os-ne-carlton-palms-closes-20181025 -story.html.

Husyar, Andrew. "Tim Geithner and the Revolving Door," *New Yorker* Nov. 20, 2013. https://www.newyorker.com/business/currency/tim-geithner-and-the -revolving-door.

Idzelis, Christine. "Buyout Firms Will Make the Next Downturn Worse, Moody's Says," *Institutional Investor*, Dec. 4, 2018. https://www.institutional investor.com/article/b1c3425ctmh8gz/Buyout-Firms-Will-Make-the-Next -Downturn-Worse-Moody-s-Says.

———. "Everything about Private Equity Reeks of Bubble, Party On," *Institutional Investor*, July 22, 2018. https://www.institutionalinvestor.com/article /b195s0y2vfll69/Everything-About-Private-Equity-Reeks-of-Bubble-Party-On.

———. "The Most Aggressive Buyout Firms Taking Debt-Financed Dividends," *Institutional Investor*, Oct. 18, 2018. https://www.institutionalinvestor.com /article/b1bfrk75zvtz9d/The-Most-Aggressive-Buyout-Firms-Taking-Debt -Financed-Dividends#:~:text=Carlyle%20Group%2C%20Golden%20Gate% 20Capital,aggressive%20in%20taking%20large%20dividends.&text=Priva te%20equity%20firms%20have%20been,%2C%20debt%2Dfinanced%20div idend%20deals.

———. "Watch Out for This Ballooning Pool of Private Equity-Owned Companies," *Institutional Investor*, Sept. 6, 2019. https://www.institutional investor .com/article/blhljrn5gqq9g8/watch-out-for-this-ballooning-pool-of-private -equity-owned-companies.

Ingraham, Christopher. "CDC Releases Grim New Opioid Overdose Figures: We're Talking about More than Exponential Increases," *Washington Post*, Dec. 21, 2017.

Institutional Investor. "Private Equity Managers Are 'Running a Grift,' Pennsylvania Treasury Says," *Institutional Investor*, Aug. 26, 2019. https:// www.institutionalinvestor.com/article/blgwp2v4dpg4d8/private-equity managers-are-running-a-grift-pennsylvania-treasury-says.

Ivory, Danielle, Ben Protess, and Kitty Bennett. "When You Dial 911 and Wall Street Answers," *New York Times*, June 25, 2016.

Ivory, Danielle, Ben Protess, and Jennifer Daniel. "What Can Go Wrong when Private Equity Takes over a Public Service," *New York Times*, June 25, 2016.

Jain, Nirad, Kara Murphy, and Jeremy Martin. "Why Private Equity Loves Retail Healthcare," *Forbes*, Apr. 4, 2018. https://www.forbes.com/sites /baininsights/2018/04/04/why-private-equity-loves-retail-healthcare.

Kelly, Jason. "Everything Is Private Equity Now," *Bloomberg Businessweek*, Oct. 3, 2019. https://www.bloomberg.com/news/features/2019-10-03/how -private-equity-works-and-took-over-everything.

Kincaid, Ellie. "Envision Healthcare Infiltrated America's ERs: Now It's Facing a Backlash," *Forbes*, May 15, 2018. https://www.forbes.com/site/elliekincaid /2018-05-15/envision-healthcare-infiltrated-america's-er-now-its-facing-a -backlash.

Klein, Naomi. "James Baker's Double Life," *Nation*, Oct. 12, 2004. https://www .thenation.com/article/james-baker's-double-life.

Knopper, Steve. "How Wickenburg, Arizona, a Town of 7,000, Became the Rehab Capital of the US," *Mic*, May 12, 2018. https://www.mic.com/articles/189305 /how-wickenburg-arizona-a-town-of-7,000-became-the-rehab-capital-of-the -us.

Kodjak, Alison. "Investors Seek to Buy Opioid Treatment Facilities," *National Public Radio*, Oct. 6, 2016. https://www.npr.org/sections/health-shots/2016 /06/10/480663056/investors-seek-to-buy-opioid-treatment-facilities.

Kosman, Josh. "Nursing Home CEO Wants $100M Payout amid Bankruptcy Threat," *New York Post*, June 2, 2017.

Krouse, Sarah. "State and Local Pension Woes Are Starting to Bite—The Shortfall Is Hitting Retirees with Little Time to Engineer a Plan B," *Wall Street Journal*, July 2018, A1.

Lebherz, James E. "The Lord of the Manor: Nursing Home, Hotel Magnate Bainum Ponders Run for MD. Governor," *Washington Post*, Apr. 5, 1994.

Levine, Art. "Dark Side of a Bain Success," *Salon*, July 18, 2012. https://www.salon.com/2012/07/18/dark-side-of-a-bain-success.

Levine, Dan, and Martha Graybow. "Special Report: Dial 911-for-Profit—Just Don't Tell a Firehouse," *Reuters*, Apr. 15, 2011. https://www.reuters.com/article/us-ambulance/special-report-dial-911-for-profit-just-dont-tell-a-firehouse-idINTRE73E3D720110415.

Lipton, Eric, and Kenneth P. Vogel. "Biden Aides' Ties to Consulting and Investment Firms Pose Ethics Test," *New York Times*, Nov. 28, 2020.

Lopez, German. "Trump Just Signed a Bipartisan Bill to Confront the Opioid Epidemic," *Vox*, Oct. 24, 2018. https://www.vox.com/policy-and-politics/2018/9/28/17913938/trump-just-signed-bipartisan-bill-to-confront-the-opiod-epidemic.

Lurie, Julia. "Mom, When They Look at Me, They See Dollar Signs," *Mother Jones*, Mar.–Apr. 2019. https://www.motherjones.com/crime-justice/2019/02/opioid-epidemic-how-rehab-recruiters-are-luring-recovery-addicts-into-a-deadly-cycle.

"Manor Care Plans Restructure after Takeover by Carlyle," *Washington Post*, Mar. 6, 2000, C24.

Mathis, Will, and Tom Metcalf. "Private Equity Is Pouring Money into a Dental Empire," *Bloomberg News*, June 28, 2018. https://www.bloombergquint.com/business/wall-street-transforms-dentistry-into-a-credit-fueled-gold-rush.

McCann, David. "Two CFOs Tell a Tale of Fraud at HealthSouth," *CFO Magazine*, Mar. 27, 2017. https://www.cfo.com/fraud/2017/03/two-cfos-tell-a-tale-of-fraud-at-healthsouth.

McDermott, Colin, and Corey Palasota. "Visiting the Home Health Marketplace: Observations of the Current Transaction Environment," *VMG Health*, Feb. 16, 2018. https://vmghealth.com/blog/home-health-current-transactions/.

McElhaney, Alicia. "Private Equity Investments Are Going to Lose Value: How Much Is Anyone's Guess," *Institutional Investor*, Apr. 3, 2020. https://www.institutionalinvestor.com/article/b111dhbfqz1pp3/Private-Equity-Investments-Are-Going-to-Lose-Value-How-Much-Is-Anyone-s-Guess.

Mclean, Bethany. "Too Big to Fail, COVID-19 Edition: How Private Equity Is Winning the Coronavirus Crisis," *Vanity Fair*, Apr. 9, 2020. https://www.vanityfair.com/news/2020/04/how-private-equity-is-winning-the-coronavirus-crisis.

McNeill, Jim. "New Report Reveals Major Problems in Behavioral Care at UHS, Further Expansion of Federal Probe," *Behind Closed Doors at UHS*, Mar. 17, 2015. https://closed1293.rssing.com/chan-56427609/all_p1.html.

Meier, Barry. "Air Ambulances Are Multiplying and Costs Rise," *New York Times*, May 3, 2005.

Miller, Carol Marbin, and Monique O. Madan. "Beset by Rapes, Rats, Scalding, Florida Homes for Disabled Lose License," *Tampa Bay Times*, Apr. 27, 2018. https://www.tampabay.com/news/health/Beset-by-rapes-rats-scalding -Florida-home-for-disabled-could-lose-license_167743670/#:~:text=Health -,Beset%20by%20rapes%2C%20rats%2C%20scalding%2C%20Florida%20 home,for%20disabled%20could%20lose%20license&text=Since%20at%20 least%202013%2C%20when,vainly%20to%20shut%20it%20down.

Mokhiber, Russell, ed. "Evercare Hospice to Pay $18 Million to Settle False Claims Charges," *Corporate Crime Reporter*, July 13, 2016. https://www .corporatecrimereporter.com/news/200/evercare-hospice-to-pay-$18 -million-to-settle-false-claims-charges.

Monk, Ashby. "Having Skin in the Game Isn't So Easy Anymore for Private Equity Managers," *Institutional Investor*, Feb. 19, 2019. https://www.institutionalinves tor.com/article/b1d6m27r19str5/having-skin-in-the-game-isnt-so-easy-any more-for-private-equity-managers/.

Monk, John. "SC Woman Charged in Alleged $9 Million Fraud involving Autism Cases," *State* (SC), Jan. 16, 2019. https://www.thestate.com/news/local/crime /article224618415.html.

Morgenson, Gretchen, and Lillian Rizzo. "Who Killed Toys 'R' Us? Hint: It Wasn't Only Amazon," *Wall Street Journal*, Aug. 23, 2018.

Mullenkamp, Carrick. "HCA Pays Owners $2 Billion," *Wall Street Journal*, Nov. 10, 2010.

Murphy, H. Lee. "Rush Ortho Group Scopes Out Private-Equity Infusion," Nov. 6, 2018, *Crain's Chicago Business*. https://www.chicagobusiness.com /health-care/rush-ortho-group-scopes-out-private-equity-infusion.

Nakamoto, Chris. "Major Problems Found at Group Home after Specialized Needs Resident Allegedly Beaten, Sexually Assaulted," *WBRZ News*, July 9, 2018. https://www.wbrz.com/news/major-problems-found-at-group-home -after-special-needs-resident-allegedly-beaten-sexually-assaulted.

News 4. "Castlewood Treatment Center and Mark Schwartz Sued for Malprac- tice," *News 4 Investigates*, YouTube, Dec. 6, 2016. https://www.youtube.com /watch?V=BUkegWLBBPA.

Nilsen, Ella. "Methadone—National Issues and Lack of Regulation," *Sentinel Source*, Nov. 10, 2014. https://www.sentinelsource.com/methadone-national -issues-and-lack-of-regulation.

Nolan, Hamilton. "The Worker Person's Guide to the Industry That Might Kill Your Company," *Splinter News*, Apr. 2, 2018. https://splinternews.com/the -worker-persons-guide-to-the-industry-that-might-kill-your-company/.

Oliver, John. "Rehab," *Last Week Tonight*, HBO, May 20, 2018.

Olmos, David R. "Federal Agents Raid Offices of Western Dental," *Los Angeles Times*, June 7, 1997. https://wwwlatimes.com/archives/la-xpm-1997-06-07-fi -941-story.

Or, Amy. "McCallum Pursues Sale amid PE Interest in Eating Disorder Treat- ment," *Wall Street Journal*, June 16, 2014.

———. "Webster Capital Explores Sale of Epic Health Services," *Wall Street Journal*, Apr. 21, 2016.

Oran, Olivia. "Obamacare Helps Private Equity Get Its Rehab Clinic Fix," *Thomson Reuters*, Dec. 8, 2014. https://www.reuters.com/article

/rehabclinics-ma-privateequity/dealtalk-obamacare-helps-private-equity
-get-its-rehab-clinic-fix-idUSL2N0TI0SQ20141208.

ParentAdvocates. "Schools for Children with Autism Are Expensive, So Parents
in NYC Sue and Have NYC Board of Education Pay for the Schooling,"
ParentAdvocates, Oct. 2018. http://www.parentadvocates.org/nicecontent
/dsp_printable.cfm?articleID=7199.

Parr, Olivia. "DermOne Brand May Be Exiting Healthcare, but Local Doctors Stay
in Business," *Port City Daily* (NC), Mar. 8, 2018. https://portcitydaily.com
/healthcare/2018/03/08/dermone-brand-is-exiting-healthcare-market
-nationwide/#:~:text=Healthcare-,DermOne%20brand%20may%20be%20
exiting%20healthcare%2C%20but,doctors%20to%20stay%20in%20
business&text=WILMINGTON%20%E2%80%94%20DermOne%20has%20
decided%20to%20exit%20the%20healthcare%20market%20nationwide
.&text=The%20DermOne%20dermatology%20offices%20in,Town%20
Center%20will%20be%20closing.

———. "DermOne to Close Six Locations on Friday," *Port City Daily* (NC), Mar. 7,
2018. https://portcitydaily.com/business/2018/03/07/dermone-to-close-6
-locations-on-friday.

Pearlstein, Steven. "The $786 Million Question: Does Steve Schwarzman—or
Anyone Else—Deserve to Make That Much," *Washington Post*, Jan. 4, 2019.

Perkes, Courtney. "As Demand for ABA Therapy Increases, Investors Buy In,"
DisabilityScoop, Oct. 23, 2018. https://www.disabilityscoop.com/2018/10/23
/as=demand-for-aba-therapy-increases-investors-buy-in.

Perlberg, Heather. "Private Equity's Backdoor Path to PPP Cash Revealed in Data
Dump," *Washington Post*, July 9, 2020. https:www.washingtonpost.com
/business/on-small-businesses/private-equity's-backdoor-path-to-ppp-cash
-revealed-in-data-dump.

———. "Rescue Cash Too Hot for KKR Proves Irresistible to Many PE Peers,"
Bloomberg News, July 2, 2020. https://news.bloombergtax.com/coronavirus
/private-equity-on-edge-with-u-s-plan-to-name-relief-recipients.

Perlberg, Heather, and Benjamin Bain. "Private Equity Wields More Power than
Ever as Warren Picks Fight," *Bloomberg Businessweek*, Oct. 3, 2019. https://
www.bloomberg.com/businessweek/private-equity-wields-more-power
-than-ever-as-warren-picks-fight.

Perlberg, Heather, Tom Metcalf, and Sabrina Willmer. "Private Equity Poised to
Face a Reckoning after Gilded Decade," *Bloomberg News*, May 1, 2020.
https://www.bloomberg.com/news/articles/2020-05-01/private-equity
-poised-to-face-a-reckoning-after-gilded-decade.

Picchi, Aimee. "Private Equity Rushed into Health Care—Now, a Nurse Warns,
'Be Scared,'" *CBS News*, July 29, 2019. https://cbsnews.com.news/private
-equity-rushed-into-health-care-now-a-hospital-fate-raises-fears.

Pollack, Andrew. "Eating Disorders a New Front in Insurance Fight," *New York
Times*, Oct. 13, 2011.

Primack, Dan. "Trimaran Claws at Its Own Investors: Dying Private Equity
Firm Tries for One More Score," *Fortune Magazine*, Mar. 12, 2012. https://
fortune.com/2012/03/12/trimaran-claws-at-its-own-investors/.

Private Equity Stakeholder Project. "H. I. G. Capital's Mental Health Company
Files for Bankruptcy amid Fraud Litigation," Jan. 19, 2021. https://pestake

holder.org/h-i-g-capitals-mental-health-company-files-for-bankruptcy-amid
-fraud-litigation/#:~:text=Capital's%20mental%20health%20company%20
Community,its%20ownership%20of%20the%20company.&text=Despite%20H
.I.G.'s%20exit%2C%20Community,owned%20by%20private%20equity%20
firms.

———. "Private Equity Health Care Acquisitions—November 2020," Dec. 8, 2020. https://pestakeholderproject.org/private-equity-health-care -acquisitions-november-2020.

———. "Private Equity: How Wall Street Firms Are Pillaging American Retail," July 25, 2019. https://www.pestakeholder.org/report/private-equity-how -wall-street-firms-are-pillaging-american-retail/.

PR Newswire. "American Capital Receives $97 Million from Sale of Portfolio Company the Meadows and Generates a 28% Equity Return on its Investment," PR Newswire, May 20, 2016. https://www.prnewswire.com/news -releases-american-capital-receives-$97-million-from-sale-of-portfolio -company-the-meadows-and-generates-a-28%-equity-return-on-its -investment.

———. "Jeffrey Newman Law Announces $4 Million Settlement in Whistleblower Fraud Case against South Bay Mental Health Center, Inc.," PR Newswire, Feb. 9, 2018. https://www.prnewswire.com/news-release/jeffrey -newman-law-announces-$4-million-settlement-in whistleblower-fraud-case-against-south-bay-mental-health-center.

———. "Ovation Fertility Announces New Private Equity Investor: Morgan Stanley Capital Partners," Yahoo!, June 17, 2019. https://finance.yahoo.com /news/ovation-fertility-announces-new-private-equity-investor-morgan -stanley-capital-partners.

Protess, Ben, Jessica Silver-Greenberg, and Rachel Abrams. "How Private Equity Found Power and Profit in State Capitals," New York Times, July 15, 2016.

Quinn, Audrey. "New Jersey Halts Admissions for Troubled Group Home Company," WNYC, Aug. 3, 2018. https://www.wnyc.org/story/new-jersey -halts-admissions-for-troubled-group-home-company.

Rice, Mark. "How, Why MCSD Camelot Education Plan Failed . . . and Lessons Learned," Ledger-Enquirer (GA), May 29, 2017. https://www.ledger-enquirer .com/news/local/education/article153277639.html.

Robbins, Rebecca. "Investors See Big Money in Infertility and They're Transforming the Industry," STAT News, Dec. 4, 2017. https://www.statnews .com2017/12/04/infertility-industry-investment/.

Roche, Walter F. "New Life Lodge Whistleblower Acted after Death of Patient," Tennessean, Apr. 22, 2014. https://tennessean.com/story/news/health/2014 /04/21/woman-whose-complaints-led-state-federal-investigation.

Rochester, Mark J., John Wisely, and Elisha Anderson. "Centria Healthcare Accused of Fraud, Targeting Poor in Metro Detroit," Detroit Free Press, Nov. 2, 2018. https://www.freep.com/story/news/local/michigan/2018/02/11/.

Rosenbaum, Jill, and David Heath. "Patients, Pressure and Profits at Aspen Dental: Dollars and Dentists," Frontline, June 26, 2012. https://www.pbs.org .wgbh/frontline/film/dollars-and-dentists.

Rothstein, Matthew. "How One Hospital's Bankruptcy Shows the Downside of Institutionalized Healthcare Real Estate," *Bisnow*, Sept. 12, 2019. https://www.bisnow.com/philadelphia/news/healthcare/hahnemann-private-equity-healthcare-real-estate-issues-100786.

Roumeliotis, Greg. "Carlyle Group Hires Former FCC Chairman as Dealmaker," *Reuters*, Jan. 6, 2014. https://www.reuters.com/articles/us-carlyle-genachowski.

Rowland, Christopher. "Why the Flight to the Hospital Is More Costly than Ever," *Washington Post*, July 1, 2019.

Rubin, Allan. "Nursing Home Bankruptcies," *Rubins*, Mar. 14, 2018. http://www.therubins.com/homes/gettingin.htm.

Rucinski, Tracy. "A Bid to Save $300 Million at HCR ManorCare, and Disrupt U.S. Healthcare," *Reuters: Business News*, May 15, 2018. https://www.reuters.com/article/us-hcrmanorcare-m-a-welltower-focus/a-bid-to-save-300-million-at-hcr-manorcare-and-disrupt-u-s-healthcare-idUSKCN1IG1IP.

Rush, Mariah. "Hahnemann University Hospital's Inner Turmoil: A Timeline of Changes, Layoffs, Closing," *Philadelphia Inquirer*, July 1, 2019.

Sabella, Giuseppe. "Teen's Death Comes amid Complaints at ResCare's WV Facilities," *West Virginia Gazette Mail*, Apr. 15, 2017. https://www.wvgazettemail.com/business/teen-s-death-comes-amid-complaints-at-res-cares-wv-facilities.

SC&H Capital. "How Private Equity Is Helping to Underwrite the Transformation of Healthcare," *SCH Group*, Mar. 28, 2018. https://www.schgroup.com/resources/blog-post/how-private-equity-is-helping-to-underwrite-the-transformation-of-healthcare.

Segal, David. "A Doctor with a Phone and a Mission," *New York Times*, Dec. 27, 2017.

Sellers, Patricia. "The New Siege at RJR Nabisco," *Fortune Magazine*, Oct. 16, 2015. https://www.fortune.com/2015/10/16/the-new-siege-at-RJR-Nabisco/.

Sergent, Don. "Workforce Board Terminates Contract with ResCare," *Bowling Green Daily News*, Apr. 10, 2018. https://www.bgdailynews.com/news/workforce-board-terminates-contract-with-res-care.

Sforza, Terri. "Lawmakers Resolve to Control Rogue Rehabs This Year," *Press Enterprise* (CA), Jan. 31, 2018. https://www.ocregister.com/2018/01/31/lawmakers-resolve-to-control-rogue-rehabs-this-year/.

Sforza, Terri, et al. "How Some California Drug Rehab Centers Exploit Addicts, Part 1," *Mercury News* (CA), May 22, 2017. https://www.ocregister.com/2017/05/21/how-some-southern-california-drug-rehab-centers-exploit-addiction/.

Shepherd, Julianne Escobedo. "Are Wall Street's For-Profit Eating Disorder Clinics Fleecing Patients and Providing Shoddy Treatment," *Jezebel*, Mar. 16, 2016. https://jezebel.com/are-wall-streets-for-profit-eating-disorder-clinics-fleecing-patients-and-providing-shoddy-treatment.

Sherman, Alex, and Lauren Hirsch. "Private Equity Eyes Industries Crippled by Coronavirus: 'They Have Been Waiting for This,'" *CNBC*, Mar. 25, 2020. https://www.cnbc.com/2020/03/25/private-equity-eyes-coronavirus-hit-industries-theyve-been-waiting.html.

Shulas, Greg. "Private Equity Poised to Reshape Home Health Care Industry?," *Home Care Magazine*, Oct. 31, 2018. https://www.homecaremag.com/home -health-private-equity-poised-to-reshape-home-health-care-industry/.

Shulman, Robyn D. "Only a Fool Would Try to Build a Business on Public-Private Partnerships in Education," *Huffington Post*, Dec. 6, 2017. https:// www.huffpost.com/entry/only-a-fool-would-try-to-build-a-business-on -public-private-partnerships-in-education.

Smith, Yves. "CalPERS Chief Investment Officer Ben Meng Made False Felonious Financial Disclosure Report: More Proof of Lack of Compliance under Marcie Frost," *Naked Capitalism*, Aug. 2, 2020. https:www.nakedcapitalism.com/2020 /08/calpers-chief-investment-officer-ben-meng-made-false-felonious -financial-disclosure-report-more-proof-of-lack-of-compliance-under-marcie -frost.html.

———. "Private Equity Flouts State Regulations by Buying Medical Practices," *Naked Capitalism*, Aug. 8, 2017. https://www.nakedcapitalism.com/2017/08 /private-equity-flouts-state-regulations-buying-medical-practices.html.

———. "Private Equity: The Perps behind Destructive Hospital Surprise Billing," *Naked Capitalism*, Aug. 1, 2019. https://www.nakedcapitalism.com/2019/08 /private-equity-the-perps-behind-destructive-hospital-surprise-billing.

Snyder, Andrew. "Ophthalmology Investments Spread across America: Part 1—The Northeast," *Physician First Healthcare Partners*, June 8, 2018. https:// www.physiciansfirst.com/blog/ophthalmology-investments-spread-across -america-part-1-the-northeast.

Solo Building Blogs. "Private Equity and Ophthalmology," *Solo Building Blogs*, July 3, 2018. https://solobuildingblogs.com/2018/03/12/private-equity-and -ophthalmology.

"The Southern California Rehab Industry Spans the Nation," *Orange County Register*, May 21, 2017. https://www.ocregister.com/2017/05/21/the-southern -california-rehab-industry-spans-the-nation.

Span, Paula. "In the Nursing Home, Empty Beds and Quiet Halls," *New York Times*, Sept. 28, 2018.

Spinger, L., et al. "Private Equity Pursues Profits in Keeping the Elderly at Home," *New York Times*, Aug. 20, 2016.

Springer, Patrick. "ND Defends Lawsuit Challenging State's Regulation of Air Ambulance Charges," *Bismarck Tribune* (ND), Apr. 2, 2018. https://bismarck tribune.com/news/state-and-regional/nd-defends-lawsuit-challenging-states -regulation-of-air-ambulance-charges.

Steele, Melissa. "AdvoServ: From Humble Beginnings to Rational Operation," *Cape Gazette* (DE), Aug. 23, 2013. https://www.capegazette.com/node/52199.

Sterngold, James. "Shaking Billions from Beatrice," *New York Times*, June 9, 1987.

Sutherland, Brooke. "It's the Greatest Health-Care Buyout Shuffle," *Washington Post*, June 11, 2018.

Swisher, Skyler. "Methadone Treatment Raises Questions about Profit Motive, Patient Care," *Daytona Beach News Journal* (FL), Apr. 21, 2013. https://www .news-journalonline.com/news/20130420/methadone-treatment-raises -questions-about-profit-motive-patient-care.

Taibbi, Matt. "Greed and Debt: The True Story of Mitt Romney and Bain Capital," *Rolling Stone* 1165, Sept. 13, 2020, 42–50.

Taub, Stephen. "Coming Downturn, Cranking Leverage: What Could Go Wrong?," *Institutional Investor*, Feb. 12, 2019. htpp://institutionalinvestor .com/article/b1d3gx71r89d7m/coming-downturn-cranking-leverage-what -could-go-wrong/.

Taylor, Kate. "Education Company to Pay $4.3 Million in Settlement," *New York Times*, Oct. 20, 2016.

Tozzi, John. "Air Ambulances Are Flying More Patients than Ever, and Leaving Massive Bills Behind," *Bloomberg News*, June 11, 2018. https://www.bloomberg .com/news/features/2018-06-11/private-equity-backed-air-ambulances-leave -behind-massive-bills.

———. "Prognosis: How Private Equity Keeps States Invested in Medical Billing Practices They've Banned," *Bloomberg*, July 3, 2018. https://www.bloomberg .com/news/articles/2018-07-03/how-private-equity-keeps-states-invested-in -medical-billing-practies-they've-banned.

Trainer, Dave. "Not Buying Acadia Healthcare's Roll-Up Story," *Forbes*, Aug. 8, 2016. https://www.forbes.com/sites/greatspeculations/.

Tribble, Sarah Jane. "Air Ambulances Woo Rural Consumers with Memberships That May Leave Them Hanging," NPR, Sept. 14, 2019. https://www.npr.org /sections/health-shots/2019/09/14/760680901/air-ambulances-woo-rural -consumers-with-memberships-that-may-leave-them-hanging#:~:text=Air%20 Ambulances%20Woo%20Rural%20Consumers%20With%20Memberships%20 That%20May%20Leave%20Them%20Hanging,-Listen%C2%B7%204%3A29 &text=Kaiser%20Health%20News-,Visitors%20and%20park%20rangers%20 at%20historic%20Fort%20Scott%20check%20out,town's%20Good%20Ol'%20 Days%20festival.

Tse, Crystal, and Liana Baker. "Private Equity Firms Fight for Lifeline Deals in Buffet-Goldman Redux," *Bloomberg News*, Apr. 27, 2020. https://www .bloomberg.com/news/articles/2020-04-27/buffet-goldman-redux-buyout -shops-fight-for-lifeline-deals.

Tully, Joseph. "ResCare Whistleblowers Have Evidence of ResCare Misconduct," *Tully & Weiss*, July 15, 2017. https://www.tully-weiss.com/blog.php ?article=rescare-whistleblowers-have-evidence-of-res-care-misconduct.

Turner, Ford. "How a Pa. Treatment Center Allegedly Made Millions from Drug Addicts," *Reading Eagle* (PA), Mar. 25, 2019. https://www.readingeagle.com /news/article/the-business-of-addiction-how-a-pa-treatment-center -allegedly-made-millions-from-drug-addicts.

———. "Liberation Way Drug Treatment Operation to Merge," *Reading Eagle* (PA), Sept. 14, 2018. https://www.readingeagle.com/news/article/liberation -way-drug-treatment-operation-to-merge.

Varney, Sarah. "Private Equity Pursues Profits in Keeping the Elderly at Home," *New York Times*, Aug. 20, 2016.

Veillette, Patrick. "How to Develop Helicopter-Centric IFR," *Aviation Week*, Jan. 29, 2016. https://www.avaiationweek.com/bca/how-to-develop -helicopter-centric-ifr.

Vogell, Heather. "Unrestrained," *ProPublica*, Dec. 10, 2015. https://www
.propublica.org/article/advoserv-profit-and-abuse-at-homes-for-the
-profoundly-disabled.

———. "What Happened to Adam," *New Republic*, Dec. 11, 2015.

Whalen, Jeanne, and Laura Cooper. "Private Equity Pours Cash into Opioid-
Treatment Sector," *Wall Street Journal*, Sept. 2, 2017.

Whorisky, Peter, and Dan Keating. "Overdoses, Bedsores, Broken Bones: What
Happened when a Private-Equity Firm Sought to Care for Society's Most
Vulnerable," *Washington Post*, Nov. 25, 2018.

Wikipedia. "Gentiva Health Services." https://en.wikipedia.org/wiki/Gentiva
_Health_Services.

Williams, James. "Air Methods Sold to American Securities in $2.5bn Deal,"
Financier Worldwide, May 2, 2017. https://www.financierworldwide.com/fw
-news/2017/5/2/air-methods-sold-to-american-securities-in-25bn-deal.

Willmer, Sabrina. "Wall Street Corners Cancer Care on Florida's Paradise
Coast," *Bloomberg News*, Oct. 26, 2020. https://bloomberg.com/news/articles
/2020-10-28/how-private-equity-helped-corner-the-market-in-naples-florida.

———. "When Wall Street Took Over This Nursing Company, Profits Grew and
Patients Suffered," *Bloomberg News*, Oct. 22, 2019. https://www.bloomberg
.com/news/features/2019-10-22/when-wall-street-took-over-this-nursing
-company-profits-grew-and-patients-suffered.

Willmer, Sabrina, and Heather Perlberg. "TPG Joins Apollo, Blackstone in
Raising Fees as Money Flows," *Bloomberg News*, July 17, 2017. https://www
.bloomberg.com/news/articles/2018-07-17/tpg-joins-Appolo-blackstone-in
-raising-fees-as-money-flows.

Wisely, John, and Elisha Anderson. "How Michigan's Largest Autism Therapy
Provider Lost $8M Grant," *Detroit Free Press*, May 9, 2018. https://www.freep
.com/story/news/2018/05/09/centria-healthcare-autism-therapy/572285002/.

Zarling, Patti. "Forefront Dermatology Adds Space, 200 Jobs," *Herald Times
Reporter* (CA), Apr. 13, 2017. https://www.htrnews.com/story/money/2017/04
/13/manitowoc-jobs-economy-wisconsin-economic-development-council
-forefront-dermatology/100414438/.

Government Documents

Chopra, Rohit. Letter to the House Energy and Commerce Committee and
Commerce Subcommittee on Oversight and Investigations, US House of
Representatives, Washington, DC, July 24, 2018. https://www.ftc.gov/system
/files/documents/public_statements/1395538/cmr_chopra_letter_to_congress
_on_opioid_treatment.pdf.

Joint Staff Report on the Corporate Practice of Medicine in the Medicaid
Program. Prepared by the Staff of the Committee on Finance, and the
Committee on the Judiciary, US Senate, 2013.

National Institute on Alcohol Abuse and Alcoholism. "Alcohol Facts and
Statistics," National Institutes of Health, 2016. https://niaaa.nih.gov
/publications/brochures-and-fact-sheets/alcohol-facts-and-statistics.

New York Attorney General. "A. G. Schneiderman, Acting Tax Commissioner
Manion and Comptroller Dinapoli Announce $4.3 Million Settlement with

Owners of For-Profit School Network for Overcharging State; Failing to Pay Taxes," Oct. 2016. https://ag-ny-gov-press-release/ag-schneiderman-acting -tax-commissioner-manion-and-comptroller-dinapoli-announce-$4.3 -million-settlement-with-owners-of-for-profit-school-network-for -overcharging-state-failing-to-pay-taxes.

———. "A. G. Schneiderman Announces Settlement with Aspen Dental Management That Bars Company from Making Decisions about Patient Care in New York Clinics," June 18, 2015. https://ag.ny.gov/press-release/ag -schneiderman-announces-settlement-with-aspen-dental-management-that -bars-company-from-making-decisions-about-patient-care-in-new-york -clinics.

US Department of Health and Human Services, Office of Inspector General. "OIG Excludes Pediatric Dental Management Chain from Participation in Federal Health Care Programs," Apr. 3, 2014.

———."Vulnerabilities in the Medicare Hospice Program Affect Quality Care and Program Integrity: An OIG Portfolio," July 2018, OEI-02-16-00570.

US Department of Justice. "Dental Management Company Benevis and Its Affiliate Kool Smiles Dental Clinics to Pay $23.9 Million to Settle False Claims Act Allegations relating to Medically Unnecessary Pediatric Dental Services," Justice News, Jan. 10, 2018. https://www.justice-gov/opa/pr/dental -management-company-beneves-and-its-affiliated-kool-smiles-dental-to-pay -$23.9-million-to-settle-false-claims-act-allegations-related-to-medically -unnecessary-dental-services.

———. "Long-Term Care Pharmacy to Pay $31.5 Million to Settle Lawsuit Alleging Violations of Controlled Substance Act and False Claims Act," May 14, 2015. https://wwwjustice.gov/opa/pr/long-term-care-pharmacy-to -pay-$31.5-million-to-settle-lawsuit-alleging-violations-of-controlled -substance-act-and-false-claims-act.

———. "Pediatric Services of America and Related Entities to Pay $6.88 Million to Resolve False Claims Act Allegations," Aug. 4, 2015. https://www.justice.gov /usao-sdga/pr/pediatric-services-america-and-related-entities-pay-688 -million-resolve-false-claims#:~:text=SAVANNAH%20%E2%80%93%20 The%20U.S.%20Attorney's%20Office,resolve%20allegations%20that%20 PSA%2C%20a.

US Government Accountability Office. "Air Ambulance: Effects of Industry Changes on Services Are Unclear," Sept. 30, 2010. https://www.gao.gov /products/GAO-10-907.

———. Case Studies of Selected Leveraged Buyouts, no. 91-107 (Washington, DC: US Government Printing Office, Sept. 1991).

Interviews

Anonymous. Owner, dermatology practice sold to PE firm, Aug. 19, 2019.
Anonymous. Eating disorders specialist, Oct. 9, 2019.
Anonymous. Principal, unnamed private equity firm, Oct. 16, 2019.
Attia, Evelyn. Former director, Eating Disorders Research Program, New York State Psychiatric Institute; director, Columbia Center for Eating Disorders, Columbia University Medical Center; professor of psychiatry at Columbia

University Medical Center; professor of psychiatry at Weill Cornell Medical College, NY, Oct. 24, 2019.

Baida, J. Mark. Founder, Bayada Home Care, Moorestown, NJ, Dec. 4, 2019.

Brennan, Timothy K. Vice president for Medical Academic Affairs, American College of Academic Addiction Medicine, Chevy Chase, MD; assistant professor and director of Addiction Institute at Mount Sinai, NY, Oct. 28, 2019.

Brooks, Christopher. CEO, Dermatology Solutions Group, Brentwood, TN, July 16, 2019.

Carey, Marni Jameson. Author, journalist, and executive director, Association of Independent Doctors, Winter Park, FL, July 11, 2019.

Casalino, Lawrence Peter. Professor of healthcare policy and research, Weill Cornell Medical College, NY, Oct. 9, 2019.

Casamassimo, Paul. Professor emeritus, pediatric dentistry, Ohio State University College of Dentistry, Columbus; chief policy officer, American Academy of Pediatric Dentistry, Chicago, IL, July 25, 2019.

Costin, Carolyn. Cofounder, Monte Nido, Miami, FL, Oct. 15, 2019.

Crittendon, Julie. Clinical psychologist and founder, Autism Center for Children, Woodstock, GA, July 22, 2019.

D'Aunno, Thomas. Professor of management and director, Health Policy and Management Program, Robert F. Wagner Graduate School of Public Service, New York University, NY, Nov. 1, 2019.

Davis, Michael W. General dentistry practice, Santa Fe, NM; writer for Dentistry Today, July 24, 2019.

Dobrowolski, Richard. Retired, general dentistry practice, Bethlehem, PA, July 22, 2019.

Frea, William. Cofounder, Autism Spectrum Therapies, Burbank, CA, June 2, 2019.

Fritts, Lani. Cofounder, Trumpet Behavioral Health, Lakewood, CO, July 8, 2019.

Guarda, Angela. Medical director, Eating Recovery Program, Johns Hopkins University, Baltimore, MD, Oct. 9, 2019.

Heilveil, Ira. Founder, Pacific Child and Family Associates/Autism Learning Partners, Glendale, CA, June 13, 2019.

Jacofsky, David. Cofounder, chair, and CEO, Center for Orthopedic Research and Education, Phoenix, AZ, Sept. 24, 2019.

Kantor, Lisa. Attorney, Kantor and Kantor, eating disorders specialist, Northridge, CA, Nov. 8, 2019.

Koegel, Lynn Kern. Author, researcher, and clinical professor of psychiatry and behavioral sciences, Department of Psychiatry and Child Development, Stanford School of Medicine, Stanford, CA, July 3, 2019.

Kolodner, George. Founder, Kolmac Outpatient Recovery Centers, Morrisville, PA, Oct. 23, 2019.

Lerz, Bobby. Cofounder, Castlewood Victims Unite, Middletown, NY, Nov. 12, 2019.

McBurnie, Michael. Founder, MyTherapyCompany/Stepping Stones Group, Lafayette, CO, June 19, 2019.

McClain, Mary. Cofounder, Invo Healthcare Associates, Jamison, PA, June 21, 2019.

McEachin, John. Cofounder, Autism Partnership, Seal Beach, CA, June 25, 2019.

Medoff, Ari. Founder, Nurse Care, Durham, NC, and CEO, Arosa+LivHome, Los Angeles, CA, Nov. 19 and 24, 2019.

Molko, Ronit. Author, advisor to PE investors, and cofounder, Autism Spectrum Therapies, Burbank, CA, July 8, 2019.

Mostaghimi, Arash. Dermatologist and researcher, Brigham and Women's Hospital, Boston, MA, Sept. 26, 2019.

Niager, Kathy. Founder, Trellis Services, Sparks, MD, July 1, 2019.

Page, Steve. Founder, president, and CEO, SUN Behavioral Health, Red Bank, NJ, Oct. 18, 2019.

Rice, Matt. Founder and CEO, Recovery Works Drug and Alcohol Rehabilitation Center, Georgetown, KY, Oct. 25, 2019.

Robinson, Jeff R. Founder, CEO, and president, Behavioral Concepts, Inc., Mansfield, MA, June 19, 2019.

Ross, Peter. Cofounder, Senior Helpers, Towson, MD, Nov. 19, 2019.

Schinfeld, Jay. Retired partner, Abington Reproductive Medicine, Abington, PA, Sept. 9, 2019.

Snyder, Nate. Cofounder and CEO, Ovation Fertility, Los Angeles, CA, Sept. 6, 2019.

Somkuti, Stephen G. Partner, Abington Reproductive Medicine, Abington, PA, Sept. 10, 2019.

Stanberry, Mike. Founder, president, and CEO, Metro Aviation, Shreveport, LA, Aug. 16, 2018.

Tanzi, Jill. Dentist and founder, Dentist at Hopkinton, Hopkinton, MA; president, Massachusetts Dentists Alliance for Quality Care, Sept. 13, 2019.

Taylor, Bridget A. Founder, Alpine Learning Group, Paramus, NJ, June 21, 2019.

Zang, Tiana. Founder and president, Sage Hospice and Palliative Care, Scottsdale, AZ, Nov. 21, 2019.

Zepp, Kevin. Founder and CEO, Liberty Healthcare Services, Mt. Laurel, NJ, Nov. 5, 2019.

Doctor Patient Unity, 125, 325n93
Dodd-Frank Act, 9, 60
DPMS/Kool Smiles, 43, 142, 341n68
Drexel Burnham Lambert, 49, 321n21, 357n60
dry powder, 27, 64; record levels, 53–54, 65, 67, 80, 100, 147, 152, 286–87, 295
due diligence, 23, 37, 209
DW Healthcare Partners, 253, 299, 334n133, 355n21
DynCorp, 62

Eagle Private Capital, 143, 330n63, 331n76, 333n100
Early Autism Project, 241
eating disorders treatment, 10, 17, 189, 210–18, 220, 273, 276; Eating Recovery Center, 216, 273, 285, 353n110; marketing techniques, 211–13; Monte Nido, 211, 217–18, 353n113; multispecialty companies, 218–20; quality of care, 212–16; single-specialty companies, 214–18; Veritas Collaborative, 218, 353n115
Eating Recovery Center, 216, 273, 285, 353n110
"echo buyouts," 27
Edgemont Partners, 104
Edmands, Benjamin, 65, 69, 73
Educational Services of America, 226, 240
Elara Caring, 169–71, 284, 285
Eli Global, 99, 331n77
EmCare, 122–23, 125, 261, 337n176
emergency medical services, 273. See also air medical transport; ground ambulance services
Emergency Medical Services Corporation (EMS), 123, 256, 261–62
emergency room care, 1, 23, 67, 79, 104, 120, 266, 288; outsourcing, 122, 123, 337nn175–76
Encompass Health, 153, 168–69, 284
endowments, 20, 35–36, 278, 315n16, 366n39
enterprise value (EV), 23
Envision Healthcare, 14, 75, 122–24, 125, 288, 322n47

Envision Healthcare Holdings, 261–62
EOS Partners, 181, 300
Epic Health Services, 162, 345n58
Epprecht, Liz, 82
equity sources, 278–79. See also limited partners; pension funds
Eureka Capital Partners, 170, 300
Evans, Colby, 86
Evans, Emily, 150
Evercare Hospice, 172, 272
Everyware, 46, 321nn10–11
executives: earnings, 30–31; payoffs to, 42, 47, 48, 56, 62, 293
EyeCare Services Partners, 102, 272
EyeSouth Partners, 103

Fair Labor Standards Act, 166, 272
False Claims Act, 142–43, 160, 241
Famakinwa, Joyce, 152, 166–67
Family Treatment Network, 250–51
Farmer, Kristin, 253
Federal Aviation Administration, 259, 269
Federal Communications Commission, 59
Federal Reserve, 54, 289, 291, 293
Federal Trade Commission, 194, 294, 335n133, 348n110
Federal Trade Commission Act, 294
Ferguson, Daniel, 45–46
fertility treatment services, 15, 116–19
FFL Partners, 102, 142, 205, 232, 300, 336n166
fiduciary duty, 37, 291, 294–95
Fields, Robin, 113
financial crises, 34–35, 58, 283. See also recessions
financialization, 2–3, 5, 11, 20, 154–58, 251
Five Arrows Capital Partners, 237, 300, 325n4, 355n21
Flatt, Bruce, 289
Florida Autism Center, 252, 356n46
Fontana, Robert, 137
Food and Drug Administration (FDA), 57, 335n141, 350n11
FORBA Holdings, 135
Forefront Dermatology, 86, 93–94, 285, 330n57

Formation Capital, 171–72, 272
Fornear, James R., 165
founder-owners, 18, 68–69, 271, 282;
  adverse effects of PE ownership on,
  278–79; incentives for sale to PE
  shops, 278–79; majority rights, 25;
  management role, 39
Francis, Joseph, 87
Frank, Fred, 177
fraudulent and illegal practices: air
  medical transport, 260; autism
  spectrum disorder services, 242–43,
  249; dental services, 132, 135, 138,
  139, 140, 141–42, 144, 147–48, 294; of
  GPs, 1–2, 4, 294; home health care,
  166, 187–88, 272; hospice care, 157,
  158, 172, 185, 187–88; hospital chains,
  66–67; medical staff outsourcing,
  123; pharmacy services, 167–68;
  physician practice management
  companies, 294; public pension
  funds and, 278; rebranding response
  to, 167, 272–73; substance abuse
  rehabilitation, 194–96, 198, 199–201,
  202, 209. See also child mistreatment / abuse; Medicaid fraud;
  Medicare fraud
Frazier Healthcare Partners, 105,
  108–9, 171
Frea, William, 228, 230, 239–40,
  356n48
Freedman, Joel, 73–74
Fresenius Medical Care, 112, 113–14,
  115–16
Fritts, Lani, 243–44
Fulcrum Equity Partners, 209, 300
Futures Behavioral Therapy Center,
  243, 357n64

Gada, Ravi, 117
Galperin, Lori, 214, 215
gastroenterology practices, 15, 79, 107–9
Geithner, Timothy, 60, 324n82
Gemini Investors, 176, 202–3, 300
Genachowski, Julius, 59
General Atlantic, 67, 253, 289, 300
general partners (GPs), 65, 271; access
  to government funding, 7; attitudes
  toward health services acquisitions,

65, 66; commission fees, 23;
COVID-19 pandemic and, 19;
fraudulent and illegal practices,
1–2, 4, 294; in government, 58, 64;
growth equity investing, 13, 24–25;
investment pools, 121; management
fees, 37; in PE process, 21, 22; political
activities, 62; segment-specific
expertise, 28–29
Genesis HealthCare, 74–75, 172, 327n43
Gentiva, 160, 161–62
Girling Health Care, 161, 345n56
Glass House (Alexander), 45–46
Global Medical Response, 255, 261,
  262, 265, 284
Global Private Equity Barometer, 38
Godfread, Jon, 260
GoHealth Urgent Care, 121
Goldberg, Stephanie, 153
Golden Gate Capital, 55, 236, 300,
  355n21
Gottfried, Miriam, 288
government, relationship with PE
  industry, 14, 58–63, 64
government funding: autism spec-
  trum disorder therapy, 223–25; GPs'
  access to, 7, 8–9. See also Medicaid
  coverage; Medicare coverage
government policies affecting PE
  industry, 18, 68, 279–81; regulatory
  restrains affecting specific
  industries / practices, 62, 81–82,
  125–27, 129, 134–36, 158, 258–59.
  See also tax laws and policies
GPs. See general partners
Granpeesheh, Doreen, 251
Grassley, Chuck, 130, 135, 342n80
Great Expressions Dental Centers,
  143–44, 342n80
Great Lakes Caring, 169–71
Great Lakes Dental Partners, 145–46
Great Point Partners, 124, 231–33
Great Recession, 33–34, 50–51, 54, 64,
  68
ground ambulance services, 18, 255–56,
  265–66, 269–70, 284; American
  Medical Response, 122–23, 255,
  261–62, 263, 265, 284; Rural / Metro
  Corporation, 255, 256, 262–63

Group for Research of Corporatization and Private Equity in Dermatology, 87

growth equity investing, 13, 24–25, 326n18

Gryphon Investors, 146, 239

GTCR Private Equity, 161, 301, 331n71

Gymboree, 1, 14, 55, 128, 323n60, 345n53

Gynecology practices, 119–20

Hahnemann University Hospital, 73–74

Haines, Avril, 61

Halifax Group, 174, 204, 242, 301, 355n21

Harden Healthcare, 161–62

Hart-Scott-Rodino Antitrust Improvements Act, 294

Harvest Partners, 92, 102, 145, 301, 342n83

Harvey, David, 2, 4

HCA. See Health Corporation of America

health care costs, 5, 10, 78, 84; consolidation-related increase, 70, 71–72; control strategies, 9–10; price-based, 9

Healthcare Innovations, 168, 347n87

health care–related companies, PE-owned, 3; adverse effects of ownership, 10, 77; alleged benefits, 284; ancillary services companies, 77; customer preferences and, 6; deficiencies, 14; diversity, 76; middle-market companies, 14; patient volume maximization, 6; public funding, 7; "roll-up" acquisition strategy, 5; scope, 14–15. See also names of individual companies

health care sector: PE industry's focus on, 1, 66, 273–74; as percentage of GDP, 9, 292

health care system: effects of PE industry on, 15; malfunctioning, 10, 14

Health Corporation of America (HCA), 14, 66–67

health food alternatives, 14–15, 77

health insurance coverage, 18, 68, 284–85; ABA therapy coverage, 224, 225–26, 228; air medical transport, 258; autism spectrum disorders treatment, 279, 281; behavioral and mental health, 190–91; coinsurance, 10; deductibles, 10; dentistry, 134; dialysis, 114; eating disorders, 210–11, 213, 221; founder-owners' complaints about, 279; ground emergency medical services, 255; home health care, 152; in vitro fertilization, 116, 117; medical staff outsourcing companies and, 123, 124; premiums, 10; substance addiction rehabilitation, 192, 204, 206; underinsurance, 10. See also Medicaid coverage; Medicare coverage

health savings accounts, 9–10

HealthSouth, 168–69, 346n84

HealthView Capital Partners, 161, 301, 345n54

Heartland Dental, 130, 139–40, 272

Heartland Hospice, 183–86

Hedgeye Risk Management, 150

Heilveil, Ira, 231–33, 355n33

Helyar, John. See Barbarians at the Gate

Hensley-Clancy, Molly, 245

Hercules Capital, 231, 335n151

Heritage Group, 171, 301

HHAs. See home health care agencies

H. H. Franchising Systems, Inc., 176

H. I. G. Capital, 75, 178–79, 301, 332n89

H. I. G. Growth Partners, 242–43, 301, 355n21

Hillhaven Corp., 159

Holden, W. Blake, 30

Holder, Robert, 171

holding periods, 33–34, 170, 285–86, 318n51

home- and community-based services (HCBS), 150

Home Care, 180, 181

home health care agencies, 11, 12, 149–55, 284; Abode Healthcare, 91, 171, 285, 347n89; AccentCare, 173–74, 347n98; annual growth rate, 149;

Aveanna Healthcare, 162–65, 277, 284; Bayada Home Health Care, 186–87; BrightSpring Health Services/ResCare, 165–68, 272, 284, 327n47, 348n116; during COVID-19 pandemic, 289–90; Elara Caring, 169–71, 284, 285; Encompass Health, 153, 168–69, 284; Epic Health Services, 162–63, 345n58; financial model, 151–56; Gentiva Health Services, 161–62; GPs, 150; Great Lakes Caring, 169–71; Interim HealthCare, 174; Jordan Health Services, 169–71; Kindred Health-care, 14, 40, 76, 159–60, 167, 284, 344n48; National Home Healthcare, 169, 170–71; nonprofit, 183–87; PACE program, 16, 154–55, 187; pediatric services, 162, 163–65, 179; profit margin, 150; PSA Healthcare, 162, 163–65; publicly traded companies, 180–81; quality of care, 153, 164, 166, 167; Senior Helpers, 175–76; Sim-plura Health Group/All Metro Health Care, 172–73; social impact investing, 181–82

HOPCo, 105

hospice, 10, 16, 153, 155–61, 170, 273, 281, 284; Abode Healthcare, 91, 171, 285, 347n89; bankruptcies, 159, 184–86; Bayada Home Health Care, 186–87; Compassus, 171–72; during COVID-19 pandemic, 289–90; Curo Health Services, 76, 160, 161, 285; Encompass Health, 153, 168–69, 284; Gentiva, 160, 161–62; Heartland Hospice, 183–86; Kindred Health-care, 14, 76, 159–61, 167, 284, 344n48; lack of regulatory restraints, 158; nonprofit, 183, 186; publicly traded companies, 180; quality of care, 157–58, 159, 178–79; Sage Hospice and Palliative Care, 177–79; Simplura Health Group/All Metro Health Care, 172–73

Hospice Advantage, 172, 347n93

Hospice of North Alabama, 171

hospital chains, 66–67

hospital health systems, 282

hospitalists, 79

hospital-owned medical practices, 78

hospitals: bankruptcy, 73–74; non-profit, 78; PE-owned, 71; staff outsourcing, 122–27

hostile takeovers, 38–39, 44

House Ways and Means Committee, Oversight Subcommittee, 292

Hsia, Renee, 256

Humana, 121, 160

ICG Enterprise Trust, 171

index funds, 30–31

Individuals with Disabilities Act, 223–24

Individuals with Disabilities Educa-tion Act, 280–81

information technology (IT), 65, 77

initial public offerings (IPOs), 30–31, 33, 40, 51, 66, 75, 346n69; air medical transport, 262–63, 266, 267; behav-ioral health care, 199; cancer care network, 74; dental services, 147; ground ambulance services, 261, 262; home health care, 162, 165, 180, 181, 345n62; medical staffing services, 123, 124; nursing homes, 183; rehabilita-tive services, 346n84; substance abuse treatment services, 199

InnovAge, 154–55

Inside Rehab (Fletcher), 192, 194

institutional investors, 36, 37, 38, 49, 50, 366n39

Institutional Limited Partners Association, 291

Integrated Medical Professionals, 110

interest: carried, 21, 40–41, 61, 62, 87, 186, 241, 283, 292, 316n6, 366n37; rates, 49, 289; tax deductibility, 62, 292

internal rate of return (IRR), 5, 32–33, 37–38, 53

Internal Revenue Service, 293

investment banks, 25, 40, 44, 48, 49, 53, 58, 64, 320n6; complicit with PEs, 18

Invo Healthcare Associates, 233–36, 274

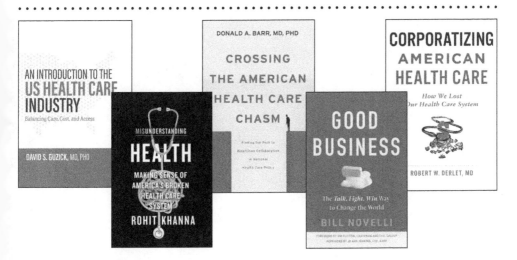
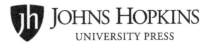
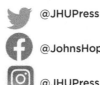